T0280223

Hypothyroidism: Novel Perspectives

Hypothyroidism: Novel Perspectives

Edited by **Benjamin Copes**

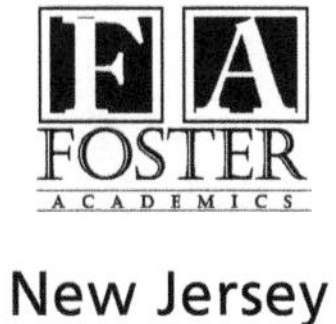

New Jersey

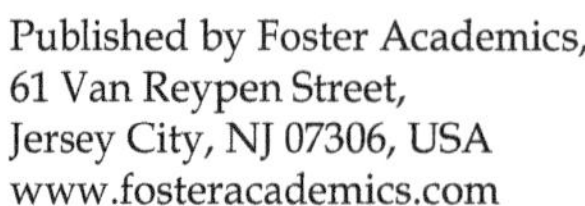
Published by Foster Academics,
61 Van Reypen Street,
Jersey City, NJ 07306, USA
www.fosteracademics.com

Hypothyroidism: Novel Perspectives
Edited by Benjamin Copes

© 2015 Foster Academics

International Standard Book Number: 978-1-63242-239-2 (Hardback)

This book contains information obtained from authentic and highly regarded sources. Copyright for all individual chapters remain with the respective authors as indicated. A wide variety of references are listed. Permission and sources are indicated; for detailed attributions, please refer to the permissions page. Reasonable efforts have been made to publish reliable data and information, but the authors, editors and publisher cannot assume any responsibility for the validity of all materials or the consequences of their use.

The publisher's policy is to use permanent paper from mills that operate a sustainable forestry policy. Furthermore, the publisher ensures that the text paper and cover boards used have met acceptable environmental accreditation standards.

Trademark Notice: Registered trademark of products or corporate names are used only for explanation and identification without intent to infringe.

Printed in the United States of America.

Contents

Preface

Hypothyroidism is described as abnormally low activity of the thyroid gland, resulting in retardation of growth and mental development in children and adults. It is the most prevalent thyroid disorder. It can lead to a diverse amount of changes in women's menstrual periods, decrease their chances of conceiving, and affect both the course of pregnancy and the neuropsychological development of babies. Throughout pregnancy, there is a considerably increased requirement of thyroid hormones and a substantial risk that a previously unnoticed, subclinical or latent hypothyroidism will develop into overt hypothyroidism. The thyroid inflammation because of patient's own immune system may shape autoimmune thyroiditis (Hashimoto's thyroiditis). Congenital hypothyroidism (CH) happens in approximately 1:2,000 to 1:4,000 newborns. Almost all of the developed countries of the world presently exercise newborn screening to diagnose and cure congenital hypothyroidism in the first weeks of life. This book includes various crucial specifications and innovations for endocrine practice.

The information shared in this book is based on empirical researches made by veterans in this field of study. The elaborative information provided in this book will help the readers further their scope of knowledge leading to advancements in this field.

Finally, I would like to thank my fellow researchers who gave constructive feedback and my family members who supported me at every step of my research.

Editor

Part 1

Introduction

1

Hypothyroidism

Osama M. Ahmed[1] and R. G. Ahmed[2,3]
[1]*Physiology Division, Zoology Department, Faculty of Science, Beni-Suef University,*
[2]*Lab of Comparative Endocrinology, Catholic University, Leuven,*
[3]*Zoology Department, Faculty of Science, Beni-Suef University,*
[1,3]*Egypt*
[2]*Belgium*

1. Introduction

Hypothyroidism is caused by insufficient secretion of thyroid hormones by the thyroid gland or by the complete loss of its function. The share of hypothyroidism among other endocrine diseases is gradually increasing. It is encountered in females more than in males. The idiopathic form of hypothyroidism occurs mainly in females older than 40 years. Hypothyroidism is usually progressive and irreversible. Treatment, however, is nearly always completely successful and allows a patient to live a fully normal life (Potemkin, 1889; Thomas, 2004; Roberts and Ladenson, 2004).

2. History

Hypothyroidism was first diagnosed in the late nineteenth century when doctors observed that surgical removal of the thyroid resulted in the swelling of the hands, face, feet, and tissues around the eyes. The term myxoedema (mucous swelling; myx is the Greek word for mucin and oedema means swelling) was introduced in 1974 by Gull and in 1878 by Ord. On the autopsy of two patients, Ord discovered mucous swelling of the skin and subcutaneous fat and linked these changes with the hypofunction or atrophy of the thyroid gland. The disorder arising from surgical removal of the thyroid gland (cachexia strumipriva) was described in 1882 by Reverdin of Geneva and in 1883 by Kocher of Berne. After Gull's description, myxoedma aroused enormous interest, and in 1883 the Clinical Society of London appointed a committee to study the disease and report its findings. The committee's report, published in 1888, contains a significant portion of what is known today about the clinical and pathologic aspects of myxoedema (Wiersinga, 2010).

3. Causes and incidence

Many permanent or temporary conditions can reduce thyroid hormone secretion and cause hypothyroidism. About 95% of hypothyroidism cases occur from problems that start in the thyroid gland. In such cases, the disorder is called primary hypothyroidism (Potemkin, 1889). Secondary and tertiary hypothyroidism is caused by disorders of the pituitary gland and hypothalamus respectively (Lania et al., 2008). Only 5% of hypothyroid cases suffer from secondary and tertiary hypothyroidism (Potemkin, 1889). The two most common causes of primary hypothyroidism are (1) Hashimoto's thyroiditis which is an autoimmune condition and (2) overtreatment of hyperthyroidism (an overactive thyroid) (Simon, 2006; Aminoff, 2007; Elizabeth and Agabegi, 2008). Primary hypothyroidism may also occur as a result of insufficient introduction of iodine into body (endemic goiter). In iodine-replete communities, the prevalence of spontaneous hypothyroidism is between 1 % and 2 %, and it is more common in older women and ten times more common in women than in men (Vanderpump, 2005 and 2009). Radioiodine therapy may lead to hypothyroidism (Potemkin, 1989). Primary hypothyroidism may also occur as a result of hereditary defects in the biosynthesis of thyroid hormones (due to defect in the accumulation of iodine by the thyroid gland or defect in the transformation of monoiodotyrosine and diiodotyrosines into triiodothyronine and thyroxine) or may be caused by hypoplasia and plasia of the thyroid gland as a result of its embryonic developmental defect, degenerative changes, total or subtotal thyroidectomy (Potemkin, 1889). Hypothalamic and pituitary hypothyroidism, or central hypothyroidism results from a failure of the mechanisms that stimulate thyroid-stimulating hormone (TSH) and TSH releasing hormone (TRH) synthesis, secretion, and biologic action (Thomas, 2004). The most prevalent cause of central hypothyroidism, including secondary and tertiary subtypes, is a defective development of the pituitary gland or hypothalamus leading to multiple pituitary hormone deficiencies, while defects of pituitary and hypothalamic peptides and their receptors only rarely have been identified as the cause of central congenital hypothyroidism (Grueters et al., 2002; Ahmed et al., 2008).

Type	Origin	Description
Primary	Thyroid gland	The most common forms include Hashimoto's thyroiditis (an autoimmune disease) and radioiodine therapy for hyperthyroidism.
Secondary	Pituitary gland	It occurs if the pituitary gland does not create enough thyroid-stimulating hormone (TSH) to induce the thyroid gland to produce enough thyroxine and triiodothyronine. Although not every case of secondary hypothyroidism has a clear-cut cause, it is usually caused by damage to the pituitary gland, as by a tumor, radiation, or surgery. Secondary hypothyroidism accounts for less than 5% or 10% of hypothyroidism cases.
Tertiary	Hypothalamus	It results when the hypothalamus fails to produce sufficient thyrotropin-releasing hormone (TRH). TRH prompts the pituitary gland to produce thyroid-stimulating hormone (TSH). Hence may also be termed hypothalamic-pituitary-axis hypothyroidism. It accounts for less than 5% of hypothyroidism cases.

Table 1. Classification of hypothyroidism according to the origin of cause (Simon, 2006; Aminoff, 2007; Elizabeth and Agabegi, 2008).

4. Grades of hypothyroidism

Hypothyroidism ranges from very mild states in which biochemical abnormalities are present but the individual hardly notices symptoms and signs of thyroid hormone deficiency, to very severe conditions in which the danger exists to slide down into a life-threatening myxoedema coma. In the development of primary hypothyroidism, the transition from the euthyroid to the hypothyroid state is first detected by a slightly elevated serum TSH, caused by a minor decrease in thyroidal secretion of T4 which doesn't give rise to subnormal serum T4 concentrations. The reason for maintaining T4 values within the reference range is the exquisite sensitivity of the pituitary thyrotroph for even very small decreases of serum T4, as exemplified by the log-linear relationship between serum TSH and serum FT4. A further decline in T4 secretion results in serum T4 values below the lower normal limit and even higher TSH values, but serum T3 concentrations remain within the reference range. It is only in the last stage that subnormal serum T3 concentrations are found, when serum T4 has fallen to really very low values associated with markedly elevated serum TSH concentrations (Figure 1). Hypothyroidism is thus a graded phenomenon, in which the first stage of subclinical hypothyroidism may progress via mild hypothyroidism towards overt hypothyroidism (Table 2) (Reverdin, 1882).

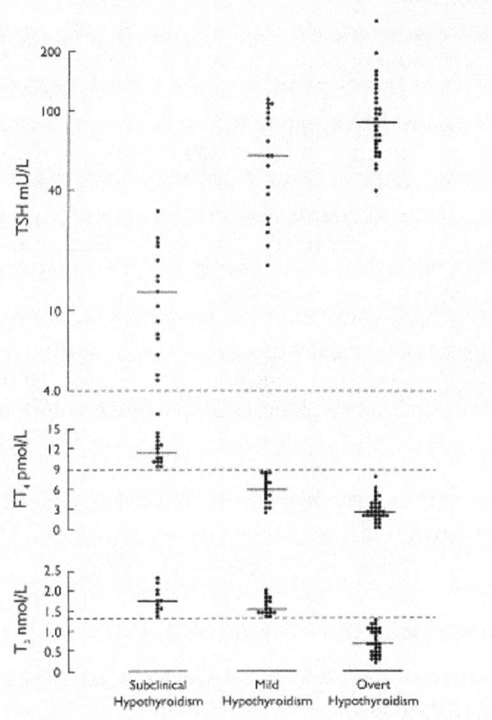

Fig. 1. Individual and median values of thyroid function tests in patients with various grades of hypothyroidism. Discontinuous horizontal lines represent upper limit (TSH) and lower limit (FT4, T3) of the normal reference ranges (Wiersinga, 2010).

Grade 1	Subclinical hypothyroidism	TSH +	FT4 N	T3 N(+)
Grade 2	Mild hypothyroidism	TSH +	FT4 -	T3 N
Grade 3	Overt hypothyroidism	TSH +	FT4 -	T3 -
+, above upper normal limit; N, within normal reference range; -, below lower normal limit.				

Table 2. Grades of hypothyroidism (Reverdin, 1882).

Taken together, hypothyroidism can be classified based on its time of onset (congenital or acquired), severity (overt [clinical] or mild [subclinical]), and the level of endocrine aberration (primary or secondary) (Roberts and Ladenson, 2004). Primary hypothyroidism follows a dysfunction of the thyroid gland itself, whereas secondary and tertiary hypothyroidism results from either defect in the development or dysfunction of pituitary gland and hypothalamus (Grueters et al., 2002; Ahmed et al., 2008).

5. Hypothyroidism and metabolic defects

The thyroid hormones act directly on mitochondria, and thereby control the transformation of the energy derived from oxidations into a form utilizable by the cell. Through their direct actions on mitochondria, the hormones also control indirectly the rate of protein synthesis and thereby the amount of oxidative apparatus in the cell. A rationale for the effects of thyroid hormone excess or deficiency is based upon studies of the mechanism of thyroid hormone action. In hypothyroidism, slow fuel consumption leads to a low output of utilizable energy. Many of the chemical and physical features of these diseases can be reduced to changes in available energy (Hoch, 1968 & 1988; Harper and Seifert, 2008).

Thyroid dysfunction is characterized by alterations in carbohydrate, lipid and lipoprotein metabolism, consequently changing the concentration and composition of plasma lipoproteins. In hyperthyroid patients, the turnover of low-density-lipoprotein apoprotein is increased, and the plasma cholesterol concentration is decreased. Hypothyroidism in man is associated with an increase in plasma cholesterol, particularly in low-density lipoproteins and often with elevated plasma VLD lipoprotein, and there is a positive correlation with premature atherosclerosis. Although it is known that myxoedemic patients have decreased rates of low-density lipoprotein clearance from the circulation, it is not known with certainty if the elevated concentration of VLD lipoprotein is due to increased secretion by the liver or to decreased clearance by the tissues (Laker and Mayes, 1981).

6. Symptoms associated with hypothyroidism

Hypothyroidism produces many symptoms related to its effects on metabolism. Physical symptoms of hypothyroidism-related reduced metabolic rate include fatigue, slowed heart rate, intolerance to cold temperatures, inhibited sweating and muscle pain. Depression is a key psychological consequence of hypothyroidism and slow metabolism as well. For women, slow metabolism can cause increased menstruation and even impair fertility. Weight gain and metabolic rate are intimately related. A slow metabolism interferes with the body's ability to burn fat, so those with hypothyroidism often experience weight gain when their condition is not treated properly. Since the metabolism keeps muscles functioning properly and controls body temperature, hypothyroidism can impair these essential metabolic processes. The weight gain can then lead to obesity, which carries its own serious health risks, including for diabetes, heart disease and certain types of cancer. Other side effects include impaired memory, gynecomastia, impaired cognitive function, puffy face, hands and feet, slow heart rate, decreased sense of taste and smell, sluggish reflexes, decreased libido, hair loss, anemia, acute psychosis, elevated serum cholesterol, difficulty swallowing, shortness of breath, recurrent hypoglycemia, increased need for sleep, irritability, yellowing of the skin due to the failure of the body to convert beta-carotene to vitamin A, and impaired renal function (Onputtha, 2010).

Hypothyroidism is frequently accompanied by diminished cognition, slow thought process, slow motor function, and drowsiness (Bunevičius and Prange Jr, 2010). Myxedema is associated with severe mental disorders including psychoses, sometimes called 'myxematous madness'. Depression related to hypothyroidism, even subclinical hypothyroidism may affect mood (Haggerty and Prange, 1995). Thyroid deficits are frequently observed in bipolar patients, especially in women with the rapid cycling form of the disease (Bauer et al., 2008). Both subclinical hypothyroidism and subclinical hyperthyroidism increase the risk for Alzheimer's disease, especially in women (Tan et al., 2008). However, most hypothyroid patients do not meet the criteria for a mental disorder. A recent study evaluated brain glucose metabolism during T4 treatment of hypothyroidism (Bunevičius and Prange Jr, 2010). A reduction in depression and cognitive symptoms was associated with restoration of metabolic activity in brain areas that are integral to the regulation of mood and cognition (Bauer et al., 2009). In hypothyroidism, replacement therapy with T4 remains the treatment of choice and resolves most physical and psychological signs and symptoms in most patients. However, some patients do not feel entirely well despite doses of T4 that are usually adequate (Saravanan et al., 2002). In T4-treated patients, it was found that reduced psychological well being is associated with occurrence of polymorphism in the D2 gene (Panicker et al., 2009), as well as in the OATP1c1 gene (van der Deure et al., 2008). Thyroid hormone replacement with a combination of T4 and T3, in comparison with T4 monotherapy, improves mental functioning in some but not all hypothyroid patients (Bunevicius et al., 1999; Nygaard et al., 2009), and most of the patients subjectively prefer combined treatment (Escobar-Morreale et al., 2005). It was concluded that future trials on thyroid hormone replacement should target genetic polymorphisms in deiodinase and thyroid hormone transporters (Wiersinga, 2009).

7. Hypothyroidism and development

7.1 Congenital hypothyroidism

Traditionally, research on the role of the thyroid hormones in brain development has focused on the postnatal phase and on identifying congenital hypothyroidism, which is the final result of the deficiency suffered throughout the pregnancy (Pérez-López, 2007). Iodine deficit during pregnancy produces an increase in perinatal mortality and low birth weight which can be prevented by iodated oil injections given in the latter half of pregnancy or in other supplementary forms (European Commission, 2002). The epidemiological studies suggest that hypothyroxinemia, especially at the beginning of pregnancy, affects the neurological development of the new human being in the long term (Pérez-López, 2007). Full-scale clinical studies have demonstrated a correlation between maternal thyroid insufficiency during pregnancy and a low neuropsychological development in the neonate (Haddow et al., 1999). Maternal hypothyroxinemia during the first gestational trimester limits the possibilities of postnatal neurodevelopment (Pop et al., 2003; Kooistra et al., 2006). The most serious form of brain lesion corresponds to neurological cretinism, but mild degrees of maternal hypothyroxinemia also produce alterations in psychomotor development (Morreale de Escobar et al., 2004; Visser, 2006). The thyroid function of neonates at birth is significantly related to the brain size and its development during the first two years of life (Van Vliet, 1999). Screening programs for neonatal congenital hypothyroidism indicate that it is present in approximately one case out of 3000 to 4000 live births (Klein et al., 1991). Seventy-eight percent were found to have an intelligence quotient (IQ) of over 85 when congenital hypothyroidism was diagnosed within the first few months after birth, 19% when it was diagnosed between 3 and 6 months, and 0% when the diagnosis was made 7 months after birth (Pérez-López, 2007). In a meta-analysis of seven studies (Derksen-Lubsen and Verkerk, 1996), a decrease of 6.3 IQ points was found among neonates who suffered hypothyroidism during pregnancy in comparison to the control group. Long-term sequelae of hypothyroidism also affect intellectual development during adolescence. The affected children show an average of 8.5 IQ points less than the control group, with deficits in memory and in visuospatial and motor abilities related to the seriousness of congenital hypothyroidism and due to inadequate treatment in their early childhood (Rovet, 1999).

Untreated congenital hypothyroidism (sporadic cretinism) produces neurologic deficits having predominantly postnatal origins (Porterfield, 2000). Although mental retardation can occur, it typically is not as severe as that seen in neurologic cretinism. Untreated infants with severe congenital hypothyroidism can lose 3-5 IQ points per month if untreated during the first 6-12 months of life (Burrow et al., 1994). If the children are treated with thyroid hormones soon after birth, the more severe effects of thyroid deficiency are alleviated (Porterfield, 2000). However, these children are still at risk for mild learning disabilities. They may show subtle language, neuromotor, and cognitive impairment (Rovet et al., 1996). They are more likely to show attention deficit hyperactivity disorder (ADHD), have problems with speech and interpretation of the spoken word, have poorer fine motor coordination, and have problems with spatial perception (Rovet et al., 1992). The severity of these effects is correlated with the retardation of bone ossification seen at birth. This would suggest that the damage is correlated with the mild hypothyroidism they experience in utero. Rovet and Ehrlich (1995) have proposed that the sensitive periods for thyroid hormones vary for verbal and nonverbal skills. The critical period for verbal and memory skills appears to be in the first 2 months postpartum, whereas for visuospatial or visuomotor skills it is prenatal (Porterfield, 2000). Thyroid hormone deficiency impairs learning and memory, which depend on the structural integrity of the hippocampus (Porterfield, 2000). Maturation and synaptic development of the pyramidal cells of the hippocampus are particularly sensitive to thyroid hormone deficiency during fetal/perinatal development (Madeira et al., 1992). Early in fetal development (rats), thyroid hormone deficiency decreases radial glial cell maturation and therefore impairs cellular migration (Rami and Rabie, 1988), which can lead to irreversible changes in the neuronal population and connectivity in this region. Animals with experimentally induced congenital hypothyroidism show delayed and decreased axonal and dendritic arborization in the cerebral cortex, a decrease in nerve terminals, delayed myelination, abnormal cochlear development, and impaired middle ear ossicle development (Porterfield and Hendrich, 1993).

7.2 Endemic cretinism

The most severe neurologic impairment resulting from a thyroid deficiency is an endemic cretinism caused by iodine deficiency (Porterfield, 2000). In fact, iodine deficiency represents the single most preventable cause of neurologic impairment and cerebral palsy in the world today (Donati et al., 1992; Morreale de Escobar et al., 1997). These individuals suffer from hypothyroidism that begins at conception because the dietary iodine deficiency prevents synthesis of normal levels of thyroid hormones (Porterfield, 2000). It is more severe than that seen in congenital hypothyroidism because the deficiency occurs much earlier in development and results in decreased brain thyroid hormone exposure both before and after the time the fetal thyroid gland begins functioning (Porterfield, 2000). Problems with endemic cretins include mental retardation that can be profound, spastic dysplasia, and problems with gross and fine motor control resulting from damage to both the pyramidal and the extrapyramidal systems (Porterfield, 2000). These problems include disturbances of gait, and in the more extreme forms, the individuals cannot walk or stand (Pharoah et al., 1981; Donati et al., 1992; Stanbury, 1997). If postnatal hypothyroidism is present, there is growth retardation and delayed or absent sexual maturation (Porterfield and Hendrich, 1993). Damage occurs both to structures such as the corticospinal system that develop relatively early in the fetus and structures such as the cerebellum that develop predominantly in the late fetal and early neonatal period (Porterfield, 2000). The damage is inversely related to maternal serum thyroxine (T4) levels but not to triiodothyronine (T3) levels (Calvo et al., 1990; Donati et al., 1992; Porterfield and Hendrich, 1993). Delong (1987) suggests that the neurologic damage occurs primarily in the second trimester, which is an important period for formation of the cerebral cortex, the extrapyramidal system, and the cochlea, areas damaged in endemic cretins. Maternal T3 levels are often normal and the mother therefore may not show any overt symptoms of hypothyroidism (Porterfield, 2000). Early development of the auditory system appears to be dependent upon thyroid hormones (Bradley et al., 1994). The greater impairment characterized by endemic cretinism relative to congenital hypothyroidism is thought to result from the longer period of exposure of the developing brain to hypothyroidism in endemic cretinism (Donati et al., 1992; Porterfield and Hendrich, 1993; Morreale de Escobar et al., 1997).

7.3 Thyroid function during pregnancy and iodine deficiency

Glinoer and his group showed that, in conditions of mild iodine deficiency, the serum concentrations of free thyroxine decrease steadily and significantly during gestation (Glinoer, 1997a,b). Although the median values remain within the normal range, one third of pregnant women have free thyroxine values near or below the lower limit of normal. This picture is in clear contrast with thyroid status during normal pregnancy and normal iodine intake, which is characterised by only a slight (15%) decrease of free thyroxine by the end of gestation. After an initial blunting of serum thyroid stimulating hormone (TSH) caused by increased concentrations of human chorionic gonadotrophin, serum TSH concentrations increase progressively in more than 80% of pregnant Belgian women, although these levels also remain within the normal range. This change is accompanied by an increase in serum thyroglobulin, which is directly related to the increase in TSH. This situation of chronic thyroid hyperstimulation results in an increase in thyroid volume by 20% to 30% during gestation, a figure twice as high as that in conditions of normal iodine supply. The role of the lack of iodine in the development of these different anomalies is indicated by the fact that a daily supplementation with physiological doses of iodine (150 µg/day) prevents their occurrence (Glinoer et al., 1995). In moderate iodine deficiency, the anomalies are of the same nature but more marked. For example, in an area of Sicily with an iodine intake of 40 µg/day, Vermiglio et al reported a decline of serum free thyroxine of 31% and a simultaneous increase of serum TSH of 50% during early (8th to 19th weeks) gestation (Vermiglio et al., 1995). Only a limited number of studies are available on thyroid function during pregnancy in populations with severe iodine deficiency (iodine intake below 25 µg iodine/day). Moreover, because of the extremely difficult conditions in which these studies were performed, the results are necessarily only partial. The most extensive data are available from New Guinea (Choufoer et al., 1965; Pharoah et al., 1984) and the Democratic Republic of Congo (DRC, formerly Zaire) (Thilly et al., 1978; Delange et al., 1982). The studies conducted in such environments show that the prevalence of goitre reaches peak values of up to 90% in females of child bearing age 20 and that during pregnancy, serum thyroxine is extremely low and serum TSH extremely high. However, it has been pointed out that for a similar degree of severe iodine deficiency in the DRC and New Guinea, serum thryoxine in pregnant mothers is much higher in the DRC (103 nmol/l) than in New Guinea (38.6–64.4 nmol/l) (Morreale de Escobar et al., 1997). The frequency of values below 32.2 nmol/l is only 3% in the DRC while it is 20% in New Guinea. This discrepancy was understood only when it was demonstrated that in the DRC, iodine deficiency is aggravated by selenium deficiency and thiocyanate overload (see later section) (Delange et al., 1982; Vanderpas et al., 1990; Contempre et al., 1991). Also, during pregnancy, iodine deficiency produces hypothyroxinemia which consequently causes (1) thyroid stimulation through the feedback mechanisms of TSH, and (2) goitrogenesis in both mother and fetus (Pérez-López, 2007). For this reason, it seems that moderate iodine deficiency causes an imbalance in maternal thyroid homeostasis, especially toward the end of pregnancy, leading to isolated hypothyroxinemia suggestive of biochemical hypothyroidism. Uncontrolled hypothyroidism in pregnancy can lead to preterm birth, low birth weight and mental retardation (Drews and Seremak-Mrozikiewicz, 2011).

7.4 Perinatal thyroid function and iodine deficiency

In mild iodine deficiency, serum concentrations of TSH and thyroglobulin are still higher in neonates than in mothers (Glinoer, 1997a,b), indicating that neonates are more sensitive than adults to the effects of iodine deficiency. Again, the role of iodine deficiency is demonstrated by the fact that neonates born to mothers who have been supplemented with iodine during pregnancy have a lower thyroid volume and serum thyroglobulin and higher urinary iodine than newborns born to untreated mothers (Glinoer et al., 1995). Other evidence of chronic TSH overstimulation of the neonatal thyroid is the fact that there is a slight shift towards increased values of the frequency distribution of neonatal TSH on day 5, which is the time of systematic screening for congenital hypothyroidism (Delange, 2001). The frequency of values above 5 mU/l blood is 4.5%, while the normal value is below 3%. In moderate iodine deficiency, the anomalies are of the same nature but more drastic than in conditions of mild iodine deficiency (Delange, 2001). Transient hyperthyrotrophinaemia or even transient neonatal hypothyroidism can occur. The frequency of the latter condition is approximately six times higher in Europe than in the United States where the iodine intake is much higher (Delange et al., 1983). The shift of neonatal TSH towards increased values is more marked and the frequency of values above 20–25 mU/l blood, that is above the cut off point used for recalling the neonates because of suspicion of congenital hypothyroidism in programmes of systematic screening for congenital hypothyroidism, is increased (Delange, 2001). There is an inverse relationship between the median urinary iodine of populations of neonates used as an index of their iodine intake and the recall rate at screening (Delange, 1994 & 1998). It has to be pointed out that these changes in neonatal TSH frequently occur for levels of iodine deficiency that would not affect the thyroid function in non-pregnant adults (Delange, 2001). The hypersensitivity of neonates to the effects of iodine deficiency is explained by their very small intrathyroidal iodine pool, which requires increased TSH stimulation and a fast turnover rate in order to maintain normal secretion of thyroid hormones (Delange, 1998). In severe iodine deficiency, as in the mothers, the biochemical picture of neonatal hypothyroidism is caricatural, especially in the DRC where mean cord serum thyroxine and TSH concentrations are 95.2 nmol/l and 70.7 mU/l respectively and where as many as 11% of the neonates have both a cord serum TSH above 100 mU/l and a cord thyroxine below 38.6 nmol/l, that is a biochemical picture similar to the one found in thyroid agenesis (Delange et al., 1993).

7.5 Hypothyroidism and brain development in humans

The neonatal period of development in humans is known to be sensitive to thyroid hormone, especially as revealed in the disorder known as congenital hypothyroidism (CH) (Krude et al., 1977; Dussault and Walker, 1983; Miculan et al., 1993; Foley, 1996; Kooistra et al., 1994; van Vliet, 1999; Rovet, 2000). CH occurs at a rate of approximately 1 in 3,500 live births (Delange, 1997). Because CH infants do not present a specific clinical picture early, their diagnosis based solely on clinical symptoms was delayed before neonatal screening for thyroid hormone (Zoeller et al., 2002). In fact, only 10% of CH infants were diagnosed within the first month, 35% within 3 months, 70% within the first year, and 100% only after age 3 (Alm et al., 1984). The intellectual deficits as a result of this delayed diagnosis and treatment were profound. One meta-analysis found that the mean full-scale intelligence quotient (IQ) of 651 CH infants was 76 (Klein, 1980). Moreover, the percentage of CH infants with an IQ above 85 was 78% when the diagnosis was made within 3 months of birth, 19% when it was made between 3 and 6 months, and 0% when diagnosed after 7 months of age (Klein, 1980; Klein and Mitchell, 1996). Studies now reveal that the long-term consequences of CH are subtle if the diagnosis is made early and treatment is initiated within 14 days of birth (Mirabella et al., 2000; Hanukoglu et al., 2001; Leneman et al., 2001), which can be accomplished only by mandatory screening for thyroid function at birth. This medical profile has become the principal example illustrating the importance of thyroid hormone for normal brain development (Zoeller et al., 2002). Recent studies indicate that thyroid hormone is also important during fetal development. Thyroid hormones are detected in human coelomic and amniotic fluids as early as 8 weeks of gestation, before the onset of fetal thyroid function at 10–12 weeks (Contempre et al., 1993). In addition, human fetal brain tissues express thyroid hormone receptors (TRs), and receptor occupancy by thyroid hormone is in the range known to produce physiological effects as early as 9 weeks of gestation (Ferreiro et al., 1988). Finally, the mRNAs encoding the two known TR classes exhibit complex temporal patterns of expression during human gestation (Iskaros et al., 2000), and the mRNAs encoding these TR isoforms are expressed in the human oocyte (Zhang et al., 1997). These data indicate that maternal thyroid hormone is delivered to the fetus before the onset of fetal thyroid function, and that the minimum requirements for thyroid hormone signaling are present at this time (Zoeller et al., 2002). Two kinds of pathological situations reveal the functional consequences of deficits in thyroid hormone during fetal development (Zoeller et al., 2002). The first is that of cretinism, a condition usually associated with severe iodine insufficiency in the diet (Delange, 2000). There are two forms of cretinism based on clinical presentation: neurological cretinism and myxedematous cretinism (Delange, 2000). Neurological cretinism is characterized by extreme mental retardation, deaf-mutism, impaired voluntary motor activity, and hypertonia (Delange, 2000). In contrast, myxedematous cretinism is characterized by less severe mental retardation and all the major clinical symptoms of persistent hypothyroidism (Delange, 2000). Iodide administration to pregnant women in their first trimester eliminates the incidence of neurological cretinism (Zoeller et al., 2002). However, the initiation of iodine supplementation by the end of the second trimester does not prevent neurological damage (Cao et al., 1994; Delange, 2000). Several detailed studies of endemias occurring in different parts of the world have led to the proposal that the various symptoms of the two forms of cretinism arise from thyroid hormone deficits occurring at different developmental windows of vulnerability (Cao et al., 1994; Delange, 2000). Therefore, thyroid hormone appears to play an important role in fetal brain development, perhaps before the onset of fetal thyroid function (Zoeller et al., 2002). The second type of pathological situation is that of subtle, undiagnosed maternal hypothyroxinemia (Zoeller et al., 2002). The concept and definition of maternal hypothyroxinemia were developed in a series of papers by Man et al. (Man and Jones, 1969; Man and Serunian, 1976; Man and Brown, 1991). Low thyroid hormone was initially defined empirically - those pregnant women with the lowest butanol-extractable iodine among all pregnant women (de Escobar et al., 2000). This work was among the first to document an association between subclinical hypothyroidism in pregnant women and neurological function of the offspring. After the development of radioimmunoassay for thyroid hormone, Pop et al. (1995) found that the presence of antibodies to thyroid peroxidase in pregnant women, independent of thyroid hormone levels per se, is associated with significantly lower IQ in the offspring. Subsequent studies have shown that children born to women with thyroxine (T4) levels in the lowest 10th percentile of the normal range had a higher risk of low IQ and attention deficit (Haddow et al., 1999). Excellent recent reviews discuss these studies in detail (de Escobar et al., 2000). Taken together, these studies present strong evidence that maternal thyroid hormone plays a role in fetal brain development before the onset of fetal thyroid function, and that thyroid hormone deficits in pregnant women can produce irreversible neurological effects in their offspring (Gupta et al., 1995; Klett, 1997).

7.6 Hypothyroidism and brain development in experimental animals

Considerable research using experimental animals has provided important insight into the mechanisms and consequences of thyroid hormone action in brain development (Zoeller et al., 2002). The body of this work is far too extensive to review here but has been reviewed at critical times during the past 50 years (de Escobar et al., 2000; Oppenheimer et al., 1994;

Oppenheimer and Schwartz, 1997; Pickard et al., 1997). Several themes have emerged that provide a framework in which to begin to understand the role of thyroid hormone in brain development. First, the majority of biological actions of thyroid hormone appear to be mediated by TRs, which are ligand-dependent transcription factors (Mangelsdorf et al., 1995). There are two genes, encoding TRα and TRβ, although these two receptors do not exhibit different binding characteristics for T4 and for triiodothyronine (T3) (Zoeller et al., 2002). Second, based on considerable work in the cerebellum, there appear to be critical periods of thyroid hormone action during development. As originally defined (Brown et al., 1939), the critical period was that developmental stage where thyroid hormone replacement to CH children could improve their intellectual outcome. This definition was also applied to experimental studies to identify the developmental period during which thyroid hormone exerts a specific action (Zoeller et al., 2002). It is now generally accepted that there is no single critical period of thyroid hormone action on brain development, either in humans (Delange, 2000) or in animals (Dowling et al., 2000). Rather, thyroid hormone acts on a specific development process during the period that the process is active. For example, thyroid hormone effects on cellular proliferation would necessarily be limited to the period of proliferation for a specific brain area. Because cells in different brain regions are produced at different times (Bayer and Altman, 1995), the critical period for thyroid hormone action on cell proliferation would differ for cells produced at different times.

7.7 Thyroid hormone deficiency and neuronal development

Thyroid hormone deficiency during a critical developmental period can impair cellular migration and development of neuronal networks. Neuronal outgrowth and cellular migration are dependent on normal microtubule synthesis and assembly and these latter processes are regulated by thyroid hormones (Nunez et al., 1991). During cerebral development, postmitotic neurons forming near the ventricular surface must migrate long distances to reach their final destination in the cortical plate where they form a highly organized 6-layer cortical structure (Porterfield, 2000). Appropriate timing of this migration is essential if normal connectivity is to be established. This migration depends not only upon specialized cells such as the radial glial cells that form a scaffolding system but also on specific adhesion molecules in the extracellular matrix that are associated with the focal contacts linking migrating neurons with radial glial fibers (Mione and Parnavelas, 1994). These neurons migrate along radial glial fibers, and following neuronal migration, the radial glial cells often degenerate or become astrocytes (Rakic, 1990). Migration also depends on adhesive interactions involving extracellular matrix proteins such as laminin and the cell-surface receptor integrin (Porterfield, 2000). Disorders of neuronal migration are considered to be major causes of both gross and subtle brain abnormalities (Rakic, 1990). Hypothyroidism during fetal and neonatal development results in delayed neuronal differentiation and decreased neuronal connectivity (Nunez et al., 1991).

8. References

Ahmed OM, El-Gareib, AW, El-bakry, AM, Abd El-Tawab, S.M, Ahmed, RG. Thyroid hormones states and brain development interactions. Int J Devl Neurosc 2008; 26: 147–209.

Alm J, Hagenfeldt L, Larsson A, Lundberg K. Incidence of congenital hypothyroidism: retrospective study of neonatal laboratory screening versus clinical symptoms as indicators leading to diagnosis. Br Med J 1984; 289: 1171–1175.

Aminoff MJ. Neurology and General Medicine: Expert Consult: Online and Print. Edinburgh: Churchill Livingstone, 2007.

Bauer M, Goetz T, Glenn T, Whybrow PC. The thyroid-brain interaction in thyroid disorders and mood disorders. J Neuroendocrinol 2008; 20: 1101–1114.

Bauer M, Silverman DH, Schlagenhauf F, et al. Brain glucose metabolism in hypothyroidism: a positron emission tomography study before and after thyroid hormone replacement therapy. J Clin Endocrinol Metab 2009; 94: 2922–2929.

Bayer SA, Altman J. Neurogenesis and neuronal migration. In: The Rat Nervous System, 2nd ed. (Paxinos G, ed). San Diego, CA:Academic Press, 1995; 1079–1098.

Bradley DJ, Towle HC, Young WS Ill. a and P thyroid hormone receptor (TR) gene expression during auditory neurogenesis: evidence for TR isoform-specific transcriptional regulation in vivo. Proc NatI Acad Sci USA 1994; 91:439-443.

Brown AW, Bronstein IP, Kraines R. Hypothyroidism and cretinism in childhood. VI. Influence of thyroid therapy on mental growth. Am J Dis Child 1939; 57:517–523.

Bunevicius R, Kazanavicius G, Zalinkevicius R, Prange AJ. Effects of thyroxine as compared with thyroxine plus triiodothyronine in patients with hypothyroidism. N Engl J Med 1999; 340: 424–429.

Bunevičius, R., Prange, A.J. Thyroid disease and mental disorders: cause and effect or only comorbidity? Current Opinion in Psychiatry 2010; 23: 363–368.

Burrow, GN, Fisher, DA, Larsen, PR. Maternal and fetal thyroid function. N Engl J Med 1994; 331:1072-1078.

Calvo R, Obregon MJ, Ruiz de Ona C, Escobar del Rey F, Morreale de Escobar G. Congenital hypothyroidism as studied in rats. J Clin Invest 1990; 86:889-899.

Cao XY, Jiang XM, Dou ZH, Murdon AR, Zhang ML, O'Donnell K, Ma T, Kareem A, DeLong N, Delong GR. Timing of vulnerability of the brain to iodine deficiency in endemic cretinism. N Engl J Med 1994; 331:1739–1744.

Choufoer JC, Van Rhijn M, Querido A. Endemic goiter in western New Guinea. II. Clinical picture, incidence and pathogenesis of endemic cretinism. J Clin Endocrinol Metab 1965; 25: 385–402.

Contempre B, Dumont JE, Bebe N, et al. Effect of selenium supplementation in hypothyroid subjects of an iodine and selenium deficient area: the possible danger of indiscriminate supplementation of iodine deficient subjects with selenium. J Clin Endocrinol Metab 1991; 73: 213–15.

Contempre B, Jauniaux E, Calvo R, Jurkovic D, Campbell S, de Escobar GM. Detection of thyroid hormones in human embryonic cavities during the first trimester of pregnancy. J Clin Endocrinol Metab 1993; 77:1719–1722.

de Escobar GM, Obregon MJ, Escobar del Rey F. Is neuropsychological development related to maternal hypothyroidism or to maternal hypothyroxinemia? J Clin Endocrinol Metab 2000; 85: 3975–3987.

Delange F, Bourdoux P, Ketelbant-Balasse P, et al. Transient primary hypothyroidism in the newborn. In: Dussault JH,Walker P, eds. Congenital hypothyroidism. New York:M Dekker, 1983; 275–301.

Delange F, Bourdoux P, Laurence M, et al. Neonatal thyroid function in iodine deficiency. In: Delange F, Dunn JT, Glinoer D, eds. Iodine deficiency in Europe.A continuing concern. New York: Plenum Press, 1993; 199–210.

Delange F, Thilly C, Bourdoux P, et al. Influence of dietary goitrogens during pregnancy in humans on thyroid function of the newborn. In: Delange F, Iteke FB, Ermans AM, eds. Nutritional factors involved in the goitrogenic action of cassava. Ottawa: International Development Research Centre, 1982; 40–50.

Delange F. Neonatal screening for congenital hypothyroidism: results and perspectives. Horm Res 1997; 48:51–61.

Delange F. Screening for congenital hypothyroidism used as an indicator of the degree of iodine deficiency and of its control. Thyroid 1998; 8: 1185–92.

Delange F. The disorders induced by iodine deficiency. Thyroid 1994; 4: 107–128.

Delange FM. Endemic cretinism. In: Werner and Ingbar's The Thyroid: A Fundamental and Clinical Text, 8th ed. (Braverman LE, Utiger RD, eds). Philadelphia:Lippincott Williams and Wilkins, 2000; 743–754.

Delange, F. Iodine deficiency as a cause of brain damage. Postgrad Med J 2001; 77: 217–220.

DeLong GR, Ma T, Cao XY, Jiang XM, Dou ZH, Murdon AR, Zhang ML, Heinz ER. The neuromotor deficit in endemic cretinism. In: The Damaged Brain of Iodine Deficiency (Stanbury JB, ed). New York:Cognizant Communications, 1994; 9-17.

DeLong R. Neurological involvement in iodine deficiency disorders. In: The Prevention and Control of Iodine Deficiency Disorders IHetzel BS, Dunn JT, Stanbury JB, eds). Amsterdam:Elsevier, 1987;49-63.

Derksen-Lubsen G, Verkerk PH. Neuropsychologic development in early treated congenital hypothyroidism: analysis of literature data. Pediatric Res 1996; 39: 561–566.

Donati 1, Antonelli A, Bertoni F, Moscogiuri D, Andreani M, Venturi S, Filippi T, Gasperinin 1, Neri S, Baschieri L. Clinical picture of endemic cretinism in central Apennines (Montefeltro). Thyroid 1992; 2:283-290.

Dowling ALS, Martz GU, Leonard JL, Zoeller RT. Acute changes in maternal thyroid hormone induce rapid and transient changes in specific gene expression in fetal rat brain. J Neurosci 2000; 20: 2255–2265.

Drews K, Seremak-Mrozikiewicz A. The Optimal Treatment of Thyroid Gland Function Disturbances During Pregnancy. Curr Pharm Biotechnol. 2011 Feb 22. [Epub ahead of print].

Dussault JH, Walker P. Congenital Hypothyroidism. New York:Marcel Dekker, 1983.

Elizabeth DA, Agabegi, SS. Step-Up to Medicine (Step-Up Series). Hagerstwon, MD. Lippincott Williams & Wilkins, 2008.

Escobar-Morreale HF, Botella-Carretero JI, Escobar del Rey F, Morreale de Escobar G. Review: Treatment of hypothyroidism with combinations of levothyroxine plus liothyronine. J Clin Endocrinol Metab 2005; 90: 4946–4954.

European Commission, Health & Consumer Protection Directorate-General. Opinion of the Scientific Committee on Food on the tolerable upper intake level of iodine. SCF/CS/NUT/UPPLEV/26 Final. Brussels: European Union, 2002. pp 1–25.

Ferreiro B, Bernal J, Goodyer CG, Branchard CL. Estimation of nuclear thyroid hormone receptor saturation in human fetal brain and lung during early gestation. J Clin Endocrinol Metab 1988; 67:853–856.

Foley TP. Congenital hypothyroidism. In: Werner and Ingbar's The Thyroid, 7th ed. (Braverman LE, Utiger RD, eds). Philadelphia:Lippincott-Raven, 1996; 988–994.

Glinoer D, De Nayer P, Delange F, et al. A randomized trial for the treatment of excessive thyroid stimulation in pregnancy: maternal and neonatal effects. J Clin Endocrinol Metab 1995; 80: 258–69.

Glinoer D. Maternal and fetal impact of chronic iodine deficiency. Clin Obstet Gynecol 1970a; 40: 102–16.

Glinoer D. The regulation of thyroid function in pregnancy: pathways of endocrine adaptation from physiology to pathology. Endocr Rev 1970b; 18: 404–33.

Grueters A, Biebermann H, Krude H. Molecular pathogenesis of congenital hypothyroidism, 2002; September, No. 4 (www.hotthyroidology.com).

Gull WW. On a cretinoid state supervening in adult life in women. Trans Clin Soc London 1874; 7: 180.

Gupta RK, Bhatia V, Poptani H, Gujral RB. Brain metabolite changes on *in vivo* proton magnetic resonance spectroscopy in children with congenital hypothyroidism. J Pediatr 1995; 126:389–392.

Haddow JE, Palomaki GE, Allan WC, Williams JR, Knight GJ, Gagnon J, O'Heir CE, Mitchell ML, Hermos RJ, Waisbren SE, et al. Maternal thyroid deficiency during pregnancy and subsequent neuropsychological development of the child. N Engl J Med 1999; 341: 549–555.

Haddow JE, Palomaki GE, Allen WC, Williams JR, Knight GJ, Gagnon J, O'Heir CE, Mitchell ML, Hermos RJ, Waisbren SE, et al. Maternal thyroid deficiency during pregnancy and subsequent neuropsychological development of the child. N Engl J Med 1999; 341:549–555.

Haggerty JJ Jr, Prange AJ Jr. Borderline hypothyroidism and depression. Annu Rev Med 1995; 46: 37–46.

Hanukoglu A, Perlman K, Shamis I, Brnjac L, Rovet J, Daneman D. Relationship of etiology to treatment in congenital hypothyroidism. J Clin Endocrinol Metab 2001; 86:186–191.

Harper M, Seifert EL. Thyroid Economy—Regulation, Cell Biology, Thyroid Hormone Metabolism and Action: The Special Edition: Metabolic Effects of Thyroid Hormones Thyroid Hormone Effects on Mitochondrial Energetics. Thyroid 2008; 18 (2): 145-156.

Hoch FL. Lipids and thyroid hormones. Prog Lipid Res 1988; 27: 199-270.

Hoch FL. Biochemistry of hyperthyroidism and hypothyroidism. Postgrad Med J 1968; 44:347-362.

Iskaros J, Pickard M, Evans I, Sinha A, Hardiman P, Ekins R. Thyroid hormone receptor gene expression in first trimester human fetal brain. J Clin Endocrinol Metab 2000; 85:2620–2623.

Klein R. History of congenital hypothyroidism. In: Neonatal Thyroid Screening (Burrow GN, Dussault JH, eds). New York:Raven Press, 1980; 51–59.

Klein RZ, Haddow JE, Faix JD, Brown RS, Hermos RJ, Pulkkinen A, Mitchell ML. Prevalence of thyroid deficiency in pregnant women. Clin Endocrinol (Oxf) 1991; 35: 41–46.

Klein RZ, Mitchell ML. Neonatal screening for hypothyroidism. In: Werner and Ingbar's The Thyroid, 7th ed. (Braverman LE, Utiger RD, eds). Philadelphia:Lipponcott- Raven, 1996;984–988.

Klett M. Epidemiology of congenital hypothyroidism. Exp Clin Endocrinol Diabetes 1997; 105 (suppl 4):19–23.

Kocher T. Ueber Kropfexstirpation und ihre Folgen. Arch Klin Chir 1983; 29:254.

Kooistra L, Crawford S, van Baar AL, Brouwers EP, Pop VJ. Neonatal effects of maternal hypothyroxinemia during early pregnancy. Pediatrics 2006; 117: 161–167.

Kooistra L, Laane C, Vulsma T, Schellekens JMH, van der Meere JJ, Kalverboer AF. Motor and cognitive development in children with congenital hypothyroidism. J Pediatr 1994; 124:903–909.

Krude H, Biebermann H, Krohn HP, Gruters A. Congenital hyperthyroidism. Exp Clin Endocrinol Diabetes 1977; 105:6–11.

Laker ME, Mayes PA. Effect of hyperthyroidism and hypothyroidism on lipid and carbohydrate metabolism of the perfused rat liver. Biochem. J 1981; 196: 247-255

Lania A, Persani L, Beck-Peccoz P. Central hypothyroidism. Pituitary 2008; 11(2):181-6.

Leneman M, Buchanan L, Rovet J. Where and what visuospatial processing in adolescents with congenital hypothyroidism. J Int Neuropsychol Soc 2001; 7:556–562.

Madeira MD, Sousa N, Lima-Andrade MT, Calheiros F, Cadete-Leite A, Paula-Barbosa MM. Selective vulnerability of the hippocampal pyramidal neurons to hypothyroidism in male and female rats. J Comp Neurol 1992; 322:501-518.

Man EB, Brown JF, Serunian SA. Maternal hypothyroxinemia: psychoneurological deficits of progeny. Ann Clin Lab Sci 1991; 21:227–239.

Man EB, Jones WS. Thyroid function in human pregnancy. Part V. Am J Obstet Gynecol 1969; 104:898–908.

Man EB, Serunian SA. Thyroid function in human pregnancy. IX: Development or retardation of 7-year-old progeny of hypothyroxinemic women. Am J Obstet Gynecol 1976; 125:949.

Mangelsdorf DJ, Evans RM. The RXR heterodimers and orphan receptors. Cell 1995; 83:841–850.

Miculan J, Turner S, Paes BA. Congenital hypothyroidism: diagnosis and management. Neonatal Netw 1993; 12:25–34.

Mione MC, Parnavelas JG. How do developing cortical neurons know where to go? Trends Neurosci 1994; 17:443-445.

Mirabella G, Feig D, Astzalos E, Perlman K, Rovet JF. The effect of abnormal intrauterine thyroid hormone economies on infant cognitive abilities. J Pediatr Endocrinol Metab 2000; 13:191–194.

Morreale de Escobar G, Obrego´n MJ, Escobar del Rey F. Role of thyroid hormone during early brain development. Eur J Endocrinol 2004; 151(Suppl 3): U25–U37.

Morreale de Escobar G, Obregon MJ, Calvo R, Pedraza P, Escobar del Rey F. Iodine deficiency, the hidden scourge: the rat model of human neurological cretinism. In: Recent Research Developments in Neuroendocrinology (Hendrich CE, ed). Kerala State, India: Research Signpost, 1997; 55-70.

Nunez J, Couchie D, Aniello F, Bridoux AM. Regulation by thyroid hormone of microtubule assembly and neuronal differentiation. Neurochem Res 1991; 16: 975-982

Nygaard B, Jensen E, Kvetny J, et al. Effect of combination therapy with thyroxine (T4) and 3,5,3-triiodothyronine (T3) versus T4 monotherapy in patients with hypothyroidism, a double blind, randomized cross-over study. Eur J Endocrinol 2009; 161: 895–902.

Onputtha DC. Effects of Hypothyroidism on the Body, 2010. EzineArticles.com.

Oppenheimer JH, Schwartz HL, Strait KA. Thyroid hormone action 1994: the plot thickens. Eur J Endocrinol 1994; 130:15–24.

Oppenheimer JH, Schwartz HL. Molecular basis of thyroid hormone-dependent brain development. Endocr Rev 1997; 18:462–475.

Ord WM. On myxedema, a term proposed to be applied to an essential condition in the "cretinoid" affection occasionally observed in middle-aged women. Medico-Chir Trans 1978; 61: 57.

Panicker V, Saravanan P, Vaidya B, et al. Common variation in the DIO2 gene predicts baseline psychological well being and response to combination thyroxine plus triiodothyronine therapy in hypothyroid patients. J Clin Endocrinol Metab 2009; 94: 1623–1629.

Pérez-López, F.R.. Iodine and thyroid hormones during pregnancy and postpartum. Gynecological Endocrinology, 2007; 23(7): 414–428.

Pharoah P, Connolly K, Hetzel B, Ekins R. Maternal thyroid function and motor competence in the child. Dev Med Child Neurol 1981; 23: 76-82.

Pharoah POD, Connolly KJ, Ekins RP, et al. Maternal thyroid hormone levels in pregnancy and the subsequent cognitive and motor performance of the children. Clin Endocrinol (Oxf) 1984; 21: 265–70.

Pickard MR, Evans IM, Bandopadhyay R, Leonard AJ, Sinha AK, Ekins RP. Thyroid hormone action in rat brain from fetal to adult life. In: Recent Research Developments in Neuroendocrinology—Thyroid Hormone and Brain Maturation (Hendrich CE, ed). Research SignPost, 1997; 15–29.

Pop VJ, Brouwers EP, Vader HL, Vulsma T, van Baar AL, de Vijlder JJ. Maternal hypothyroxinemia during early pregnancy and subsequent child development: a 3-year follow-upstudy. Clin Endocrinol (Oxf) 2003; 59: 282–288.

Pop VJ, de Vries E, van Baar AL, Waelkens JJ, de Rooy HA, Horsten M, Donkers MM, Komproe IH, van Son MM, Vander HL. Maternal thyroid peroxidase antibodies during pregnancy: a marker of impaired child development? J Clin Endocrinol Metab 1995; 80: 3560–3566.

Potemkin V. Endocrinology. Russian edition, Mir publishers, Moscow, 1989.

Porterfield SP, Hendrich CE. The role of thyroid hormones in prenatal and neonatal neurological development-current perspectives. Endocr Rev 1993; 14:94-106.

Porterfield, S.P. Thyroidal Dysfunction and Environmental Chemicals Potential Impact on Brain Development. - Environ Health Perspect 2000; 108(suppl 3): 433-438.

Rakic P. Principles of neural cell migration. Experientia 1990; 46:882-891.

Rami A, Rabie A. Effect of thyroid deficiency on the development of glia in the hippocampal formation of the rat: an immunocytochemical study. GLIA 1988; 1:337-345.

Report of a Committee of the Clinical Society of London to Investigate the Subject of Myxedema. London, Longmans. Green & Co. Ltd. 1888.

Reverdin JL: In discussion. Société médicale de Genève. Rev Med Suisse Romande 1882; 2: 537.

Roberts CGP, Ladenson PW. Hypothyroidism. Lancet 2004; 363 (9411): 793–831.

Rovet J, Ehrlich R, Altmann D. Psychoeducational outcome in children with early-treated congenital hypothyroidism. American Thyroid Association, 1996.

Rovet JF, Ehrlich Rm, Sorbara DL. Neurodevelopment in infants and preschool children with congenital hypothyroidism: etiological and treatment factors affecting outcome. J Pediatr Psychol 1992; 2: 187-213.

Rovet JF, Ehrlich RM. Long-term effects of L-thyroxine therapy for congenital hypothyroidism. J Pediatr 1995; 126:380-386.

Rovet JF. Congenital hypothyroidism: long-term outcome. Thyroid 1999; 9: 741–748.

Rovet JF. Neurobehavioral consequences of congenital hypothyroidism identified by newborn screening. In: Therapeutic Outcome of Endocrine Disorders (Stabler B, Bercu BB, eds). New York:Springer-Verlag, 2000; 235–254.

Saravanan P, Chau WF, Roberts N, et al. Psychological well being in patients on 'adequate' doses of l-thyroxine: results of a large, controlled community based questionnaire study. Clin Endocrinol (Oxf) 2002; 57: 577–585.

Simon H. "Hypothyroidism". University of Maryland Medical Center, 2006.University of Maryland Medical System, 22 S. Greene Street, Baltimore, MD 21201.

Stanbury JB. The pathogenesis of endemic cretinism. J Endocrinol Invest 1997; 7: 409-419.

Tan ZS, Beiser A, Vasan RS, et al. Thyroid function and the risk of Alzheimer disease: the Framingham Study. Arch Intern Med 2008; 168: 1514–1520.

Thilly CH, Delange F, Lagasse R, et al. Fetal hypothyroidism and maternal thyroid status in severe endemic goiter. J Clin Endocrinol Metab 1978; 47: 354–60.

Thomas, PF. Hypothyroidism. Pediatrics in Review 2004; 25 (3): 94-100.

van der Deure WM, Appelhof BC, Peeters RP, et al. Polymorphisms in the brain-specific thyroid hormone transporter OATP1C1 are associated with fatigue and depression in hypothyroid patients. Clin Endocrinol (Oxf) 2008; 69: 804–811.

Van Vliet G. Neonatal hypothyroidism: treatment and outcome. Thyroid 1999; 9: 79–84.

Vanderpas JB, Contempre B, Duale NL, et al. Iodine and selenium deficiency associated with cretinism in northern Zaire. Am J Clin Nutr 1990; 52: 1087–93.

Vanderpump MPJ. Epidemiology of Thyroid Dysfunction - Hypothyroidism and Hyperthyroidism. Thyroid International 2009; 2: 1-12.

Vanderpump MPJ. The epidemiology of thyroid diseases. In: Braverman LE, Utiger RD, eds. Werner and Ingbar's The Thyroid: A Fundamental and Clinical Text. 9th edn, 2005; pp 398-406. JB Lippincott-Raven, Philadelphia.

Vermiglio F, Lo Presti VP, Scaffidi Argentina G, et al. Maternal hypothyroxinemia during the first half of gestation in an iodine deficient area with endemic cretinism and related disorders. Clin Endocrinol (Oxf) 1995; 42: 409–415.

Visser TJ. The elemental importance of sufficient iodine intake: a trace is not enough. Endocrinology 2006; 147: 2095–2097.

Wiersinga WM. Adult hypothyroidism. In: Thyroid Gland and its Diseases. Thyroid disease manager organization, 2010.

Wiersinga WM. Do we need still more trials on T4 and T3 combination therapy in hypothyroidism? Eur J Endocrinol 2009; 161: 955–959.

Zhang SS, Carrillo AJ, Darling DS. Expression of multiple thyroid hormone receptor mRNAs in human oocytes, cumulus cells, and granulosa cells. Mol Hum Reprod 1997; 3: 555–562.

Zoeller, R.T., A.L.S. Dowling, Herzig, C.T.A., Iannacone, E.A., Gauger, K.J., Bansal, R. Thyroid Hormone, Brain Development, and the Environment. Environ Health Perspect 2002; 110(suppl 3): 355–361.

2

Environmental Thyroid Disruptors and Human Endocrine Health

Francesco Massart[1], Pietro Ferrara[2] and Giuseppe Saggese[1]
[1]*St. Chiara University Hospital of Pisa,*
[2]*Sacro Cuore Catholic University of Rome,*
Italy

1. Introduction

In the last 30 years, there is increasing concern about chemical pollutants that have the ability to act as hormone mimics. Because of structural similarity with endogenous hormones, their ability to interact with hormone transport proteins, or their ability to disrupt hormone metabolism, these environmental chemicals have the potential mimic, or in some cases block, the effects of endogenous hormones (Safe, 2000). In either case, these chemicals serve to disrupt the normal actions of endogenous hormones and thus have become known as "*endocrine disruptors*". An endocrine disruptor is defined as "an exogenous agent which interferes with the synthesis, secretion, transport, binding, action or elimination of natural hormones in the body which are responsible for maintenance of homeostasis, reproduction, development or behavior" (Massart et al., 2006a). This wide definition includes all substances that can affect endocrine function via interference with estrogen, androgen or thyroid hormone (TH) signaling pathways.

Chemicals such as dioxins, furans and organohalogens are widespread, man-made and persistent environmental pollutants, causing a variety of toxic effects. These environmental pollutants tend to degrade slowly in the environment, to bioaccumulate and to bioconcentrate in the food chain having long half-lives in mammalian fatty tissues. Animals fats and breastfeeding are the most important human dietary sources (Kavlock et al., 1996). Several biomonitoring studies have detected many environmental pollutants in adults, children, pregnant women and in the fetal compartments (Massart et al., 2005; Takser et al., 2005). Adverse effects induced by these compounds are due to their potentially toxic effects on physiological processes, particularly through direct interaction with nuclear receptors or affecting hormone metabolism (Moriyama et al., 2002).

In humans, adverse health outcomes such as neurodevelopmental toxicity, goiter and thyroid diseases are associated with TH disruption (Massart et al., 2007). Polychlorinated dibenzo-*p*-dioxins (PCDDs), polychlorinated dibenzo-*p*-furans (PCDFs), polychlorinated biphenyls (PCBs) and polybrominated diphenylethers (PBDEs) can adversely affect thyroid function mainly resulting in hypothyroidism, which is known to cause permanent cognitive deficiencies (Guo et al., 2004; Stewart et al., 2003; Walkowiak et al., 2001). Indeed, their chemical effects on the brain development may be attributable, at least in part, to their ability to affect the thyroid system (Zoeller et al., 2002). This hypothesis is supported in part by the overlap in neurological deficits observed in humans associated with chemical exposure and those deficits observed in the offspring to hypothyroxinemic women (Hagmar et al., 2001a; Koopman-Esseboom et al., 1994; Mirabella et al., 2000; Rogan et al., 1986).

2. Chemical interferences with the thyroid system

Several environmental pollutants (i.e. thyroid disruptors (TDs)) have high degree of structural resemblance to the endogenous thyroxine (T4) and triiodothyronine (T3) (Figure 1), and therefore, may interfere with binding to TH receptors (TRs) (Howdeshell, 2002; Massart et al., 2006b).

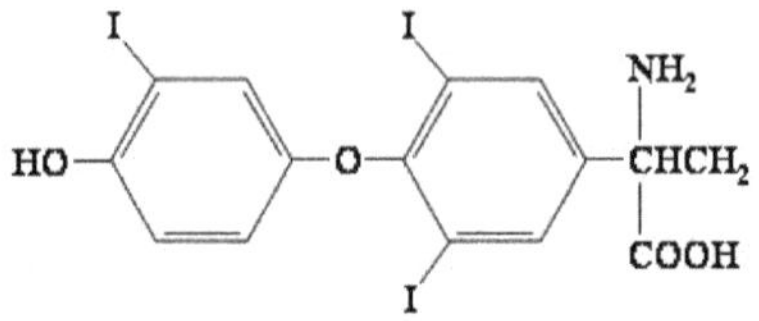

(a)

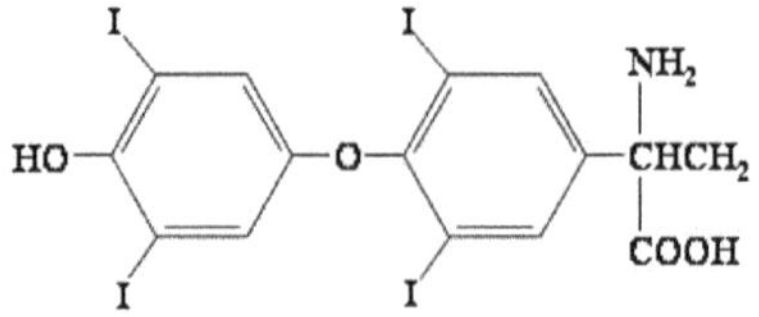

(b)

Fig. 1. Chemical structure of triiodothyronine (a) and thyroxine (b).

Moreover, because the mechanisms involved in the thyroid system homeostasis are numerous and complex (Figure 2), TDs may interfere with TH signaling at many levels (Howdeshell, 2002; Massart et al., 2006b).

A broad range of synthetic chemicals is known to affect the thyroid system at different points of regulation disrupting nearly every step in the production and metabolism of THs (Table 1) (Brouwer et al., 1998; Brucker-Davis, 1998). Chemical interference with uptake of iodide by the thyroid gland and, more specifically with the sodium/iodide symporter (which facilitates the iodide uptake), can result as decrease in the circulating levels of T4/T3 (Wolff, 1998). Chemical exposure can also lead to a decrease in serum protein-bound iodide levels, perhaps largely due to inhibition of the thyroid peroxidase enzyme, which disrupts the normal production of THs (Marinovich et al., 1997).

The displacement of T4/T3 from the transport proteins (e.g. thyroid binding globulin, transthyretin and albumin) may result in decreased ability of THs to reach its target tissue and then, may facilitate the transport of the chemicals into the fetus (Brouwer et al., 1998; Van den Berg et al., 1991).

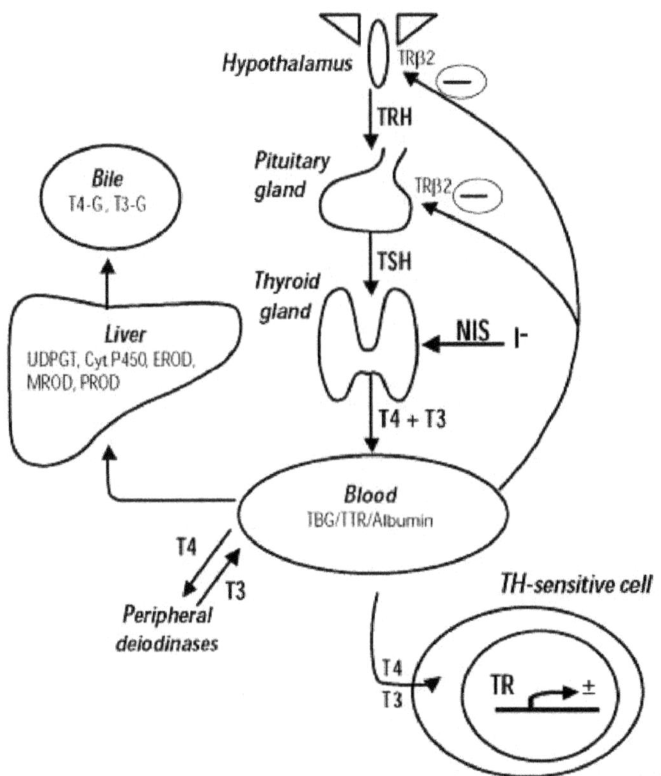

Fig. 2. Feedback mechanisms of thyroid system homeostasis (*modified from Boas M et al. European Journal of Endocrinology 2006;154:599-611*).

Chemical disruption of T4/T3 metabolism can influence deiodinase, glucuronidase and sulfatase activity, and may ultimately result in increased biliary elimination of T4/T3. Inhibition of deiodinase enzymes can result as decrease in T3 available to elicit thyroid action at tissue level (Maiti & Kar, 1997). Conversely, deiodinase activity may increase in response to TD exposure, either as direct effect or in response to increased clearance of T4/T3 by the chemical stimulation of glucuronidase or sulfatase enzymes (Spear et al., 1990; van Raaij et al., 1993). Brucker-Davis (Brucker-Davis, 1998) suggested that such increases in the metabolism and in the clearance of T3 could result in goiter as the thyroid gland increases production to maintain proper TH levels.

The TD list in Table 1 capable of disrupting normal TH production, transport, and metabolism is by no means exhaustive; further discussion of the effects of disruption of these processes can be found in specific reviews (Brouwer et al., 1998; Brucker-Davis, 1998). There are many more chemicals that have effects on the thyrotrophin-stimulating hormone (TSH) and T4/T3 levels, and thyroid histopathology for which no mechanism has been tested (Brucker-Davis, 1998). It is unlikely that these are working as T4/T3 agonists or antagonists at level of TR binding, as no chemical tested this far has demonstrated high affinity binding to the mammalian TRs (Cheek et al., 1999).

Uptake of iodide by thyroid gland
Aldrin
Amitrole
3-Amino-1,2,4-triazole
Aroclor
Catechol
4-Chlororesorcinol
Clofentezine
Cresol
Cythion
2,4-Dichlorophenoxyacetic Acid
Dihydroxynaphthalene
2,4-Dihydroxybenzaldehyde
2,4-Dihydroxybenzoic Acid
Ethiozin
Ethylene thiourea
Fipronil
Hexachlorobenzene
Hexadrin
4-Hexylresorcinol
Hydroxyquinol
Hydroxyquinol Triacetate
Lead
Mancozed
Mercuric Chloride
3-Methylcholanthrene
Methylmercuric Chloride
Methylparathion
2-Methylresorcinol
Mull-Soy
Nabam
Orcinol
Pendimethalin
Pentachloronitrobenzene
Phenobarbital
Phenol
Phloroglucinol
Polybrominated Biphenyls
Pregnenolone-16α-carbonitrile
Propylthiouracil
Pyrogallol
Pyrimenthanil
Resorcinol
Saligenin
Selenium
Thiocyanate

Sodium/iodide symporter
Perchlorate
Perrhenate

Serum protein-bound iodide level
Amitrole
Aroclor
Cythion
2,4-Dichlorophenoxyacetic Acid
1,1-Dichloro-2,2-bis (p-chlorophenyl) ethane
2,4-Dinitrophenol
Hexadrin
Malathion
Mancozeb
Mercuric Chloride
3-Methylcholanthrene

Thyroid peroxidase reactions
Aminotriazole
Amitrole
Ammonia
Cadmium Chloride
Endosulfan
Ethylene Thiourea
Fipronil
Lindane
Malathion
Mancozeb
Mercury Chloride
Methamizole
4,4′-Methylenedianiline
Polybrominated Biphenyls
Thiocyanate
Thiourea

Binding to albumin
Pentachlorophenol

Binding to thyroglobulin
1,1-Dichloro-2,2-bis(p-chlorophenyl)ethane
Pentachlorophenol

Binding to transthyretin
Bromoxynil (3,5-bibromo-4-hydroxybenzonitril)
4-(Chloro-o-tolyloxy)acetic Acid
4-(4-Chloro-2-methylphenoxy) butyric Acid
Chlorophenol
Chlororoxuron
1,1-Dichloro-2,2-bis(p-chlorophenyl)ethanes
2,4-Dichlorophenoxyacetic Acid
2,4-Dichlorophenoxybutric Acid
Dioxtylphthalate
Dichlorophenols
Dichloroprop
Difocol
2,4-Dinitrophenol
2,4-Dinitro-6-methylphenol
Ethyl-bromophos
Ethyl-parathion
Fenoprop
Hexachlorobenzene
Hexachlorophene
Hydroxybiphenyls
Lindane
Linuron
Malathion
Pentachlorophenol
Phenol
Pyrogallol
Polybrominated Biphenyl 77
1,4-Tetrachlorophenol
Trichloroacetic Acid
Trichlorobenzene
Trichlorophenols
2,4,5-Trichlorophenoxyacetic Acid

Type I & II 5′-deiodinase catabolism
Aminotriazole
Amiodarone
Aroclor
Cadmium Chloride
Dimethoate
Fenvalerate
Hexachlorobenzene
3,3′,4,4′,5,5′-Hexachlorobiphenyl
Lead
3-Methylcholanthrene
Phenobarbital
Propylthiouracil
Polybrominated Biphenyl 77
TCDD

Glucuronidation of T4/T3
Acetochlor
Aroclor 1254
3,4-Benzopyrene
Clofentenzine
Clofibrate
DDT
Fenbuconazole
3,3′,4,4′,5,5′-Hexabromobiphenyl
Hexacholorobenzene
Hexacholorobiphenyls
3-Methylcholanthrene
Pendimethalin
Phenobarbital
Polybrominated Biphenyls
Pregnenolone-16□-carbonitrile
Promadiamine
Pyrimethanil
TCDD
Thiazopyr

Catabolism & biliary T4/T3 elimination
Aroclor
3,4-Benzopyrene
DDT
Hexachlorobenzene
3-Methylcholanthrene
Phenobarbital
Polybrominated Biphenyls

Table 1. Environmental chemical pollutants interfering with the normal production, transport, metabolism, and excretion of thyroid hormones (*modified from Howdeshell KL. Environmental Health Perspects 2002;110:337-348*).

Relatively few studies evaluated the mechanism of TD action in the fetal/neonatal organism. Darnerud et al. (Darnerud et al., 1996) reported that developmental exposure to 4-OH-3,5,3′,4′-tetracholorobiphenyl, a major metabolite of polychlorinated biphenyl (PCB) congener 3,3′,4,4′-tetrachlorobiphenyl (PCB77), binds to fetal and maternal transthyretin in mice on the gestation day 17 (GD17); significant decrease in the fetal T4 (free and total) was reported. Aminotriazole inhibited the catabolism of T4 to T3 in renal primary cell cultures from 4 to 5 months of gestation in human fetuses, indicating an interference with type 1 iodothyronine deiodinase function in the kidney (Ghinea et al., 1986). *In utero* exposure to PCB congener 3,3′,4,4′,5,5′-hexachlorobiphenyl alone or in combination with PCB77 increased type II deiodinase activity in whole-brain homogenates from fetal (GD20) and neonatal rats; total T4 levels in plasma were decreased by both treatments (Morse et al., 1992). Uridine diphosphoglucuronosyl transferase (UDP-GT) activity was increased in neonatal rats at postnatal day 21 (PND21) weanlings exposure to PCB congeners or TCDD (2,3,7,8-tetrachlorodibenzo-*p*-dioxin) on the GD10 (Seo et al., 1995). The increase in UDP-GT activity was seen in the near absence of significant decreases in T4 concentration on the PND21 (Seo et al., 1995). Gestational exposure to Aroclor 1254 depressed UDP-GT activity in GD20 rat fetuses, while increasing the enzyme in PND21 rats (Morse et al., 1996). The total and free T4 levels in GD20 fetuses were significantly suppressed by both levels of Aroclor 1254 exposure during development, whereas the total T4 and total T3 were significantly depressed on the PND21 only by the highest dose of Aroclor 1254 (Morse et al., 1996).

In addiction, as reviewed by Zoeller et al. (Zoeller et al., 2002), many TDs can disrupt TH signaling without affecting circulating levels of THs. Many studies use circulating levels of THs as the sole indicator of an effect on the thyroid system by pollutants, or focus on mechanisms by which chemicals affect TH levels (Zoeller et al., 2002). Therefore, the prevailing view is that TDs interfere with TH signaling by reducing circulating levels of THs, thereby limiting the hormone available to act on the target tissues (Brouwer et al., 1998). However, the developmental effects of TD exposure in experimental animals are not fully consistent with mechanism attributable to hypothyroidism. For example, PCB exposure induces hearing loss in rats (Goldey et al., 1995) similarly to that observed in hypothyroid rats. Moreover, this PCB-induced hearing loss can be at least partially restored in PCB-treated rats by TH replacement (Goldey et al., 1998). On the other hand, circulating levels of TSH were not elevated by PCB exposure as it is after exposure to the goitrogen propylthiouracil (Goldey et al., 1995; Hood & Klaassen, 2000). Moreover, the timing of eye opening was advanced by PCB exposure, rather than delayed after exposure to the goitrogen 6-*n*-propyl-2 thiouracil (Goldey et al., 1995). These and other observations suggest that different TDs or their mixtures may produce heterogeneous disrupting effects on the thyroid system also without affecting circulating T4/T3 levels.

3. Thyroid toxicants

From the earliest reports in 1950s (Wyngaarden et al., 1952), many TDs have been identified by improving analytical methods. Here, we focused on some historical and emerging TDs.

3.1 Perchlorate

Over 50 years ago, Wyngaarden and colleagues (Wyngaarden et al., 1952; Stanbury & Wyngaarden, 1952) reported the inhibitory effect of perchlorate (ClO_4^-) (Figure 3) upon the accumulation and retention of iodide by human thyroid gland. Such observation had immediate therapeutic application for thyrotoxicosis using 250-500 mg/day doses of potassium perchlorate (Loh, 2000).

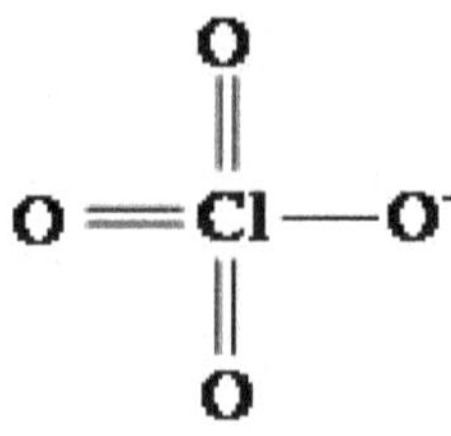

Fig. 3. Perchlorate

Because of its chemical properties, perchlorate is a competitive inhibitor of the process by which iodide, circulating in the blood, is actively transported into thyroid follicular cells (Clewell et al., 2004). The site of this inhibition is the sodium-iodide symporter, a membrane protein located adjacent to the capillaries supplying blood iodide to the thyroid gland (Carrasco, 1993). If sufficient inhibition of iodide uptake occurs, pharmacological effect results in subnormal levels of T4 and T3, and an associated compensatory increase in TSH secretion (Loh, 2000). Therefore, perchlorate exposure both results in hypothyroidism leading to the potential for altered neurodevelopment if observed in either dams or fetus/neonates, and increases in serum TSH leading to the potential for thyroid hyperplasia (Strawson et al., 2004).

Beside its pharmacological applications, perchlorate has been widely used as solid rocket propellants and ignitable sources in munitions, fireworks and matches (Strawson et al., 2004). Furthermore, perchlorates are laboratory waste by-products of perchloric acid. Perchlorate also occurs naturally in nitrate-rich mineral deposits used in fertilizers. An analysis of 9 commercial fertilizers revealed perchlorate in all samples tested ranging between 0.15-0.84% by weight (Collette et al., 2003).

In humans, there is clear and apparently linear relationship between perchlorate levels and inhibition of iodine uptake (Greer et al., 2002; Lawrence et al., 2000). Serum perchlorate levels of approximately 15 µg/l result in minimal inhibition of iodine uptake (about 2%) compared to serum 871 µg/l level, which results in about 70% inhibition of iodine uptake (Strawson et al., 2004). By contrast, several adult studies of differing exposure duration, reported serum T4 levels do not decrease after perchlorate exposure resulting in serum perchlorate levels up to 20,000 µg/l (Gibbs et al., 1998; Greer et al., 2002; Lamm et al., 1999; Lawrence et al., 2000).

3.2 Dioxins and furans

Dioxins (e.g. PCDDs) and furans (e.g. PCDFs) are a group of structurally related compounds (Giacomini et al., 2006) (Figure 4). PCDDs and PCDFs are not commercially produced but are formed unintentionally as by-products of various industrial processes (e.g. chlorine synthesis, production of hydrocarbons) during pyrolysis and uncompleted combustion of organic materials in the presence of chlorine.

During the last 20 years, an enormous public and scientific interest was focused on these substances, resulting in many publications on generation, input, and behavior in the environment (Giacomini et al., 2006; Lintelmann et al., 2003; US EPA, 1994). These toxicants have a potent concern for public health: several *in vitro* and *in vivo* experiments have suggested that PCDDs and PCDFs may interfere with thyroid function (Boas et al., 2006; Giacomini et al., 2006).

The 2,3,7,8-tetra-chloro-dibenzo-*p*-dioxin (TCDD), the most toxic, is the prototype among PCDD/F congeners. TCDD, used as standard for toxic equivalent (TEQ) calculation, shows high environmentally persistence and extremely long half-life in humans (seven or more years) (Michalek et al., 2002). TCDD is detectable at background levels in plasma or adipose tissues of individuals with no specific exposure to identifiable sources, usually at concentrations lower than 10 ppt (parts per trillion, lipid adjusted) (Michalek & Tripathi, 1999; Papke et al., 1996). Mean TCDD levels in subjects representative of the European and the US populations range between 2-5 ppt (Aylward et al., 2002; Papke et al., 1996). Nonetheless, Environmental Protection Agency (EPA) estimated that at least in the US population a number of people may have levels up to three-times higher than this average (Aylward et al., 2002; Flesch-Janys et al., 1996).

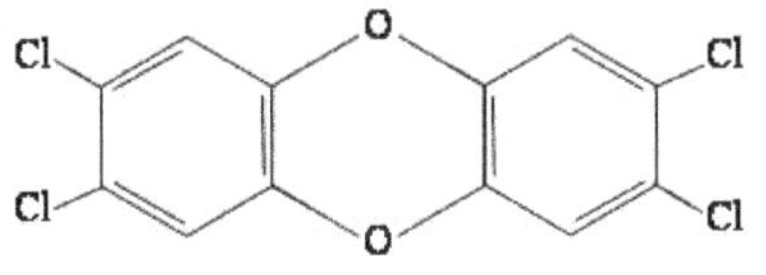

(a)

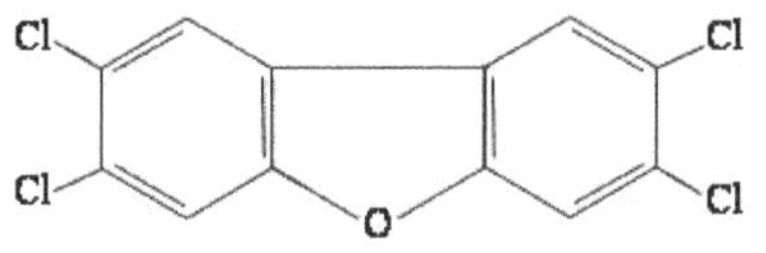

(b)

Fig. 4. Chemical structure of 2,3,7,8-tetra-chloro-dibenzo-*p*-dioxin (a) and tetrachlorodibenzo-furan (b).

3.3 Polychlorinated biphenyls

PCBs (Figure 5) comprise 209 highly environmental persistent, distinct congeners consisting of paired phenyl rings with various degrees of chlorination (Chana et al., 2002). It is estimated that since 1929, approximately 1.5 million tons of PCBs were produced.

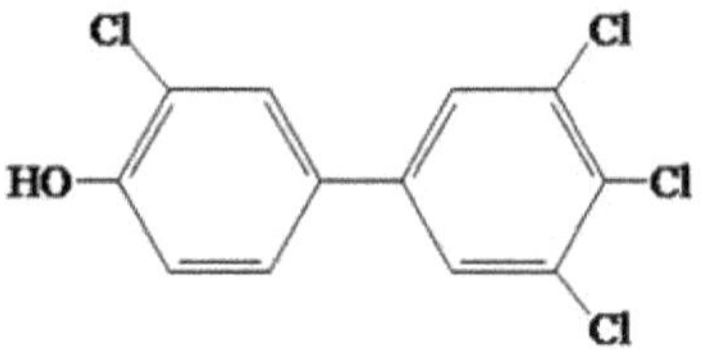

Fig. 5. 4OH-Tetrachlorobyphenyl.

The high persistence of PCBs in adipose tissues and their toxic potential for animals and humans (Breivik et al., 2002; Fisher, 1999), resulted in an almost international production stop in the 1970-80s (Lintelmann et al., 2003). However, the PCB properties, such as chemical and thermal stability, noninflammability, high boiling points, high viscosity, and low vapor pressure, are the reason for their worldwide distribution (Safe, 2000). Even after the ban of PCB production in most countries, the current world inventory of PCBs is estimated at 1.2 million tons with about one-third of this quantity circulating in the environment (Lintelmann et al., 2003).

PCBs, and especially the hydroxylated metabolites, have an high degree of structural resemblance to THs as well as thyroid-like activities (Hagmar, 2003). Laterally substituted chlorinated aromatic compounds such as *meta-* and *para-*PCBs particularly when hydroxylated, are ideally suited to serve as binding ligands to TRs and to TH-binding proteins (Arulmozhiraja et al., 2005; Cheek et al., 1999; Fritsche et al., 2005; Kitamura et al., 2005). Indeed, experimental studies indicated that PCB exposure may exert adverse effects on the developing brain by reducing circulating levels of THs, causing a state of relative hypothyroidism (Brouwer et al., 1998; Crofton, 2004). This is supported by animal data that PCBs reduce the TH levels (Gauger et al., 2004; Kato et al., 2004; Zoeller et al., 2000). PCBs may also exert direct actions on the TR independently from their effects on the TH secretion (Zoeller, 2002; Zoeller, 2003). This hypothesis is based in part on *in vitro* observations that PCBs can directly inhibit or enhance TR activity (Arulmozhiraja et al., 2005; Bogazzi et al., 2003; Iwasaki et al., 2002; Kitamura et al., 2005; Miyazaki et al., 2004; Yamada-Okabe et al., 2004) such as other TH-like actions in the developing brain (Bansal et al., 2005; Fritsche et al., 2005; Gauger et al., 2004; Zoeller et al., 2000). However, Sharlin et al. (Sharlin et al., 2006) demonstrated that PCB exposure during development does not recapitulate the full effect of hypothyroidism on the cellular composition of rat white matter.

Multiple studies regarding PCB exposure have been carried out in human populations, the majority of which raises concern that environmental PCB levels may alter thyroid homeostasis (Hagmar, 2003). In subjects from highly PCB-exposed areas, the PCB concentration in blood samples negatively correlated to circulating TH levels (Hagmar et al., 2001a; Persky et al., 2001). However, few studies also demonstrated positive correlation between PCB exposure and TSH (Osius et al., 1999; Schell et al., 2004). By contrast, other studies found no association between PCBs and thyroid secretion (Bloom et al., 2003; Hagmar et al., 2001b; Sala et al., 2001).

3.4 Bisphenols

The 4,4'-isopropylidenediphenol or bisphenol A (BPA; Figure 6), produced at a rate of over 800 million kg annually in the US alone, is extensively used in plastic manufactures including polycarbonate plastics, epoxy resins that coat food cans, and in dental sealants (Howe et al., 1998; Kang et al., 2006; Lewis et al., 1999; Zoeller, 2005).

Howe et al. (Howe et al., 1998) estimated human PBA consumption from epoxy-lined food cans alone to be about 6.6 μg/person-day. BPA has been reported in concentrations of 1-10 ng/ml in the serum of pregnant women, in the amniotic fluid of their fetus, and in the cord serum taken at birth (Ikezuki et al., 2002; Schonfelder et al., 2002). Moreover, BPA concentrations of up to 100 ng/g were reported in the placenta tissues (Schonfelder et al., 2002).

Considering human pattern of BPA exposure, it is of endocrine concern that BPA shows thyroid antagonist activities (Kang et al., 2006; Moriyama et al. 2002). Best characterized as weak estrogen, BPA binds to TR and antagonizes T3 activation of TR with K_i of approximately 10^{-4} M, but as little as 10^{-6} M BPA significantly inhibits TR-mediated gene activation (Ikezuki et al., 2002; Moriyama et al. 2002). Moreover, BPA reduces T3-mediated gene expression by enhancing the interaction with the co-repressor N-CoR (Moriyama et al. 2002). Limited human data exist regarding BPA as TD.

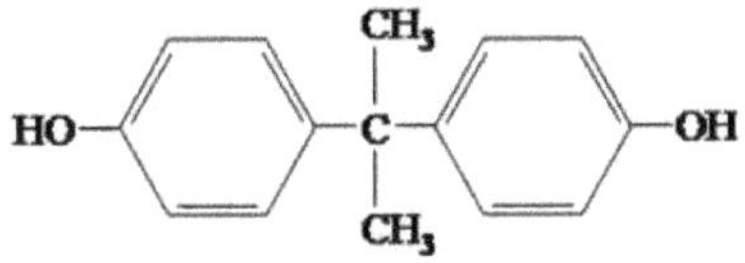

CH_3 HO— —C— —OH CH_3

(a)

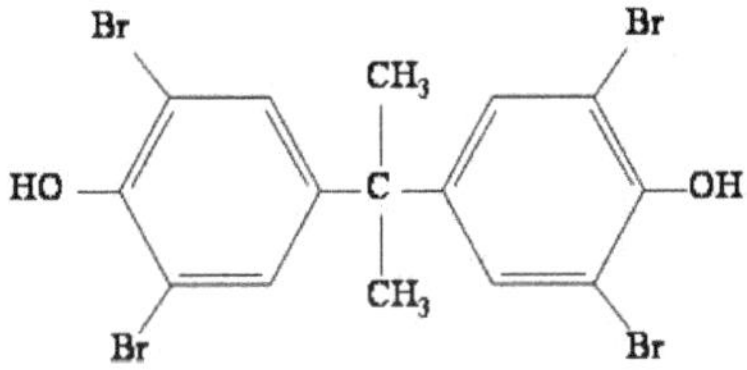

Br Br CH_3 HO —C— —OH CH_3 Br Br

(b)

Fig. 6. 4,4'-isopropylidenediphenol (a) and tetrabromo-bisphenol A (b).

Tetrabromobisphenol A (TBBPA; Figure 6), an halogenated BPA derivative, is widely used as flame retardant in electrical equipment such as televisions, computers, copying machines, video displays and laser printers (Kitamura et al., 2002) with over 60,000 tons of TBBPA annually produced (WHO EHC 1995; WHO EHC 1997). Thomsen et al. (Thomsen et al., 2002) reported that brominated flame retardants, including TBBPA, have increased in human serum from 1977 to 1999 with concentrations in adults ranging from 0.4 to 3.3 ng/g serum lipids. However, infants (0-4 years) exhibited serum concentrations that ranged from 1.6 to 3.5 times higher (Thomsen et al., 2002).

TBBPA is generally regarded a safe flame retardant because it is not readily accumulated in the environment, nor it is highly toxic (Birnbaum & Staskal, 2004). However, TBBPA and tetrachlorobisphenol A show even closer structural relationship to T4 than PCBs: both these tetrahalogenated bisphenols induce thyroid-dependent growth in pituitary GH3 cell line at concentrations 4-to-6 orders of magnitude higher than T3 (Kitamura et al., 2002). Unfortunately, no data are actually available on thyroid function in human exposed to these bisphenols.

3.5 Perfluoroalkyl acids

The perfluoroalkyl acids (PFAAs; Figure 7) are a family of synthetic, highly stable perfluorinated compounds with wide range of uses in industrial and consumer products, from stain- and water-resistant coatings for carpets and fabrics to fast-food contact materials, fire-resistant foams, paints, and hydraulic fluids (OECD, 2005).

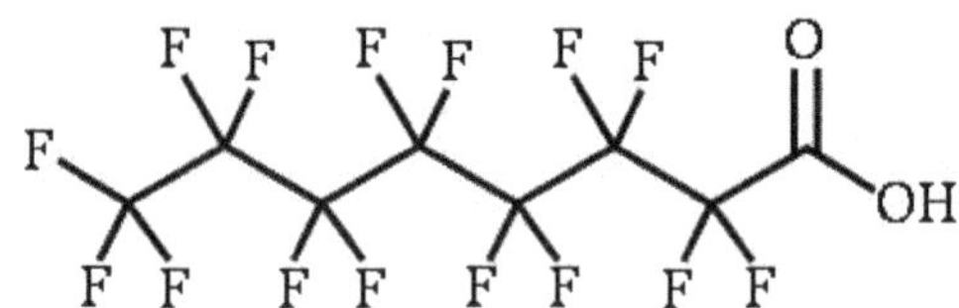

Fig. 7. Perfluoroalkyl Acids.

The carbon–fluoride bonds that characterize PFAAs and make them useful as surfactants are highly stable, and recent reports indicate the widespread persistence of certain PFAAs in the environment and in wildlife and human populations globally (Fromme et al., 2009; Giesy & Kannan, 2001; Lau et al., 2007; Saito et al., 2004). Two of the PFAAs of most concern are the eight-carbon–chain perfluorooctane sulfonate (PFOS) and perfluo-rooctanoic acid (PFOA, also known as C8).

Most persistent organic pollutants are lipophilic and accumulate in fatty tissues, but PFOS and PFOA are both lipo- and hydro-phobic, and after absorption bind to proteins in serum rather than accumulating in lipids (Hundley et al., 2006; Jones et al., 2003). The renal clearance of PFOA and PFOS is negligible in humans, leading to reported half-lives in blood serum of 3.8 and 5.4 years for PFOA and PFOS, respectively (Olsen et al., 2007).

Human biomonitoring of the general population in various countries (Calafat et al., 2006; Kannan et al., 2004; Metzer et al., 2010). has shown that, in addition to the near ubiquitous presence of PFOS and PFOA in blood, these may also be present in breast milk, liver, seminal fluid, and umbilical cord blood (Lau et al., 2007). Occupational exposure to PFOA reported in 2003 showed mean serum values of 1,780 ng/mL (range, 40–10,060 ng/mL) (Olsen et al., 2003a) and 899 ng/mL (range, 722–1,120 ng/mL) (Olsen et al., 2003b). Since then, voluntary industry reductions in production and use of other perfluorinated compounds, such as the US EPA-initiated PFOA Stewardship Program (US EPA, 2006), have contributed to a decreasing trend in human exposure for all perfluorinated compounds

(Calafat et al., 2007; Olsen et al., 2007). In May 2009, PFOS was listed under the Stockholm Convention on Persistent Organic Pollutants (Stockholm Convention on POPs, 2008).

Numerous studies have now shown PFAAs to impair thyroid homeostasis in animal studies. Depression of serum T4 and T3 in PFOS-exposed rats has been reported (Lau et al., 2003; Luebker et al., 2005; Seacat et al., 2003), without the concomitant increase in TSH that would be expected through feedback stimulation. Earlier mechanistic studies of structurally related perfluorodecanoic acid showed that it could reduce serum TH levels apparently by reducing the responsiveness of the hypothalamus-pituitary-thyroid axis and by displacing circulating THs from their plasma protein-binding sites (Gutshall et al., 1989). Although circulating hormone levels were depressed, the activities of TH–sensitive liver enzymes were elevated, suggesting that functional hypothyroidism was not occurring. A similar mechanism for PFOS has been hypothesized (Chang et al., 2008). A recent study of the mechanisms involved in PFOS-induced hypothyroxinemia in rats has indicated that increased conjugation of T4 in the liver, catalyzed by the hepatic enzyme UDP-GT 1A1, and increased thyroidal conversion of T4 to T3 by type 1 deiodinase may be partly responsible for the effects (Yu et al., 2009). Taken together, these findings suggest that the PFAA actions on the thyroid system are multiple and complex.

Disruption to TH balance was not found in previous studies of community exposure to PFOA (Emmett et al., 2006; Olsen et al., 2003c) or PFOS (Inoue et al., 2004). Modest associations between PFOA and THs (negative for free T4 and positive for T3) were reported in 506 PFOA production workers across three production facilities (Olsen & Zobel, 2007); there were no associations between TSH or T4 and PFOA, and the free TH levels were within the normal reference range. On the other hand, Metzer et al. (Metzer et al., 2010) recently determined whether increased serum PFOA or PFOS concentrations are associated with thyroid disease in a general adult US population sample (n = 3,974 individuals ≥ 20 years of age from NHANES waves 1999–2000 (n = 1,040), 2003–2004 (n = 1,454), and 2005–2006 (n = 1,480)). They found that, across all the available data from NHANES, thyroid disease associations with serum PFOA concentrations are present in women and are strongest for those currently being treated for thyroid disease (P=0.002) (Metzer et al., 2010). In men, they also found a significant association between PFOS and treated thyroid disease (P=0.043). An interaction term analysis suggested that the PFAA trends in men and women are not significantly different, despite the relative rarity of thyroid disease in men (Metzer et al., 2010).

3.6 Phthalates

Phthalates are recently proposed to be emerging TDs (Boas et al., 2006) (Figure 8). Phthalates are widely used as plastic emollients, and their amount used globally is rising (Hauser & Calafat, 2005; Latini, 2005; Schettler, 2006).

Environmental exposure to phthalates is inevitable, but for certain groups such as hospitalized subjects including neonates and infants, exposure may be massive (Shea, 2003). Phthalate exposure through necessary medical devices such as feeding tubes is correlated to the urinary content of mono(2-ethylexyl)phthalate (Green et al., 2005). Thus, an intensive phthalate exposure at potentially vulnerable point of development may cause permanent damage, despite the fast metabolism of phthalates.

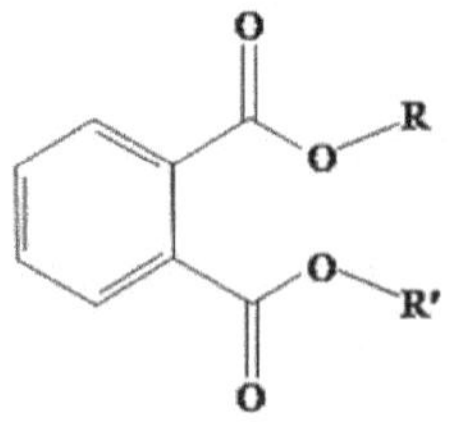

Fig. 8. Phathalates.

Rodent studies found histopathological changes in the rat thyroid glands after exposure to di(2-ethylhexyl) phthalate (DEHP), di-noctyl phthalate (DnOP) and di-n-hexyl phthalate (DnHP), corresponding to thyroid hyperactivity (Hinton et al., 1986; Howarth et al., 2001; Mitchell et al., 1985; Poon et al., 1997; Price et al., 1988). Long-term treatment with high doses of DEHP resulted in basophilic deposits in the colloid and enlargement of the lysosomes (Mitchell et al., 1985). The levels of circulating THs were not affected after oral rat exposure to DEHP (Bernal et al., 2002), whereas i.v. exposure in doses corresponding to levels of DEHP solubilized in blood bags for human transfusions resulted in significant increase in the serum T3 and T4, which returned to normal after 7 days (Gayathri et al., 2004). The thyroid glands examined in this study showed initial reactive hyperplasia. In contrast di-n-butyl phthalate (DBP) decreased T3 and T4 in rats in dose-dependent manner (O'Connor et al., 2002).

Only few data exist on the thyroid function of phthalate-exposed humans. However, recent studies reported significant associations between urine phthalate levels and altered THs (Jurewicz & Hanke, 2011; Rais-Bahrami et al., 2004).

4. Thyroid disruptors assays

Until recent years, all known TDs have been identified solely by their ability to reduce circulating TH levels, and to affect thyroid size or histopathology (e.g. colloid size, quantitative appearance of hypertrophic or hyperplastic effects) (Brucker-Davis, 1998; DeVito et al., 1999). However, TH levels vary with time and age, and then, caution must be taken in the result interpretation. In this view, histological changes in the exposed thyroid gland (particularly, increased weight and follicular cell number) are better *in vivo* markers (Janosek et al., 2006). In addition, TDs present in small amounts in the environment may not cause overt changes of TH levels but may nonetheless alter hormonal homeostasis (Boas et al., 2006). A well-established example is perchlorate, which in small amounts does not alter circulating TH levels but diminished T4 content in the thyroid gland (Isanhart et al., 2005; McNabb et al., 2004a; McNabb et al., 2004b). These data agreed with *in vitro* studies which proposed an perchlorate-induced inhibition of sodium-iodide symporter (Tonacchera et al., 2004).

Regarding *in vivo* toxicity assays for TDs, several tests have been proposed evaluating delayed eye-opening, abnormalities in the brain development, increased the sperm counts or the testes weight (DeVito et al., 1999). Perchlorate discharge test is also used as *in vivo* method for determining thyroid toxicity through TR (Atterwill et al., 1987). Finally, another *ex vivo* parameter is hepatic UDP-GT activity (a marker of enhanced TH clearance form serum) (Barter & Kòaassen, 1994; Kohn et al., 1996; Okazaki & Katayama, 2003; Sewall et al., 1995). On the other hand, many TDs that directly act on the TRs, may produce variable and perhaps unpredicted effects on the TH target tissues (Zoeller, 2005).

Several *in vitro* assays have been developed to evaluate substances that may affect specific TH-related processes such as synthesis, metabolism, protein binding and downstream effects (transcription and translation). Expert panel reports reviewed the thyroid toxicological methods (Calamandrei et al., 2006; DeVito et al., 1999; Janosek et al., 2006;). Finally, intra-thyroidal T4 content, gene transcription activity and cellular growth appear to be more sensitive endpoints when assessing the significance of thyroid disruption for various chemicals (Boas et al., 2006). With respect to multiple recognized toxicity mechanisms, several screening methods should be used to characterize chemical potencies of potential thyroid disruptors.

5. Conclusions

Industrial compounds such thyroid disruptors are now ubiquitous, persistent environmental contaminants routinely found in samples of human and animal tissues (Boas et al., 2006; Massart et al., 2005; Zoeller et al., 2002). Their potency to disrupt TH pathways has been demonstrated in both *in vitro* and *in vivo* studies, in which they have been shown to typically evoke reductions in TH levels (Massart & Meucci, 2007; Zoeller, 2005). However, most important, as synthetic chemicals can interfere with nearly every step in the thyroid system (Massart et al., 2006b), more research should be targeted at understanding how TDs may impact normal brain development and functioning. Unfortunately, a toxicological profile of many chemicals is actually too incomplete and insufficient to perform an adequate human and ecological risk assessment. Furthermore, chemicals are not currently tested specifically for their ability to mimic, disrupt, or otherwise act as hormone agonists or antagonists, except on research basis. Finally, more studies are crucial to fill in the research gaps regarding permanent endocrine and neurological outcome in next generations exposed to background TDs.

6. References

Arulmozhiraja, S.; Shiraishi, F.; Okumura, T.; Iida, M.; Takigami, H.; Edmonds, J.S. & Morita, M. (2005). Structural requirements for the interaction of 91 hydroxylated polychlorinated biphenyls with estrogen and thyroid hormone receptors. *Toxicological Sciences*, 84, 1, (March 2005), pp. 49-62.

Atterwill, C.K.; Collins, P.; Brown, C.G. & Harland, R.F. (1987). The perchlorate discharge test for examining thyroid function in rats. *Journal of Pharmacological and Toxicological Methods*, 18, 3, (November 1987), pp. 199-203.

Aylward, L.L. & Hays, S.M. (2002). Temporal trends in human TCDD body burden: decreases over three decades and implications for exposure levels. *Journal of Exposure Analysis and Environmental Epidemiology*, 12, 5, (September 2002), pp. 319-28.

Bansal, R.; You, S.H.; Herzig, C.T. & Zoeller, R.T. (2005). Maternal thyroid hormone increases HES expression in the fetal rat brain: an effect mimicked by exposure to a mixture of polychlorinated biphenyls (PCBs). *Brain Research. Developmental Brain Research*, 156, 1, (April 2005), pp. 13-22.

Barter, R.A. & Kòaassen, C.D. (1994). Reduction of thyroid hormone levels and alteration of thyroid function by four representative UDP-glucuronosyltransferase inducers in rats. *Toxicology and Applied Pharmacology*, 128, 1, (September 1994), pp. 9-17.

Bernal, C.A.; Martinelli, M.I. & Mocchiutti, N.O. (2002). Effect of the dietary exposure of rat to di(2-ethyl hexyl) phthalate on their metabolic efficiency. *Food Additives and Contaminants*, 19, 11, (November 2002), pp. 1091–1096.

Birnbaum, L.S. & Staskal, D.F. (2004). Brominated flame retardants: cause for concern? *Environmental Health Perspects*, 112, 1, (January 2004), pp. 9-17.

Bloom, M.S.; Weiner, J.M.; Vena, J.E. & Beehler, G.P. (2003). Exploring associations between serum levels of select organochlorines and thyroxine in a sample of New York state sportsmen: the New York State Angler Cohort Study. *Environmental research*, 93, 1, (September 2003), pp. 52-66.

Boas, M.; Feldt-Rasmussen, U.; Skakkebaek, N.E. & Main, K.M. (2006). Environmental chemicals and thyroid function. *European Journal of Endocrinology*, 154, 5, (May 2006), pp. 599-611.

Bogazzi, F.; Raggi, F.; Ultimieri, F.; Russo, D.; Campomori, A.; McKinney, J.D.; Pinchera, A.; Bartalena, L. & Martino, E. (2003). Effects of a mixture of polychlorinated biphenyls (Aroclor 1254) on the transcriptional activity of thyroid hormone receptor. *Journal of Endocrinological Investigation*, 26, 10, (October 2003), pp. 972-8.

Breivik, K.; Sweetman, A.; Pacyna, J.M. & Jones, K.C. (2002). Towards a global historical emission inventory for selected PCB congeners--a mass balance approach. 1. Global production and consumption. *The Science of the Total Environment*, 290, 1-3, (May 2002), pp. 181-98.

Brouwer, A.; Morse, D.C.; Lans, M.C.; Schuur, A.G.; Murk, A.J.; Klasson-Wehler, E.; Bergman, A. & Visser, T.J. (1998). Interactions of persistent environmental organohalogens with the thyroid hormone system: mechanisms and possible consequences for animal and human health. *Toxicology and Industrial Health*, 14, 1-2, (January-April 1998), pp. 59-84.

Brucker-Davis, F. (1998). Effects of environmental synthetic chemicals on thyroid function. *Thyroid*, 8, 9, (September 1998), pp. 827-56.

Calafat, A.M.; Kuklenyik, Z.; Caudill, S.P.; Reidy, J.A. & Needham, L.L. (2006). Perfluorochemicals in pooled serum samples from United States residents in 2001 and 2002. *Environmental Science & Technology*, 40, 7, (April 2006), pp. 2128–2134.

Calafat, A.M.; Wong, L.Y.; Kuklenyik, Z.; Reidy, J.A. & Needham, L.L. (2007). Polyfluoroalkyl chemicals in the U.S. population: data from the National Health and Nutrition Examination Survey (NHANES) 2003–2004 and comparisons with NHANES 1999–2000. *Environmental Health Perspects*, 115, 11, (November 2007), pp. 1596–1602.

Calamandrei, G.; Maranghi, F.; Venerosi, A.; Alleva, E. & Mantovani, A. (2006). Efficient testing strategies for evaluation of xenobiotics with neuroendocrine activity. Reproductive toxicology, 22, 2, (August 2006), pp. 164-74.

Carrasco, N. (1993). Iodide transport in the thyroid gland. *Biochimica et Biophysica Acta*, 1154, 1, (June 1993), pp. 65-82.

Chana, A.; Concejero, M.A.; de Frutos, M.; Gonzalez, M.J. & Herradon, B. (2002). Computational studies on biphenyl derivatives. Analysis of the conformational mobility, molecular electrostatic potential, and dipole moment of chlorinated biphenyl: searching for the rationalization of the selective toxicity of polychlorinated biphenyls (PCBs). *Chemical Research in Toxicology*, 15, 12, (December 2002), pp. 1514-26.

Chang, S.C.; Das, K.; Ehresman, D.J.; Ellefson, M.E.; Gorman, G.S.; Hart, J.A.; Noker, P.E.; Tan, Y.M.; Lieder, P.H.; Lau, C.; Olsen, G.W. & Butenhoff, J.L. (2008). Comparative pharmacokinetics of perfluorobutyrate in rats, mice, monkeys, and humans and relevance to human exposure via drinking water *Toxicological Sciences*,104, 1, (July 2008), pp.40-53.

Cheek, A.O.; Kow, K.; Chen, J. & McLachlan, J.A. (1999). Potential mechanisms of thyroid disruption in humans: interaction of organochlorine compounds with thyroid receptor, transthyretin, and thyroid-binding globulin. *Environmental Health Perspects*, 107, 4, (April, 1999), pp. 273-8.

Clewell, R.A.; Merrill, E.A.; Narayanan, L.; Gearhart, J.M. & Robinson, P.J. (2004). Evidence for competitive inhibition of iodide uptake by perchlorate and translocation of perchlorate into the thyroid. *International Journal of Toxicology*, 23, 1, (January-February 2004), pp. 17-23.

Collette, T.W.; Williams, T.L.; Urbansky, E.T.; Magnuson, M.L.; Hebert, G.N. & Strauss, S.H. (2003). Analysis of hydroponic fertilizer matrixes for perchlorate: comparison of analytical techniques. *The Analyst*, 128, 1, (January 2003), pp. 88-97.

Crofton, K.M. (2004). Developmental disruption of thyroid hormone: correlations with hearing dysfunction in rats. *Risk Analysis*, 24, 6, (December 2004), pp. 1665-71.

Darnerud, P.O.; Morse, D.; Klasson-Wehler, E. & Brouwer, A. (1996). Binding of a 3,3', 4,4'-tetrachlorobiphenyl (CB-77) metabolite to fetal transthyretin and effects on fetal thyroid hormone levels in mice. *Toxicology* 106, 1-3, (January 1996), pp. 105-14.

DeVito, M.; Biegel, L.; Brouwer, A.; Brown, S.; Brucker-Davis, F.; Cheek, A.O.; Christensen, R.; Colborn, T.; Cooke, P.; Crissman, J.; Crofton, K.; Doerge, D.; Gray, E.; Hauser, P.; Hurley, P.; Kohn, M.; Lazar, J.; McMaster, S.; McClain, M.; McConnell, E.; Meier, C.; Miller, R.; Tietge, J. & Tyl, R. (1999). Screening methods for thyroid hormone disruptors. *Environmental Health Perspects*, 107, 5, (May 1999), pp. 407-15.

Emmett, E.A.; Zhang, H.; Shofer, F.S.; Freeman, D.; Rodway, N.V.; Desai, C. & Sham, L.M. (2006). Community exposure to perfluorooctanoate: relationships between serum levels and certain health parameters. *Journal of Occupational and Environmental Medicine*, 48, 8, (August 2006), pp. 771–779.

Fisher, B.E. (1999). Most unwanted. *Environmental Health Perspects* , 107, 1, (January 1999), pp. A18-23.

Flesch-Janys, D.; Becher, H.; Gurn, P.; Jung, D.; Konietzko, J.; Manz, A. & Papke, O. (1996). Elimination of polychlorinated dibenzo-p-dioxins and dibenzofurans in occupationally exposed persons. *Journal of Toxicology and Environmental Health*, 47, 4, (March 1996), pp. 363-78.

Fritsche, E.; Cline, J.E.; Nguyen, N.H.; Scanlan, T.S. & Abel, J. (2005). Polychlorinated biphenyls disturb differentiation of normal human neural progenitor cells: clue for involvement of thyroid hormone receptors. *Environmental Health Perspects*, 113, 7, (July 2005), pp. 871-6.

Fromme, H.; Tittlemier, S.A.; Volkel, W.; Wilhelm, M. & Twardella, D. (2009). Perfluorinated compounds—exposure assessment for the general population in Western countries. *International Journal of Hygiene and Environmental Health*, 212, 3, (May 2009), pp. 239–270.

Gayathri, N.S.; Dhanya, C.R.; Indu, A.R. & Kurup, P.A. (2004). Changes in some hormones by low doses of di (2-ethyl hexyl) phthalate (DEHP), a commonly used plasticizer in PVC blood storage bags and medical tubing. *Indian Journal of Medical Research* 119, 4, (April 2004), pp. 139–144.

Gauger, K.J.; Kato, Y.; Haraguchi, K.; Lehmler, H.J.; Robertson, L.W.; Bansal, R. & Zoeller, R.T. (2004). Polychlorinated biphenyls (PCBs) exert thyroid hormone-like effects in the fetal rat brain but do not bind to thyroid hormone receptors. *Environmental Health Perspects*, 112, 5, (April 2004), pp. 516-23.

Ghinea, E.; Dumitriu, L.; Stefanovici, G.; Pop, A.; Oprescu, M. & Ciocirdia, C. (1986). Action of some pesticides on T4 to T3 conversion in cultured kidney and liver cells in the presence or absence of cysteine. *Endocrinologie*, 24, 3, (July-September 1986), pp. 157-66.

Giacomini, S.M.; Hou, L.; Bertazzi, P.A. & Baccarelli, A. (2006). Dioxin effects on neonatal and infant thyroid function: routes of perinatal exposure, mechanisms of action and evidence from epidemiology studies. *International Archives of Occupational and Environmental Health*, 79, 5, (May 2006), pp.396-404.

Gibbs, J.P.; Ahmad, R.; Crump, K.S.; Houck, D.P.; Leveille, T.S.; Findley, J.E. & Francis, M. (1998). Evaluation of a population with occupational exposure to airborne ammonium perchlorate for possible acute or chronic effects on thyroid function. *Journal of Occupational and Environmental Medicine*, 40, 12, (December 1998), pp. 1072-82.

Giesy, J. & Kannan, K. (2001). Global distribution of perfluorooctanoate sulfonate in wildlife. *Environmental Science & Technology*, 35, 7, (April 2001), pp. 1339–1342.

Goldey, E.S.; Kehn, L.S.; Lau, C.; Rehnberg, G.L. & Crofton, K.M. (1995). Developmental exposure to polychlorinated biphenyls (Aroclor 1254) reduces circulating thyroid hormone concentrations and causes hearing deficits in rats. *Toxicology and Applied Pharmacology*, 135, 1, (November 1995), pp. 77-88.

Goldey, E.S. & Crofton, K.M. (1998). Thyroxine replacement attenuates hypothyroxinemia, hearing loss, and motor deficits following developmental exposure to Aroclor 1254 in rats. *Toxicological Sciences* , 45, 1, (September 1998), pp. 94-105.

Green, R.; Hauser, R.; Calafat, A.M.; Weuve, J.; Schettler, T.; Ringer, S.; Huttner, K. & Hu, H. (2005). Use of di(2-ethylhexyl) phthalate-containing medical products and urinary levels of mono(2-ethylhexyl) phthalate in neonatal intensive care unit infants. *Environmental Health Perspects*, 113, 9, (September 2005), pp. 1222-5.

Greer, M.A.; Goodman, G.; Pleus, R.C. & Greer, S.E. (2002). Health effects assessment for environmental perchlorate contamination: the dose response for inhibition of thyroidal radioiodine uptake in humans. *Environmental Health Perspects*, 110, 9, (September 2002), pp. 927-37.

Guo, Y.L.; Lambert, G.H.; Hsu, C.C. & Hsu, M.M. (2004). Yucheng: health effects of prenatal exposure to polychlorinated biphenyls and dibenzofurans. *International Archives of Occupational and Environmental Health*, 77, 3, (April 2004), pp. 153-8.

Gutshall, D.M.; Pilcher, G.D. & Langley, A.E. (1989). Mechanism of the serum thyroid hormone lowering effect of perfluoro-n-decanoic acid (PFDA) in rats. *Journal of Toxicology and Environmental Health*, 28, 1, (1989), pp. 53–65.

Hagmar, L.; Rylander, L.; Dyremark, E.; Klasson-Wehler, E. & Erfurth, E.M. (2001a). Plasma concentrations of persistent organochlorines in relation to thyrotropin and thyroid hormone levels in women. *International Archives of Occupational and Environmental Health* 74, 3, (April 2001), pp. 184-8.

Hagmar, L.; Bjork, J.; Sjodin, A.; Bergman, A. & Erfurth, E.M. (2001b). Plasma levels of persistent organohalogens and hormone levels in adult male humans. Archives of Environmental Health, 56, 2, (March-April 2001), pp. 138-43.

Hagmar, L. (2003). Polychlorinated biphenyls and thyroid status in humans: a review. *Thyroid* , 13, 11, (November 2003), pp. 1021-8.

Hauser, R. & Calafat, A.M. (2005). Phthalates and human health. *Occupational and Environmental Medicine*, 62, 11, (November 2005), pp. 806-18.

Hinton, R.H.; Mitchell, F.E.; Mann, A.; Chescoe, D.; Price, S.C.; Nunn, A.; Grasso, P. & Bridges, J.W. (1986). Effects of phthalic acid esters on the liver and thyroid. *Environmental Health Perspectives*, 70, (December 1986), pp. 195–210.

Hood, A. & Klaassen, C.D. (2000). Differential effects of microsomal enzyme inducers on in vitro thyroxine (T_4) and triiodothyronine (T_3) glucuronidation. *Toxicological Sciences*, 55, 1, (May 2000), pp. 78-84.

Howarth, J.A.; Price, S.C.; Dobrota, M.; Kentish, P.A. & Hinton, R.H. (2001). Effects on male rats of di(2-ethylhexyl) phthalate and di-n-hexylphthalate administered alone or in combination. *Toxicology Letters*, 121, 1, (April 2001), pp. 35-43.

Howdeshell, K.L. (2002). A model of the development of the brain as a construct of the thyroid system. *Environmental Health Perspects*, 110, S3, (June 2002), pp. 337-48.

Howe, S.R.; Borodinsky, L. & Lyon, R.S. (1998). Potential exposure to bisphenol A from food-contact use of epoxy coated cans. *Journal of Coatings Technology*, 70, (February 1998), pp. 69-74.

Hundley, S.; Sarrif, A. & Kennedy, G. (2006). Absorption, distribution and excretion of ammonium perfluorooctanoate (APFO) after oral administration in various species. *Drug and Chemical Toxicology*, 29, 2, (2006), pp. 137–145.

Ikezuki, Y.; Tsutsumi, O.; Takai, Y.; Kamei, Y. & Taketani, Y. (2002). Determination of bisphenol A concentrations in human biological fluids reveals significant early prenatal exposure. *Human Reproduction*, 17, 11, (November 2002), pp. 2839-41

Inoue, K.; Okada, F.; Ito, R.; Kato, S.; Sasaki, S.; Nakajima, S.; Uno, A.; Saijo, Y.; Sata, F.; Yoshimura, Y.; Kishi, R. & Nakazawa, H. (2004). Perfluorooctane sulfonate (PFOS) and related perfluorinated compounds in human maternal and cord blood samples: assessment of PFOS exposure in a susceptible population during pregnancy. *Environmental Health Perspects*, 112, 11, (August 2004), pp. 1204–1207.

Isanhart, J.P.; McNabb, F.M. & Smith, P.N. (2005). Effects of perchlorate exposure on resting metabolism, peak metabolism, and thyroid function in the prairie vole (Microtus ochrogaster). *Environmental Toxicology and Chemistry*, 24, 3, (May 2005), pp. 678-84.

Iwasaki, T.; Miyazaki, W.; Takeshita, A.; Kuroda, Y. & Koibuchi, N. (2002). Polychlorinated biphenyls suppress thyroid hormone-induced transactivation. *Biochemical and Biophysical Research Communications*, 299, 3, (December 2002), pp. 384-8.

Janosek, J.; Hilscherova, K.; Blaha, L. & Holoubek, I. (2006). Environmental xenobiotics and nuclear receptors--interactions, effects and in vitro assessment. *Toxicology In Vitro*, 20, 1, (February 2006), pp. 18-37.

Jones, P.; Hu, W.; De coen, W.; Newsted, J. & Giesy, J. (2003). Binding of perfluorinated fatty acids to serum proteins. *Environmental Toxicology and Chemistry*, 22, 11, (November 2003), pp. 2639–2649.

Jurewicz, J. & Hanke, W. (2011). Exposure to phthalates: reproductive outcome and children health. A review of epidemiological studies. *International Archives of Occupational and Environmental Health* 24, 2, (June 2011), pp. 115-141.

Kang, J.H.; Kondo, F. & Katayama, Y. (2006). Human exposure to bisphenol A. *Toxicology* 226, 2-3, (September 2006), pp. 79-89.

Kannan, K.; Corsolini, S.; Falandysz, J.; Fillmann, G.; Kumar, K.S.; Loganathan, B.G.; Mohd, M.A.; Olivero, J.; Van Wouwe, N.; Yang, J.H. & Aldoust, K.M. (2004). Perfluorooctanesulfonate and related fluorochemicals in human blood from several countries. *Environmental Science & Technology*, 38, 17, (September 2004), pp. 4489–4495.

Kato, Y.; Ikushiro, S.; Haraguchi, K.; Yamazaki, T.; Ito, Y.; Suzuki, H.; Kimura, R.; Yamada, S.; Inoue, T. & Degawa, M. (2004). A possible mechanism for decrease in serum thyroxine level by polychlorinated biphenyls in Wistar and Gunn rats. *Toxicological Sciences*, 81, 2, (October 2004), pp. 309-15.

Kavlock, R.J.; Daston, G.P.; DeRosa, C.; Fenner-Crisp, P.; Gray, L.E.; Kaattari, S.; Lucier, G.; Luster, M.; Mac, M.J.; Maczka, C.; Miller, R.; Moore, J.; Rolland, R.; Scott, G.; Sheehan, D.M.; Sinks, T. & Tilson, H.A. (1996). Research needs for the risk assessment of health and environmental effects of endocrine disruptors: a report of the U.S. EPA-sponsored workshop. *Environmental Health Perspects*, 104, S4, (August 1996), pp. 715-40.

Kitamura, S.; Jinno, N.; Ohta, S.; Kuroki, H. & Fujimoto, N. (2002). Thyroid hormonal activity of the flame retardants tetrabromobisphenol A and tetrachlorobisphenol A. *Biochemical and Biophysical Research Communications* , 293, 1, (April 2002), pp. 554-9.

Kitamura, S.; Jinno, N.; Suzuki, T.; Sugihara, K.; Ohta, S.; Kuroki, H. & Fujimoto, N. (2005). Thyroid hormone-like and estrogenic activity of hydroxylated PCBs in cell culture. *Toxicology*, 208, 3, (March 2005), pp. 377-87.

Kohn, M.C.; Sewall, C.H.; Lucier, G.W. & Portier, C.J. (1996). A mechanistic model of effects of dioxin on thyroid hormones in the rat. *Toxicology and Applied Pharmacology*, 136, 1, (January 1996), pp. 29-48.

Koopman-Esseboom, C.; Morse, D.C.; Weisglas-Kuperus, N.; Lutkeschipholt, I.J.; Van der Paauw, C.G.; Tuinstra, L.G.; Brouwer, A. & Sauer, P.J. (1994). Effects of dioxins and polychlorinated biphenyls on thyroid hormone status of pregnant women and their infants. *Pediatric Research*, 36, 4, (October 1994), pp. 468-73.

Lamm, S.H.; Braverman, L.E.; Li, F.X.; Richman, K.; Pino, S. & Howearth, G. (1999). Thyroid health status of ammonium perchlorate workers: a cross-sectional occupational health study. *Journal of Occupational and Environmental Medicine*, 41, 4, (April 1999), pp. 248-60.

Latini, G. (2005). Monitoring phthalate exposure in humans. *Clinica Chimica Acta*, 361, 1-2, (November 2005), pp. 20-9.

Lau, C.; Thibodeaux, J.R.; Hanson, R.G.; Rogers, J.M.; Grey, B.E.; Stanton, M.E.; Butenhoff, J.L. & Stevenson, L.A. (2003). Exposure to perfluorooctane sulfonate during pregnancy in rat and mouse. II: Postnatal evaluation. *Toxicological Sciences*, 74, 2, (August 2003), pp. 382–392.

Lau, C.; Anitole, K.; Hodes, C.; Lai, D.; Pfahles-Hutchens, A. & Seed, J. (2007). Perfluoroalkyl acids: a review of monitoring and toxicological findings. *Toxicological Sciences*, 99, 2, (October 2007), pp. 366–394.

Lawrence, J.E.; Lamm, S.H.; Pino, S.; Richman, K. & Braverman, L.E. (2000). The effect of short-term low-dose perchlorate on various aspects of thyroid function. *Thyroid* 10, 8, (August 2000), pp. 659-63.

Lewis, J.B.; Rueggeberg, F.A.; Lapp, C.A.; Ergle, J.W. & Schuster, G.S. (1999). Identification and characterization of estrogen-like components in commercial resin-based dental restorative materials. *Clinical Oral Investigations*, 3, 3, (September 1999), pp. 107-13.

Lintelmann, J.; Katayama, A.; Kuhihara, N. & Wenzel, A. (2003). Endocrine disruptors in the environment (IUPAC Technical Report). *Pure and Applied Chemistry*, 75, 5, (2003), pp. 631-681.

Loh, K.C. (2000). Amiodarone-induced thyroid disorders: a clinical review. *Postgraduate Medical Journal*, 76, 893, (March 2000), pp. 133-40.

Luebker, D.J.; Case, M.T.; York, R.G.; Moore, J.A.; Hansen, K.J. & Butenhoff, J.L. (2005). Two-generation reproduction and cross-foster studies of perfluorooctanesulfonate (PFOS) in rats. *Toxicology*, 215, 1-2, (November 2005), pp. 126–148.

Maiti, P.K. & Kar, A. (1997). Dimethoate inhibits extrathyroidal 5'-monodeiodination of thyroxine to 3,3',5-triiodothyronine in mice: the possible involvement of the lipid peroxidative process. *Toxicology Letters*, 91, 1, (March 1997), pp. 1-6.

Marinovich, M.; Guazzetti, M.; Ghilardi, F.; Viviani, B.; Corsini, E. & Galli, C.L. (1997). Thyroid peroxidase as toxicity target for dithiocarbamates. *Archives of Toxicology*, 71, 8, (1997), pp. 508-12.

Massart, F.; Harrell, J.C.; Federico, G. & Saggese, G. (2005). Human breast milk and xenoestrogen exposure: a possible impact on human health. *Journal of Perinatology*, 25, 4, (April 2005), pp. 282-8.

Massart, F.; Parrino, R.; Seppia, P.; Federico, G. & Saggese, G. (2006a). How do environmental estrogen disruptors induce central precocious puberty ? *Minerva Pediatrica*, 58, 3, (June 2006), pp. 247-254.

Massart, F.; Massai, G.; Placidi, G. & Saggese, G. (2006b). Child thyroid disruption by environmental chemicals. *Minerva Pediatrica*, 58, 1, (February 2006), pp. 47-53.

Massart, F. & Meucci, V. (2007). Environmental thyroid toxicants and child endocrine health. *Pediatric Endocrinology Reviews*, 5, 1, (September 2007), pp. 500-509.

McNabb, F.M.; Larsen, C.T. & Pooler, P.S. (2004a). Ammonium perchlorate effects on thyroid function and growth in bobwhite quail chicks. *Environmental Toxicology and Chemistry*, 23, 4, (April 2004), pp. 997-1003.

McNabb, F.M.; Jang, D.A. & Larsen, C.T. (2004b). Does thyroid function in developing birds adapt to sustained ammonium perchlorate exposure? *Toxicological Sciences*, 82, 1, (November 2004), pp. 106-13.

Metzer, D.; Rice, N.; Deplege, M.H.; Henley, W.E. & Galloway, T.S. (2010). Association between Serum Perfluorooctanoic Acid (PFOA) and Thyroid Disease in the U.S. National Health and Nutrition Examination Survey. *Environmental Health Perspectives*, 118, 5, (May 2010), pp. 686-692.

Mirabella, G.; Feig, D.; Astzalos, E.; Perlman, K. & Rovet, J.F. (2000). The effect of abnormal intrauterine thyroid hormone economies on infant cognitive abilities. *Journal of Pediatric Endocrinology & Metabolism*, 13, 2, (February 2000), pp. 191-4.

Michalek, J.E. & Tripathi, R.C. (1999). Pharmacokinetics of TCDD in veterans of Operation Ranch Hand: 15-year follow-up. *Journal of Toxicology and Environmental Health. Part A*, 57, 6, (July 1999), pp. 369-78.

Michalek, J.E.; Pirkle, J.L.; Needham, L.L.; Patterson, D.G. Jr.; Caudill, S.P.; Tripathi, R.C. & Mocarelli, P. (2002). Pharmacokinetics of 2,3,7,8-tetrachlorodibenzo-p-dioxin in Seveso adults and veterans of operation Ranch Hand. *Journal of Exposure Analysis and Environmental Epidemiology*, 12, 1, (January-February 2002), pp. 44-53.

Mitchell, F.E.; Price, S.C.; Hinton, R.H.; Grasso, P. & Bridges, J.W. (1985). Time and dose-response study of the effects on rats of the plasticizer di(2-ethylhexyl) phthalate. *Toxicology and Applied Pharmacology*, 81, 3 Pt 1, (December 1985), pp. 371–392.

Miyazaki, W.; Iwasaki, T.; Takeshita, A.; Kuroda, Y. & Koibuchi, N. (2004). Polychlorinated biphenyls suppress thyroid hormone receptor-mediated transcription through a novel mechanism. *The Journal of Biological Chemistry*, 279, 18, (April 2004), pp. 18195-202.

Moriyama, K.; Tagami, T.; Akamizu, T.; Usui, T.; Saijo, M.; Kanamoto, N.; Hataya, Y.; Shimatsu, A.; Kuzuya, H. & Nakao, K. (2002). Thyroid hormone action is disrupted by bisphenol A as an antagonist. *The Journal of Clinical Endocrinology and Metabolism*, 87, 11, (November 2002), pp. 5185-90.

Morse, D.C.; Groen, D.; Veerman, M.; van Amerongen, C.J.; Koëter, H.B.; Smits van Prooije, A.E.; Visser, T.J.; Koeman, J.H. & Brouwer, A. (1993). Interference of polychlorinated biphenyls in thyroid hormone metabolism: Possible neurotoxic consequences in fetal and neonatal rats. *Toxicology and Applied Pharmacology*, 122, 1, (September 1993), pp. 27-33.

Morse, D.C.; Wehler, E.K.; Wesseling, W.; Koeman, J.H. & Brouwer, A. (1996). Alterations in rat brain thyroid hormone status following pre- and postnatal exposure to polychlorinated biphenyls (Aroclor 1254). *Toxicology and Applied Pharmacology*, 136, 2, (February 1996), pp. 269-79.

O'Connor, J.C.; Frame, S.R. & Ladics, G.S. (2002). Evaluation of a 15-day screening assay using intact male rats for identifying antiandrogens. *Toxicological Sciences*, 69, 1, (September 2002), pp. 92–108.

Okazaki, Y. & Katayama, T. (2003). Effects of dietary carbohydrate and myo-inositol on metabolic changes in rats fed 1,1,1-trichloro-2,2-bis (p-chlorophenyl) ethane (DDT). *The Journal of Nutritional Biochemistry*, 14, 2, (February 2003), pp. 81-9.

Olsen, G.W.; Burris, J.M.; Burlew, M.M. & Mandel, J.H. (2003a). Epidemiologic assessment of worker serum perfluorooctanesulfonate (PFOS) and perfluorooctanoate (PFOA) concentrations and medical surveillance examinations. *Journal of Occupational and Environmental Medicine*, 45, 3, (March 2003), pp. 260–270.

Olsen, G.W.; Logan, P.W.; Hansen, K.J.; Simpson, C.A.; Burris, J.M.; Burlew, M.M.; Vorarath, P.P.; Venkateswarlu, P.; Schumpert, J.C. & Mandel, J.H. (2003b). An occupational exposure assessment of a perfluorooctanesulfonyl fluoride production site: biomonitoring. *American Industrial Hygiene Association journal*, 64, 5, (September-October 2003), pp. 651–659.

Olsen, G.W.; Church, T.R.; Miller, J.P.; Burris, J.M.; Hansen, K.J.; Lundberg, J.K.; Armitage, J.B.; Herron, R.M.; Medhdizadehkashi, Z.; Nobiletti, J.B.; O'Neill, E.M.; Mandel, J.H. & Zobel, L.R. (2003c). Perfluorooctanosulfonate (PFOS) and other fluorochemicals in the serum of American Red Cross adult blood donors. *Environmental Health Perspects* , 111, 16, (December 2003), pp. 1892–1901.

Olsen, G. & Zobel, L. (2007). Assessment of lipid, hepatic and thyroid parameters with serum perfluorooctanoate (PFOA) concentrations in fluorochemical production workers. *International Archives of Occupational and Environmental Health*, 81, 2, (November 2007), pp. 231–246.

Organisation for Economic Co-operation and Development (OECD), (2005). *Results of Survey on Production and Use of PFOS and PFOA, Related Substances and Products/Mixtures Containing These Substances*. Organisation for Economic Co-operation and Development, Paris.

Osius, N.; Karmaus, W.; Kruse, H. & Witten, J. (1999). Exposure to polychlorinated biphenyls and levels of thyroid hormones in children. *Environmental Health Perspects*, 107, 10, (October 1999), pp. 843-9.

Papke, O.; Ball, M.; Lis, A. & Wuthe, J. (1996). PCDD/PCDFs in humans, follow-up of background data for Germany, 1994. *Chemosphere*, 32, 3, (February 1996), pp. 575-82.

Persky, V.; Turyk, M.; Anderson, H.A.; Hanrahan, L.P.; Falk, C.; Steenport, D.N.; Chatterton, R. Jr.; Freels, S. & Great Lakes Consortium. (2001). The effects of PCB exposure and fish consumption on endogenous hormones. *Environmental Health Perspects*, 109, 12, (December 2001), pp. 1275-83.

Poon, R.; Lecavalier, P.; Mueller, R.; Valli, V.E.; Procter, B.G. & Chu, I. (1997). Subchronic oral toxicity of di-n-octyl phthalate and di(2-ethylhexyl) phthalate in the rat. *Food and Chemical Toxicology*, 35, 2, (February 1997), pp. 225–239.

Price, S.C.; Chescoe, D.; Grasso, P.; Wright, M. & Hinton, R.H. (1988). Alterations in the thyroids of rats treated for long periods with di-(2-ethylhexyl) phthalate or with hypolipidaemic agents. *Toxicology Letters*, 40, 1, (January 1988), pp. 37–46.

Rais-Bahrami, K.; Nunez, S.; Revenis, M.E.; Luban, N.L. & Short, B.L. (2004). Follow-up study of adolescents exposed to di(2-ethylhexyl) phthalate (DEHP) as neonates on extracorporeal membrane oxygenation (ECMO) support. *Environmental Health Perspects*, 112, 13, (September 2004), pp. 1339-40.

Rogan, W.J.; Gladen, B.C.; McKinney, J.D.; Carreras, N.; Hardy, P.; Thullen, J.; Tinglestad, J. & Tully, M. (1986). Neonatal effects of transplacental exposure to PCBs and DDE. Journal of Pediatrics, 109, 2, (August 1986), pp. 335-41.

Safe, S.H. (2000). Endocrine disruptors and human health--is there a problem? An update. *Environmental Health Perspects*, 108, 6, (June 2000), pp. 487-93.

Saito, N.; Harada, K.; Inoue, K.; Sasaki, K.; Yoshinaga, T. & Koizumi, A. (2004). Perfluorooctanoate and perfluorooctane sulfonate concentrations in surface water in Japan. *Journal of Occupational Health*, 46, 1, (January 2004), pp. 49–59.

Sala, M.; Sunyer, J.; Herrero, C.; To-Figueras, J. & Grimalt, J. (2001). Association between serum concentrations of hexachlorobenzene and polychlorobiphenyls with thyroid hormone and liver enzymes in a sample of the general population. *Occupational and Environmental Medicine*, 58, 3, (March 2001), pp. 172-7.

Schell, L.M.; Gallo, M.V.; DeCaprio, A.P.; Hubicki, L.; Denham, M.; Ravenscroft, J. & The Akwesasne Task Force on the Environment. (2004). Thyroid function in relation to burden of PCBs, *p,p'*-DDE, HCB, mirex and lead among Akwesasne Mohawk youth: a preliminary study. *Environmental Toxicology and Pharmacology*, 18, 2, (November 2004), pp. 91-99.

Schettler, T. (2006). Human exposure to phthalates via consumer products. *International Journal of Andrology* 29, 1, (February 2006), pp. 134-9 and 181-5.

Schonfelder, G.; Wittfoht, W.; Hopp, H.; Talsness, C.E.; Paul, M. & Chahoud, I. (2002). Parent bisphenol A accumulation in the human maternal-fetal-placental unit. *Environmental Health Perspects*, 110, 11, (November 2002), pp. A703-7.

Seacat, A.M.; Thomford, P.J.; Hansen, K.J.; Clemen, L.A.; Eldridge, S.R.; Elcombe, C.R. & Butenhoff, J.L. (2003). Sub-chronic dietary toxicity of potassium perfluorooctanesulfonate in rats. *Toxicology*, 183, 1-3, (February 2003), pp. 117–131.

Seo, B.W.; Li, M.H.; Hansen, L.G.; Moore, R.W.; Peterson, R.E. & Schantz, S.L. (1995). Effects of gestational and lactational exposure to coplanar polychlorinated biphenyl (PCB) congeners or 2,3,7,8-tetrachlorodibenzo-p-dioxin (TCDD) on thyroid hormone concentrations in weanling rats. *Toxicology Letters*, 78, 3, (August 1995), pp. 253-62.

Sewall, C.H.; Flagler, N.; Vanden Heuvel, J.P.; Clark, G.C.; Tritscher, A.M.; Maronpot, R.M. & Lucier, G.W. (1995). Alterations in thyroid function in female Sprague-Dawley rats following chronic treatment with 2,3,7,8-tetrachlorodibenzo-p-dioxin. *Toxicology and Applied Pharmacology*, 132, 2, (June 1995), pp. 237-44.

Sharlin, D.S.; Bansal, R. & Zoeller, R.T. (2006). Polychlorinated biphenyls exert selective effects on cellular composition of white matter in a manner inconsistent with thyroid hormone insufficiency. *Endocrinology*, 147, 2, (February 2006), pp. 846-58.

Shea, K.M. (2003). American Academy of Pediatrics Committee on Environmental Health. Pediatric exposure and potential toxicity of phthalate plasticizers. *Pediatrics*, 111, 6 Pt 1, (June 2003), pp. 1467-74.

Spear, P.A.; Higueret, P. & Garcin, H. (1990). Increased thyroxine turnover after 3,3',4,4',5,5'-hexabromobiphenyl injection and lack of effect on peripheral triiodothyronine production. *Canadian Journal of Physiology and Pharmacology*, 68, 8, (August 1990), pp. 1079-84.

Stanbury, J.B. & Wyngaarden, J.B. (1952). Effect of perchlorate on the human thyroid gland. *Metabolism* 1, 6, (November 1952), pp. 533-9.

Stewart, P.; Fitzgerald, S.; Reihman, J.; Gump, B.; Lonky, E.; Darvill, T.; Pagano, J. & Hauser, P. (2003). Prenatal PCB exposure, the corpus callosum, and response inhibition. *Environmental Health Perspects*, 111, 13, (October 2003), pp. 1670-7.

Stockholm Convention on Persistent Organic Pollutants (POPs), (2008). Available: http://chm.pops.int/ [accessed 2 October 2009].

Strawson, J.; Zhao, Q. & Dourson, M. (2004). Reference dose for perchlorate based on thyroid hormone change in pregnant women as the critical effect. *Regulatory Toxicology and Pharmacology*, 39, 1, (February 2004), pp. 44-65.

Takser, L.; Mergler, D.; Baldwin, M.; de Grosbois, S.; Smargiassi, A. & Lafond, J. (2005). Thyroid hormones in pregnancy in relation to environmental exposure to organochlorine compounds and mercury. *Environmental Health Perspects*, 113, 8, (August 2005), pp. 1039-45.

Thomsen, C.; Lundanes, E. & Becher, G. (2002). Brominated flame retardants in archived serum samples from Norway: a study on temporal trends and the role of age. *Environmental Science & Technology*, 36, 7, (April 2002), pp. 1414-8.

Tonacchera, M.; Pinchera, A.; Dimida, A.; Ferrarini, E.; Agretti, P.; Vitti, P.; Santini, F.; Crump, K. & Gibbs, J. (2004). Relative potencies and additivity of perchlorate, thiocyanate, nitrate, and iodide on the inhibition of radioactive iodide uptake by the human sodium iodide symporter. *Thyroid*, 14, 12, December 2004, pp. 1012-9.

US Environmental Protection Agency (EPA), (1994). Health *Assessment Document for 2,3,7,8-Tetrachlorodibenzo- p-dioxin (TCDD) Related Compounds. External review draft.* EPA/600/BP-92/001a.

US Environmental Protection Agency (EPA), (2006). *The 2010/2015 PFOA Stewardship Program.* Available: http://www.epa.gov/oppt/pfoa/pubs/stewardship/index.html [accessed 10 October 2009].

Van den Berg, K.J.; van Raaij, J.A.; Bragt, P.C. & Notten, W.R. (1991). Interactions of halogenated industrial chemicals with transthyretin and effects on thyroid hormone levels in vivo. *Archives of Toxicology*, 65, 1, (1991), pp. 15-9.

van Raaij, J.A.; Kaptein, E.; Visser, T.J. & van den Berg, K.J. (1993). Increased glucuronidation of thyroid hormone in hexachlorobenzene-treated rats. *Biochemical Pharmacology*, 45, 3, (February 1993), pp. 627-31.

Walkowiak, J.; Wiener, J.A.; Fastabend, A.; Heinzow, B.; Kramer U.; Schmidt, E.; Steingruber, H.J.; Wundram, S. & Winneke, G. (2001). Environmental exposure to polychlorinated biphenyls and quality of the home environment: effects on psychodevelopment in early childhood. *The Lancet*, 358, 9293, (November 2001), pp. 1602-7.

Wyngaarden, J.B.; Wright, B.M. & Ways, P. (1952). The effect of certain anions upon the accumulation and retention of iodide by the thyroid gland. *Endocrinology*, 50, 5, (May 1952), pp. 537-49.

World Health Organization (WHO) E.H.C. (1995). *Tetrabromobisphenol A and derivates.* World Health Organization, Geneva, Switzerland.

World Health Organization (WHO) E.H.C. (1997). *Flame-retardants: a general introduction.* World Health Organization, Geneva, Switzerland.

Wolff, J. (1998). Perchlorate and the thyroid gland. *Pharmacological Reviews*, 50, 1, (March 1998), pp. 89-105.

Yamada-Okabe, T.; Aono, T.; Sakai, H.; Kashima, Y. & Yamada-Okabe, H. (2004). 2,3,7,8-tetrachlorodibenzo-p-dioxin augments the modulation of gene expression mediated by the thyroid hormone receptor. *Toxicology and Applied Pharmacology*, 194, 3, (February 2004), pp. 201-10.

Yu, W.G.; Liu, W. & Jin, Y.H. (2009). Effects of perfluorooctane sulfonate on rat thyroid hormone biosynthesis and metabolism. *Environmental Toxicology and Chemistry*, 28, 5, (May 2009), pp. 990–996.

Zoeller, R.T.; Dowling, A.L. & Vas, A.A. (2000). Developmental exposure to polychlorinated biphenyls exerts thyroid hormone-like effects on the expression of RC3/neurogranin and myelin basic protein messenger ribonucleic acids in the developing rat brain. *Endocrinology*, 141, 1, (January 2000), pp. 181-9.

Zoeller, T.R.; Dowling, A.L.; Herzig, C.T.; Iannacone, E.A.; Gauger, K.J. & Bansal, R. (2002). Thyroid hormone, brain development, and the environment. *Environmental Health Perspects*, 110, S3, (June 2002), pp. 355-61

Zoeller, R.T. (2003). Thyroid toxicology and brain development: should we think differently? *Environmental Health Perspects* , 111, 12, (September 2003), pp. A628.

Zoeller, R.T. (2005). Environmental chemicals as thyroid hormone analogues: new studies indicate that thyroid hormone receptors are targets of industrial chemicals? *Molecular and Cellular Endocrinology*, 242, 1-2, (October 2005), pp. 10-5.

Part 2

Autoimmune Thyroid Diseases

3

Hashimoto's Disease

Noura Bougacha-Elleuch[1], Mouna Mnif-Feki[2],
Nadia Charfi-Sellami[2], Mohamed Abid[2] and Hammadi Ayadi[1]
[1]*Unité Cibles pour le Diagnostic et la Thérapie, Centre de Biotechnologie de Sfax,*
[2]*Service Endocrinologie, CHU Hédi Chaker, Sfax,*
Tunisia

1. Introduction

The thyroid gland is one of the largest endocrine glands. It is prone to several very distinct pathologies, some of which are extremely common such as autoimmune thyroid diseases (AITDs). AITDs are conditions in which the immune system attacks the body's own thyroid gland which leads to a deregulation in thyroid hormones production. Because these hormones are used almost everywhere in the body, AITDs can have widespread, serious effects and many symptoms. AITDs can be broken down into two classes: i- Graves' disease (GD) characterized by hyperthyroidism and ii-Autoimmune Hypothyroidism, where the major clinical form is Hashimoto's thyroiditis (HT). In HT, the antibodies against thyroid peroxidase or thyroglobulin appear characteristically in the patients' sera, while tissue damage due to T cell-mediated cytotoxicity usually contributes to gradual development of hypothyroidism.

HT, described by Hakaru Hashimoto in 1912, is a common autoimmune disease, afflicting up to 10% of the population (Canaries et al., 2000). However, its etiology is still unknown. In fact, although environmental factors, such as infection, certain drugs, stress, smoking, can play a role in their progression, the HT- as AITDs - is generally hereditary in origin. Comprehension of physiopathological mechanism behind has been improved over the last few decades. In the literature, a number of excellent reviews have been published on the genetic background of AITDs (Eschler et al., 2011; Hadj Kacem et al., 2009). However, there is still a paucity concerning HT. Several parameters have contributed to this paucity. Some of them are general for AITDs such as genetic heterogeneity; others are rather specific to HT mainly clinical heterogeneity and diagnostic difficulties. This chapter examines the recent progress in our understanding of the genetic and environmental contributions to the etiology of Hashimoto's thyroiditis. We will also focus on epidemiology, clinical progression and physiopathological mechanism of the disease. We will shed light on our findings concerning a Tunisian multigenerational family "Akr" (Maalej et al., 2001a) which has benefited from a regular clinical follow-up, a complex segregation analysis as well as a genetic investigation using both genome screening and candidate genes approaches.

2. Epidemiology

Hashimoto's thyroiditis is a common form of chronic AITDs. The disorder affects from 2% (Wang et al., 1997) up to 10% (Canaries et al., 2000) of the general population. It is more common in older women and ten times more frequent in women than in men (Tunbridge et al., 2000). Based on TSH (thyroid stimulating hormone) levels or anti-thyroid auto antibodies, a population-based prevalence study has reported prevalence of 3.6% and 8.8% respectively (Tunbridge et al., 1977). In the United States, Hollowell and collaborators (2002) found that 4.6% of the population had hypothyroidism and 13.0% had anti-thyroid peroxydase auto antibodies.

In Tunisian population, a study performed on 1076 patients who resorted to the Department of Endocrinology of Sfax, Hédi Chaker Universitary Hospital at Sfax, found that prevalence of HT was 22.8% (Chabchoub et al., 2006). This high value could be explained by the fact that this study has assed sedan oriented demand. In a district from the central east of Tunisia, where "Akr" family members live, the prevalence and incidence of AITDs were 4.36% and 7.2 per 1000 inhabitants per year respectively. Particularly, the prevalence of autoimmune hypothyroidism was 2.13% (Bougacha-Elleuch et al., 2011).

3. Etiology

HT results from a complex combination of genetic, environmental, and endogenous factors which interplay to initiate thyroid autoimmunity.

3.1 Environmental factors

Several environmental factors are thought to affect the incidence and the progression of HT disease. Thus, recent studies have shown the close relationship between either excessive iodine levels (Camargo et al., 2006; Doğan et al., 2011; Teng et al., 2011) or Selenium deficiency (Toulis et al., 2010) and HT. High levels of several chemical agents have also been implicated in the incidence of goiter and autoimmune thyroiditis (de Freitas et al., 2010). Moreover, the components of several viruses (hepatitis C, human parvovirus B19, coxsackie and herpes viruses) were detected in the thyroid of Hashimoto's thyroiditis patients (Mori & Yoshida 2010). Moreover, the possible involvement of the oxidative stress profile in HT pathogenesis was also reported (Baskol et al., 2007; Lassouad et al., 2010).

3.2 Epigenetic factors

Using disease discordant twin pairs, Brix and collaborators have found that the frequency of skewed X chromosome inactivation in female twins with HT was 31% (vs 8% in control population) (Brix et al., 2005). In Tunisian population, findings reported by our team suggest a possible role for X chromosome inactivation mosaicism in the pathogenesis of AITDs (GD and HT) and may, to some extent, explain the female preponderance of these diseases (Chabchoub et al., 2009).

3.3 Endogenous factors

HT could be considered as a "sex realated disease", since women are more susceptible to develop HT than men. Indeed, the Sex ratio is 7F/1M (Duron et al., 2004), with an incidence of 3,5 cases per 1000 woman in year vs 0,8 cases per 1000 men per year (vanderpump et al.,1995). The importance of pregnancy and postpartum thyroiditis in autoimmune thyroiditis is well-established (Friedrich et al., 2008).

3.4 Genetic susceptibility to HT

Evidence for genetic susceptibility to HT is strongly shown by epidemiological data from family and twin studies.

3.4.1 Family studies

The familial occurrence of AITDs (HT and GD) has been reported by investigators for many years (Hall & Stanbury, 1967; Martin, 1945). One of the large multiplex families in the world was reported in Tunisia (Akr family) (Maalej, A. et al. 2001a). The high prevalence of both GD and HT, found in the "Akr" family (17.5%), is another argument to the contribution of genetic factors in HT pathogenesis.

3.4.2 Sibling risk ratio (λs)

The λs is a useful quantitative measure of the heritability of a disease, with a λs greater than 5 usually indicating a genetic influence on the etiology of the disease (Risch, 1990; Vyse & Todd, 1996). The risk in siblings of parents with AITDs was estimated to 28.0 for HT, giving evidence for a strong genetic component (Villanueva et al., 2003).

3.4.3 Twin studies

The use of twins is a well-established method to investigate the relative importance of genetic and environmental factors to traits and diseases (MacGregor et al., 2000). Thus, for HT, the concordance rates were 55 and 0% for Monozygotic and Dizygotic twins, respectively (Brix et al., 2000). Concerning anti thyroid antibodies, monozygotic twins had 80% concordance, and dizygotic twins had only 40% concordance (Brix et al., 2000).

4. Physiopathology

It is well known that HT results from a multistep process, requiring several genetic and environmental abnormalities to converge before disease development. Thus, thyroid follicle damage may be provoked by self-antigen presentation by antigen presenting cells and specific T lymphocyte activation. On the other hand, toxic destruction of thyroid cells possibly through the generation of oxygen radicals may participate in eclosion of autoimmunity (Bagchi et al., 1995). Both proliferation and apoptosis are involved in the pathogenesis of HT. Analysis of the mechanisms by which such autoimmune pathology arises has been facilitated by the use of animal models. These include the Obese Strain (OS) chicken and the BioBreeding (BB) and Buffalo rats as spontaneous models of HT. HT can also be experimentally induced by specific immunization protocols with target auto antigens or elevation of dietary iodine.

4.1 Autoimmunity in HT

HT is considered to be a th1-mediated disease leading to aberrant infiltration of lymphoid cells and destruction of thyroid follicles (figure1). The final outcome is fibrosis replacing normal thyroid parenchyma and hypothyroidism resulting of thyroid cell destruction (Parish & Cooke, 2004). Indeed, a central phase of HT is characterized by an apparent uncontrolled production of auto reactive CD4+ T cells, CD8+ cytotoxic T cells and immunoglobulin G auto antibodies. This immunological synapse is defined by the interface between antigen presenting cells and T-cells that is formed during T-cell activation (Chistiakov, 2005). On the other hand, existence of naturally existing CD4+ CD25+ foxp3+ T regulatory cells influencing thyroiditis development in naïve susceptible mice was recently demonstrated. Moreover, it has been shown that naturally T regulatory cells are required for induction of antigen specific tolerance, indicating that induced Murine experimental autoimmune thyroiditis tolerance is a result of activation of naturally existing T regulatory cells rather than de novo generation of induced T regulatory cells (Morris et al., 2009).

Interestingly, several of the AITDs susceptibility genes participate in the immunological synapse, suggesting that abnormalities in antigen presentation are important mechanisms leading to AITDs (Tomer, 2010).

Initially, the production of self-reactive cells and auto antibodies occurs in the draining lymph nodes. Later, the lymphoid tissue often develops directly in the thyroid gland itself. This tissue is generally very well-organized, with cords of anti-Tg-antibody- producing plasma cells in the periphery (Chistiakov, 2005). In a final, destructive step of HT, the auto reactive T cells diffusely accumulate in large numbers and infiltrate thyroid parenchyma. This phenomenon will determine clinical phenotype of the disease. In the BB-DP rat model, Th1-mediated mechanisms involving production of IL-12, tumor necrosis factor-α (TNF-α) and interferon-γ play a major role in the destruction of thyrocytes (Blüher et al., 1999a; Mooij et al., 1993). Furthermore, it has been recently shown that pro-IL18 is constitutively expressed in thyroid cells and IL18 up regulation by INF-γ is an immunological feature of HT patients with an important role in promoting the local immune response (Liu et al., 2010).

4.2 Apoptosis in HT

Apoptosis appears to play a major role in the final stage of the disease (figure1). In fact, apoptotic molecules such as Fas and Fas ligand (FasL) expression was higher in rats with lympholytic thyroiditis indicating a possible role in thyrocyte death (Blüher et al., 1999b). Theses molecules are expressed at low level by normal thyroid cells compared to patients with HT with an increasing number of apoptotic cells (Kaczmarek et al., 2011). The mechanism and regulation of apoptosis in thyroid gland are still little known. The most studied receptor mediated apoptic pathway is the Fas/Fas ligand system. Fas is substantially expressed on lymphocytes. Fas-Fas ligand interaction could lead to the thyrocyte cell death (Kaczmarek et al., 2011). Thyroid cells express constitutively Fas but these latters are normally unaffected by Fas-mediated apoptosis. In contrast, they can be sensitised to Fas-induced destruction under certain pathologic conditions such as the release of IFN-γ, TNF-α and IL-1β, by infiltrating immune cells (Giordano et al., 2001). Over the past few years, many reports have shown that mobilisation of the Fas/Fas ligand apoptotic pathway by proinflamatory cytokines plays a pivotal role in the devastation of thyroid follicular cells in HT leading to hypothyroidism. (Kaczmarek et al.,2011). Therefore, the Fas pathway is the most important mechanism of Tlymphocyte mediated apoptosis. It is just possible that this process plays an essential role in the pathogenesis of Hashimoto thyroiditis, because cytotoxic T lymphocytes are fully present in the thyroid in places where apoptosis is located (Mitsiades et al ., 1998 ; Fountoulakis et al., 2008; Chen el al ., 2004; Baker., 1999; Bretz.,2002).

Mechanisms of regulation of this pathway include probably changes in Fas expression level, and the expression of molecules that promote survival, including the Bcl-2 gene family

(Bretz et al.,1999; Mitsiades et al.,1998). This latter antiapoptotic protein and sFas system, which normally protect thyroid cells from apoptosis, are decreased in the thyroid cells of patients with HT, creating a proapoptotic phenotype (Fountoulakis & Tsatsoulis, 2004). Thus, the rate of thyrocyte apoptosis dictates the clinical outcome of thyroid autoimmunity. Though rare in normal thyroid, it markedly increases during HT, but not in GD with a divergent phenotype. Therefore, regulation of thyrocyte survival is a crucial pathogenic determinant via the balance between Th2 and Th1 response (Chistiakov, 2005).

Despite the "crucial" role played by these apoptotic molecules, they are poorly investigated in HT pathogenesis at the genetic level. Therefore, arguments of their "real" implication in HT are still missing.

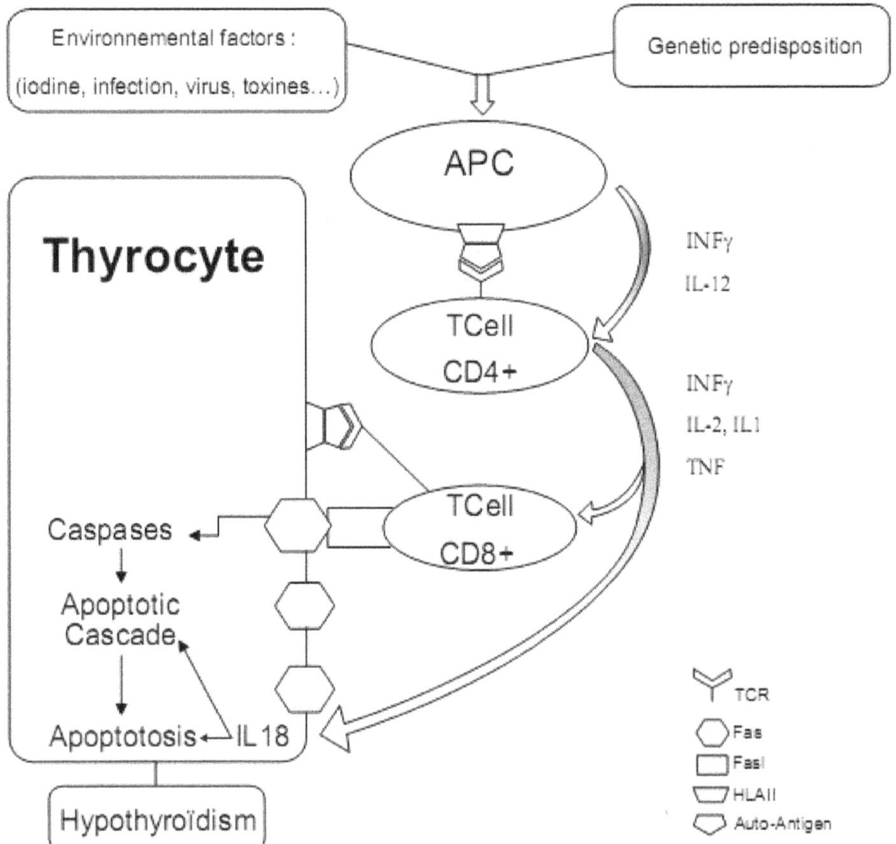

Fig. 1. Autoimmune events in Hashimoto's thyroiditis.

At the onset of disease, (HLA) class II-positive Antigen-presenting cells (APC), present thyroid-specific autoantigens to the naïve T cells, leading to the maturation of autoreactive T cells. Interaction with auto antigen leads to the production of different cytokines inducing T-helper type 1 (Th1)-mediated cell immune response. The stimulation of the Fas/Fas ligand apoptotic pathway by pro-inflammatory cytokines is the most important mechanism of

T lymphocyte mediated apoptosis. The caspase cascade ultimately induces enzymes that progressively destroy the cell, leading to thyroid cell death and hypothyroidism

5. Clinical data

HT occurs especially during the decades from 30 to 50 but no age is exempt, although the prevalence increases with age (Akamizu et al.,2008) The Sex ratio is 7F/1M, (Duron et al.,2004), with an incidence of 3.5 cases per 1000 women per year vs 0.8 cases per 1000 men per year (Vanderpump et al.,1995).

This disease is primarily associated with symptoms of altered thyroid function. Early in the course of the disease, the patient is usually euthyroid, but may show clinical hyperthyroidism, due to the inflammatory breakdown of thyroid follicles with release of thyroid hormones. Thyrotoxicosis may be present in 20% of patients when first seen (Akamizu et al.,2008),or commonly develop over a period of several years. In contrast, late in the disease, the patient is often hypothyroid because of progressive destruction of the thyroid gland. The most common eventual outcome of HT is hypothyroidism (Bottazzo & Doniach 1986).

In HT, the association of goiter with hypothyroidism is the most frequent condition of the diagnosis. Most often the gland is hypertrophic; two to four times the normal size, firm and nubbey. It is usually symmetrical, although much variation in symmetry can occur (Duron et al.,2004). Ultrasound may display an enlarged gland with normal texture, a characteristic picture with very low echogenity, or a suggestion of multiple well-defined nodules (Pedersen et al., 2000).

The goiter of HT may remain unchanged for decades (Akamizu et al., 2008), but usually it gradually increases in size. However, in some cases there is an involution of the goiter with evolution. Hence, the two major forms of the disorder are goitrous and atrophic autoimmune thyroiditis. A fast increase of the volume of the goiter and a very firm consistence of a fibrous goiter in aging patients, have to be taken with particular attention due to possible existence of a malignancy or a thyroid lymphoma (Duron et al., 2004).

Generally the progression from euthyroidism to hypothyroidism has been considered an irreversible process due to thyroid cell damage and loss of thyroidal iodine stores. However, it is now clear that up to one-fourth of patients who are hypothyroid may spontaneously return to normal function over the course of several years. This sequence may reflect the initial effect of high titers of thyroid stimulation blocking antibodies which fall with time and allow thyroid function to return (Takasu et al., 1992). Progression from subclinical hypothyroidism (normal FT4 but elevated TSH) to overt hypothyroidism occurs in a certain fraction (3-5%) each year. In Akr family, 11 patients (30%) had subclinical hypothyroidism (unpublished results).

Various auto antibodies may be present in sera of patients with HT: anti-thyroid peroxidase antibodies and, less frequently, anti-thyroglobulin antibodies. These later are positive in about 80% of patients and their prevalence increases with age. Anti- thyroid peroxidase antibodies are positive in 90% of patients; their frequency is higher in women and aging subjects. If both anti-thyroglobulin and anti-thyroid peroxidase antibodies are measured, 97% are positive. In contrast to the anti-thyroglobulin antibodies, the presence of anti-thyroid peroxidase antibody is correlated with the occurrence of hypothyroidism (duron et al.,2004).

The titles of anti -thyroid peroxidase antibodies are typically higher in atrophic form than in goitrous one.Young patients tend to have lower or occasionally negative levels. In this age group, even low titles evolve the presence of thyroid autoimmunity (Akamizu et al., 2008).

In the Tunisian study achieved by our group, 70 patients belonging to "Akr" famiy, were included. This family is actually composed of about 400 members with high level of consanguinity (60.5% vs 38.3% in controls from the same region) (Bougacha-Elleuch et al., 2011). Among these patients, 63 have benefited from a regular clinical follow up during these two last decades. Strikingly, we have found in this large family a co segregation of the two AITDs: 38 cases of HT (60.3%) and 25 cases (39.6%) of GD. Given the genetic predisposition of AITDs in this large family and occurrence of HT precisely at later ages, 115 healthy members of "Akr" family were carefully followed up by physicians, during 2 decades. We have found that 13 subjects (11,3%) developed AITDs. HT was seen in 77% of the cases while GD was found in only 23% (Charfi et al., 2009). In these patients, HT was in a hyperthyroid state in 13. 6% vs only 5% in literature (Duron et al., 2004)

6. Genetic susceptibility to HT

In complex diseases such as HT, it's well-established now that genetic susceptibility exists and represents an important piece in the general puzzle. However, determining both the "true" involved genes and the importance of contribution of each gene in the physiopathology of the disease, remains a laborious task which is not achieved yet.

To dissect the genetic component of HT, the major technologies used were mainly candidate gene analysis and whole-genome linkage screening. However, and unlike GD, at the genetic level, HT was poorly investigated as an individualized clinical entity. A general methodological problem has been disease definition. Indeed, HT encompasses a spectrum of manifestations, ranging from the simple presence of thyroid auto antibodies to the presence of goitrous or atrophic thyroiditis, characterized by gross thyroid failure (Davies et al., 1993). A second problem is lack of families composed only of HT patients. Thus, in most studies, AITDs are explored as a whole and in a second step, HT is considered aside. This situation is well encountered in genome scans where the investigated families usually comprise both GD and HT patients. This approach may identify more easily the common than the specific HT or GD gene susceptibility.

Another issue in genetic investigation of complex diseases such as HT, is search of a major gene in the general genetic entity. Possible existence of such a major gene could be evidenced by a particular type of statistical analysis: ie complex segregation analysis.

In our previous work, we have analyzed genetic susceptibility of AITDs (HT and GD) at the two levels: i-determination of involved genes using the two complementary approaches: ie whole genome screening and candidate genes analysis and ii- complex segregation analysis to search for possible major genes. In the following sections, we will focus on our findings concerning HT.

6.1 Dissection of genetic susceptibility

6.1.1 Whole genome screening

Genome-wide linkage analysis was the first approach employed to screen the genome for the genetic contribution to AITDs and particularly HT. Thus, the first genome linkage scan in AITDs was performed in 1999. There were two areas of linkage to HT, designated HT-1 and HT-2 on chromosome 13q32 and 12q22, respectively (Tomer et al., 1999). Since, many genome screenings were conducted and revealed regions with suggestive linkage (MLS<3.3), except the chromosomal region 8q23-q24 which has given a value of MLS=3.77 (Reviewed in Hadj Kacem et al., 2009). Therefore, it could be considered as "significantly linked" to HT. Indeed, according to Lander and Kruglyak, in complex diseases (such as HT) a lod score of >1.9 is suggestive of linkage, while a lod score of >3.3 indicates significant linkage in studies using the parametric approach. Linkage is confirmed if evidence for linkage is replicated in two separate data sets (Lander & Kruglyak, 1995).

Among linked regions, only 12q22 and 8q23-q24 were replicated. If we examine these replications, we will find that for the first region (12q22), we could not consider that replication was done in two separate data sets, since the second data set already contains the first one (Tomer et al., 2003; 2007). Concerning the second region (8q23-q24), replication was rather reported with AITDs and not HT (Tomer et al., 2002). In Tunisian population, genome screening, performed on Akr family, has revealed a genetic linkage of AITDs as a whole with the chromosomal region 2p.21. There were no regions linked to HT (Maalej et al., 2001a).

6.1.2 Candidate genes

Candidate genes analyzed in HT can be classified into two groups: (i) immune regulatory genes (MHC, CTLA-4, PTPN-22, cytokines..) and (ii) thyroid-specific genes (Tg, TPO, PDS..). Investigation of these genes in HT pathogenesis was done (for most of them) since they are functional candidates (they are selected by virtue of their physiological functions as possible contributors to disease pathogenesis). Among these genes, there are only two (CTLA-4 and Tg genes) which are both functional and positional genes (Table 1). In fact, they are localized in chromosomal regions found linked using the genome scan approach (2q33 and 8q23 respectively). At the statistical level, these two regions share a significant value of lod score (MLS= 4.2 and 3.77 for 2q33 and 8q23 respectively) (reviewed in Hadj Kacem et al., 2009).We have to get in mind that the chromosomal region 2q33 (harboring CTLA-4 gene) was linked with positive antibody rather than HT.

On the other hand, what we can note is that genetic associations reported with candidate genes were less definitive than in GD. Indeed, genetic investigation of AITDs since early 1990, has given arise to "significantly associated genes" either with AITDs or GD, but not HT. This could be explained by limited investigated samples. Thus, until now, there is no consortium in HT.

In table 1, we have only reported candidate genes which have been associated with HT and for which, potential mechanisms were proposed. In this regard, genes showing no association were not included. Potential mechanisms of associated genes variants were proposed by authors. They mainly involve higher production of either anti-thyroid antibody or the protein encoded by the gene itself. What we can note is that explored candidate genes are mainly those of immunoregulatory pathway. However, genes involved in apoptosis are poorly studied in HT in spite of their functional involvement in thyroid destruction in HT.

Gene	Chromosome	Associated variant (p<0.05)	Populations showing association	Potential mechanism	References
<u>Immunoregulatory genes</u>					
MHC classI genes (HLA-A, B, C)	6p21	A2, B16,B35, B46,B51,B54,C3	Asians		Chistialov, 2005
		A2-B50	Tunisian**		Bougacha-Elleuch et al., 2004
MHC classII genes (HLA-DP, DQ, DR)		DR3, DR4,	Caucasians	direct thyroid auto antigen presentation	Tandon N et al. 1991;
		DRw53	Japanese		Honda K et al. 1989
		DR9	Chinese		Hawkins et al; 1987
		DQw7 (DQB1*0301)	Caucasians		Badenhoop et al; 1990
		DRB1*04, DQB1*03	Caucasians		Zeitlin et al., 2008
		DR11, DR12	Tunisian**		Bougacha-Elleuch et al., 2004
CTLA-4*	2q33.2	-318C/T	Caucasians (Slovenians)	Higher thyroid autoantibody concentrations	zaletel et al., 2006
		49A/G	Caucasians (Slovenians)		
		CT60	Caucasians	reduced production of soluble CTLA-4	Udea et al., 2003
PTPN22	1p13	1858C/T	Slovenians (children)	Inhibition of T cell activation	Dallos et al., 2008
		R620W	Caucasians	Higher thyroid auto antibody concentrations	zaletel et al., 2010
IFN-gamma	12q15	874A/T	Japanese	High producing IFN gamma	Ito et al., 2006
			Indian		Rekha et al., 2006

Gene	Chromosome	Associated variant ($p<0.05$)	Populations showing association	Potential mechanism	References
TGF	19q13	869T/C	Japanese	Suppression of cytotoxic T cells actions and IFN-g expressions leading to thyroid destruction in HT	Yamada et al., 2008
IL6	7p15.3	-572 C/G	Japanese	High producing IL6	Inoue et al., 2011
IL4	5q31.1	-590C/T	Japanese	higher activity of inflammatory Th1 cytokines and more rapid progression of thyroid destruction	Nanba et al., 2008
TNF	6p21	-308A/G	Tunisian**	high constitutive and inducible levels of the TNFα chain	Bougacha-Elleuch et al., 2004
		−1031C/T	Japanese	high TNF-α production	Inoue et al., 2009
Thyroid specific genes					
Tg	8q24.22	Tgms2	Japanese	Interaction between HLA-DR3 and Tg polymorphisms	Ban et al., 2004
PDS	7q31	D7S2459	Tunisian	Low level of gene expression and/or protein activity in the thyroid tissue	Hadj-Kacem et al., 2003

*: Candidate genes harbored in linked regions found by genome scans.
**: The studied sample in Tunisian population is "Akr" family

Table 1. Functional and positional candidate genes associated with HT pathogenesis.

6.1.2.1 Immune regulatory genes

6.1.2.1.1 HLA

Data on HLA haplotypes in HT have been less definitive than in GD. In patients with HT, HLA associations have been found with the HLA'DR4' haplotypes (Tandon et al., 1991). Interestingly, it was shown that substitution of the neutral amino acids Ala or Gln with arginine at position beta 74 in the HLA-DR peptide-binding pocket is a key to the etiology of both GD and HT (Ban et al., 2004; Menconi et al., 2008).

In the Tunisian "Akr" family, using transmission disequilibrium test, we have reported a genetic association of AITDs with HLA-B37and HLA-DR11 alleles (Elleuch-Bougacha et al., 2001). Sequencing of the rare allele HLA-B37 in Akr family, has given evidence that it is not a new variant, but rather the known subtype HLA-B37*01 (unpublished results). In a second step, investigation of MHC (class I, II and III) genes polymorphisms has shown that TNF-308 A/G polymorphism was involved in GD and HT with different alleles.

Thus, TNFA allele was associated with GD, whereas TNFG, HLA-DR11 and DR12 were rather implicated in HT pathogenesis giving evidence for particular component for each disease (GD or HT) (Bougacha-Elleuch et al., 2004).

6.1.2.1.2 CTLA-4 gene

CTLA-4 (cytotoxic T lymphocyte-associated 4) is a cell surface immunoglobulin like receptor involved in the regulation of T-lymphocyte activation. CTLA-4 gene polymorphisms have been shown to be associated with a variety of autoimmune conditions. The most consistent reported association was with AITDs (Taylor et al., 2006). A recent investigation of patients with HT provided evidence that -318C/T promoter, 49A/G exon 1 and CT60 CTLA-4 gene SNPs were associated with higher thyroid autoantibody concentrations (Zaletel et al., 2006; 2010). In "Akr" family, CTLA-4 gene did not reveal any associated variant with HT (Maalej et al., 2001b).

6.1.2.1.3 PTPN22 gene

The PTPN22 (protein tyrosine phosphatase N22) molecule is involved in the activation of both naïve and activated T cells. The association of PTPN22 1858C/T polymorphism with HT is much weaker than the association with GD (Kahles et al., 2005). T-allele carriers were reported to be at particularly high risk of developing HT (Dultz et al., 2009). In a recent study performed in Japanese population, a novel protective effect of a haplotype containing five SNPs in this gene was observed for HT (Ban et al., 2010).

In Akr family, stratifying patients according to their phenotype (HT) did not show any significant association with PTPN22 R620W allele (Chabchoub et al., 2006).

6.1.2.1.4 VDR gene

VDR (vitamin D receptor) plays an immunoregulatory role based on the fact that the activation of human leucocytes causes the expression of VDR. The VDR gene, lies on chromosome 12q12-14 and harbors several polymorphisms and was found to be associated with several autoimmune diseases, (Huang et al., 2002; Mc Dermott et al., 1997; Pani et al., 2000; 2002)

Our previous results, in Tunisian population, showed no significant association of the Vitamin D receptor gene polymorphisms with HT in the "Akr" family (Maalej et al. 2008).

6.1.2.1.5 Cytokine genes

Local release of cytokines within the thyroid gland is important in regulating antigen presentation and lymphocyte trafficking by enhancing the expression of MHC class II and adhesion molecules on thyroid follicular cells (Kelso, 1998)

Studies, interested in cytokine gene polymorphisms with HT, are limited in literature. Thus, Ito C and collaborators (2006), have reported that the +874A/T polymorphism in the IFN-gamma gene was associated with severity of HT. Moreover, a significant association between high IFN-gamma-producing genotype TT (+874 A/T) and HT was found (Rekha et al., 2006). A recent study, exploring IL-1B, IL-1RN, IL-6 and TNFA genes polymorphisms, has given evidence that only IL-6 gene promoter (-572) C/G polymorphism could represent a potential "candidate" genetic marker to predict an individual's susceptibility to HT (Chen et al., 2006). It has been later revealed that the IL6-572G allele carriers, which have higher producibility of IL-6, were more frequent in severe HT (Inoue et al., 2011). Concerning IL4 gene, it was shown that the-590CC genotype appears to be a strong predictive factor for the development of hypothyroidism in HT (Nanba et al., 2008).

In "Akr" family, investigation of IL-1RN VNTR, IL-1B-511 C/T and IL-1A-889 C/T SNPs in the IL1 gene cluster and TNFRI ((GT)17 (GA)n microsatellite marker has not revealed any association with HT (Kammoun-Krichen et al., 2007; 2008).

6.1.2.2 IDDM6 locus

The IDDM6 locus (on 18q21 chromosome) was found to be linked to many autoimmune diseases: (Davies et al., 1994), (Cornelis et al., 1998), (Shai et al., 1999) (Vaidya et al., 2000), providing evidence that it is likely to harbor important autoimmunity loci. This locus was also examined in "Akr" family. Genetic linkage was found associated with both AITDs and HT (Hadj kacem et al., 2006) confirming again its key role in autoimmunity.

6.1.2.3 Thyroid specific genes

6.1.2.3.1 Thyroglobulin gene

Genetic-linkage studies have reported chromosome 8q24, containing the thyroglobulin (Tg) gene, as a susceptibility locus for AITDs in two different family samples (Sakai et al. 2001; Tomer et al., 2002). Later, association of the thyroglobulin intragenic marker (Tgms2) was found with HT (Ban et al., 2004). In a previous study, our group has examined the genomic region (11.5 cM) containing the Thyroglobulin gene by genotyping seven microsatellite markers and four SNPs in "Akr" family. Analysis of data did not show linkage of the Thyroglobulin gene with AITDs nor did analysis of HT and considered separately (Belguith-Maalej et al. 2008).

6.1.2.3.2 PDS gene

The PDS gene (7q31), responsible for Pendred syndrome (congenital sensorineural hearing loss and goiter), encodes a transmembrane protein known as pendrin (Everett et al., 1997). Pendrin functions as a transporter of iodide and chloride (Scott et al., 1999). In the Tunisian population,

PDS gene was reported to be associated with sporadic HT (goitrous and non goitrous forms) patients. In "Akr" family, there was an absence of linkage between HT and the PDS gene which could be explained by the reduced number of patients in the studied sample or by the weak contribution of the PDS gene in HT development (Hadj Kacem et al., 2003).

6.2 Complex segregation analysis

This kind of analysis aims to foresee whether the genetic susceptibility of complex diseases is governed by either a major gene or several minor genes. In AITDs, two previous studies have reported evidence for genetic transmission of thyroid peroxidase auto antibodies in old order Amish families using the Pointer program (Jaume et al., 1999; Pauls et al., 1993).

In "Akr" family, we have thought for a long time that segregation of both GD and HT with such prevalence could only reflect existence of at least a major gene behind. In order to decide between existence and absence of such a component, we have recently performed a complex segregation analysis of AITDs in the region harbouring Akr family. Our results gave evidence for a polygenic character of these diseases suggesting that genetic susceptibility to AITDs results from numerous loci, each contributing with small effects rather than a major one (Bougacha-Elleuch et al., 2011).

7. Conclusion

Based on "Akr" family studies, it seems that natural history but also the clinical and immunological feature of HT disease are not so different between familial and sporadic cases. Nevertheless, this multigenerational family remains a particular one with its high prevalence of AITDS, its high level of consanguinity and endogamy.

Regarding the literature, and despite extensive efforts, association studies often failed to reach consensus. Many reasons could be advanced for non replication of association studies, such as inadequate sample sizes, population stratification, variation in study design, confounding sampling bias and misclassification of phenotypes. Concerning HT, besides these parameters, there are some difficulties in disease definition. Additionally, co segregation of the two clinical forms (HT and GD) in the same family could be considered as another element making HT diagnosis more difficult. In such families, genome scan carried out tend to reveal chromosomal regions predisposing to AITDs rather than HT. Indeed, this approach may identify more easily the common than the specific HT or GD gene susceptibility. These observations might advocate setting up separate genome screening studies for GD and HT.

On the other hand, we can also postulate that among important reasons for non replication of many linked and/or associated regions/genes is that all these components of AITDs or HT "puzzle" contribute with minor effects (as it was evidenced in "Akr" family). Consequently, the appropriate approach to detect these small pieces of the puzzle would be genome wide association study in large samples. Indeed, as risk factors become more common and have smaller effect sizes, GWA studies emerge as a more powerful approach, There still is a paucity of GWAS in AITD in general and particularly in HT. A full genome-wide association analysis solely on AITD has not been published yet.

It is clear then, that we have to search for these genes in a large cohort composed only of HT patients with restricted clinical criteria to have a homogeneous sample. In this sample, investigation will not only be at the genetic level, but also at the transcriptomic one.

8. Acknowledgments

We are indebted to Akr family members for their invaluable cooperation. This work was supported by the Tunisian Ministry of High Education, Scientific Research and Technology and the International Centre for Genetic Engineering and Biotechnology ICGEB (Italy). We are grateful to Mrs Amel Mabrouk for her technical helpful in figure design. We thank Mr. Riadh Koubaa for his proof reading of the manuscript.

9. References

Akamizu T, Sale MM, Rich SS, Hiratani H, Noh JY, Kanamoto N, Saijo M, Miyamoto Y, Saito Y, Nakao K & Bowden DW. (2000). Association of autoimmune thyroid disease with microsatellite markers for the thyrotropin receptor gene and CTLA-4 in Japanese patients. *Thyroid, Vol.*10, No.10, (October 2000), pp. 851-858, ISSN 1050-7256

Akamizu T, Amino N & De Groot LJ. (2008) www.thyroidmanager.org. Chapter 8 Hashimoto's Thyroiditis Updated 15 August

Badenhoop K, Schwarz G, Walfish PG, Drummond V, Usadel KH & Bottazzo GF. (1990). Susceptibility to thyroid autoimmune disease: molecular analysis of HLA-D region genes identifies new markers for goitrous Hashimoto's thyroiditis. *J Clin Endocrinol Metab,* Vol.71, No.5, (November 1990), pp. 1131-1137, ISSN 1945-7197

Bagchi N, Brown TR & Sundick RS. (1995). Thyroid cell injury is an initial event in the induction of autoimmune thyroiditis by iodine in obese strain chickens. *Endocrinology,* Vol.136, No.11, (November 1995), pp. 5054-5060, ISSN 1945-7170

Baker JR (1999). Dying (Apoptosing?) for a consensus on the Fas death pathway in the thyroid. *J Clin Endocrinol Metab,* Vol. 84, No. 8, pp. 2593-5 ISSN 0021-972X

Ban Y, Tozaki T, Taniyama M, Nakano Y & Hirano T. (2010). Association of the protein tyrosine phosphatase nonreceptor 22 haplotypes with autoimmune thyroid disease in the Japanese population. *Thyroid,* Vol.20, No.8, (August 2010), pp. 893-899, ISSN 1050-7256

Ban Y, Davies TF, Greenberg DA, Concepcion ES, Osman R, Oashi T & Tomer Y. (2004). Arginine at position 74 of the HLA-DR beta1 chain is associated with GD. *Genes Immun,* Vol.5, No.3, (May 2004), pp. 203-208, ISSN 1466-4879

Baskol G, Atmaca H, Tanriverdi F, Baskol M, Kocer D & Bayram F. (2007). Oxidative stress and enzymatic antioxidant status in patients with hypothyroidism before and after treatment. *Exp Clin Endocrinol Diabetes,* Vol.115, No.8, (September 2007),pp. 522-526, ISSN 0947-7349

Belguith-Maalej S, Hadj Kacem H, Rebai A, Mnif M, Abid M & Ayadi H. (2008). Thyroglobulin polymorphisms in Tunisian patients with AITDs (AITD). *Immunobiology,* Vol.213, No.7, (2008), pp. 577-583, ISSN 0171-2985

Blüher M, Krohn K, Wallaschofski H, Braverman LE & Paschke R. (1999a). Cytokine gene expression in autoimmune thyroiditis in BioBreeding/Worcester rats. *Thyroid,* Vol.9, No.10, (October 1999),pp. 1049-1055, ISSN 1050-7256

Blüher M, Krohn K, Wallaschofski H, Braverman LE & Paschke R. (1999b). Fas and Fas ligand gene expression in autoimmune thyroiditis in BB/W rats. *Eur J Endocrinol*, Vol.141, No.5, (november 1999), pp. 506-511, ISSN 0804-4643

Bottazzo GF & Doniach D. (1986). Autoimmune thyroid disease. *Annu Rev Med*, Vol.37, (1986), pp. 353-359, ISSN 0066-4219

Bougacha-Elleuch N, Rebai A, Mnif M, Makni H, Bellassouad M, Jouida J, Abid M & Hammadi A. (2004). Analysis of MHC genes in a Tunisian isolate with AITDs: implication of TNF -308 gene polymorphism. *J Autoimmun*, Vol.23, No.1, (August 2004), pp. 75-80, ISSN 1740-2557

Bougacha-Elleuch N, Arab SB, Rebai A, Mnif M, Maalej A, Charfi N, Lassouad MB, Jouida J, Abid M & Ayadi H. (2011). No major genes in AITDs: complex segregation and epidemiological studies in a large Tunisian pedigree. *J Genet, Vol.*90, No.2, (August 2011), pp. 333-337, ISSN 0973-7731

Bretz JD, Arscott PL, Myc A & Baker JR Jr. (1999). Inflammatory cytokine regulation of Fas-mediated apoptosis in thyroid follicular cells. *J Biol Chem*, Vol. 274, No.36, (September 1999), pp. 25433-25438, ISSN 1083-351X

Bretz JD, Mezosi E, Giordano TJ, Gauger PG, Thompson NW & Baker JR Jr (2002). Inflammatory cytokine regulation of TRAIL-mediated apoptosis in thyroid epithelial cells. *Cell Death Differ* , Vol 9, No 3, (Mar 2002), pp. 274-86 ISSN 1350-9047

Brix TH, Kyvik KO & Hegedus L. (2000). A population-based study of chronic autoimmune hypothyroidism in Danish twins. *J Clin Endocrinol Metab*, Vol.85, No.2, (February 2000), pp. 536-539, ISSN 1945-7197

Brix TH, Knudsen GP, Kristiansen M, Kyvik KO, Orstavik KH & Hegedus L. (2005). High frequency of skewed X-chromosome inactivation in females with autoimmune thyroid disease: a possible explanation for the female predisposition to thyroid autoimmunity. *J Clin Endocrinol Metab*, Vol.90, No.11, (November 2005), pp. 5949-5953, ISSN 1945-7197

Camargo RY, Tomimori EK, Neves SC, Knobel M & Medeiros-Neto G. (2006). Prevalence of chronic autoimmune thyroiditis in the urban area neighboring a petrochemical complex and a control area in Sao Paulo, Brazil. *Clinics (Sao Paulo)*, Vol.61, No.4, (August 2006), pp. 307-312, ISSN 1807-5932

Canaris GJ, Manowitz NR, Mayor G & Ridgway EC. (2000). The Colorado thyroid disease prevalence study. *Arch Intern Med*, Vol.160, No.4, (February 2000), pp. 526-534, ISSN 0003-9926

Chabchoub G, Mnif M, Maalej A, Charfi N, Ayadi H & Abid M. (2006). [Epidemiologic study of autoimmune thyroid disease in south Tunisia]. *Ann Endocrinol (Paris)*, Vol.67, No.6, (December 2006), pp. 591-595, ISSN 0003-4266

Chabchoub G, Uz E, Maalej A, Mustafa CA, Rebai A, Mnif M, Bahloul Z, Farid NR, Ozcelik T & Ayadi H. (2009). Analysis of skewed X-chromosome inactivation in females with rheumatoid arthritis and AITDs. *Arthritis Res Ther*, Vol.11, No.4, (2009), pp. R106, ISSN 1478-6362

Chen S, Fazle Akbar SM, Zhen Z, Luo Y, Deng L, Huang H, Chen L & Li W. (2004) Analysis of the expression of Fas, FasL and Bcl-2 in the pathogenesis of autoimmune thyroid disorders. *Cell Mol Immuno, Vol. 1, No 3, pp. 224-8*

Chen RH, Chang CT, Chen WC, Tsai CH & Tsai FJ. (2006). Proinflammatory cytokine gene polymorphisms among Hashimoto's thyroiditis patients. *J Clin Lab Anal*, Vol.20, No.6, (2006), pp. 260-265, ISSN 0887-8013

Chistiakov DA. (2005). Immunogenetics of Hashimoto's thyroiditis. *J Autoimmune Dis*, Vol.2, No.1, (March 2005), pp.1, ISSN 1740-2557

Cornelis F, Fauré S, Martinez M, Prud'homme JF, Fritz P, Dib C, Alves H, Barrera P, de Vries N, Balsa A, Pascual-Salcedo D,Maenaut K, Westhovens R, Migliorini P, Tran TH, Delaye A, Prince N, Lefevre C, Thomas G, Poirier M, Soubigou S, Alibert O,Lasbleiz S, Fouix S, Bouchier C, Lioté F, Loste MN, Lepage V, Charron D, Gyapay G, Lopes-Vaz A, Kuntz D, Bardin T,Weissenbach J & ECRAF. (1998). New susceptibility locus for rheumatoid arthritis suggested by a genome-wide linkage study. *Proc Natl Acad Sci U S A*, Vol.95, No.18, (September 1998), pp. 10746-10750, ISSN 0027-8424

Dallos T, Avbelj M, Barak L, Zapletalova J, Pribilincova Z, Krajcirova M, Kostalova L, Battelino T & Kovacs L. (2008). CTLA-4 gene polymorphisms predispose to autoimmune endocrinopathies but not to celiac disease. *Neuro Endocrinol Lett*, Vol.29, No.3, (Jun 2008), pp. 334-340, ISSN 0172-780X

Davies JL, Kawaguchi Y, Bennett ST, Copeman JB, Cordell HJ, Pritchard LE, Reed PW, Gough SC, Jenkins SC, Palmer SM, et al. (1994). A genome-wide search for human type 1 diabetes susceptibility genes. *Nature*, Vol.371, No.6493, (September 1994), pp. 130-136, ISSN 0028-0836

Davies TF & Amino N. (1993). A new classification for human autoimmune thyroid disease. *Thyroid*, Vol.3, No.4, (Winter 1993), pp. 331-333, ISSN 1050-7256

de Freitas CU, Grimaldi Campos RA, Rodrigues Silva MA, Panachão MR, de Moraes JC, Waissmann W, Roberto Chacra A,Maeda MY, Minazzi Rodrigues RS, Gonçalves Belchor J, Oliveira Barbosa S & Santos RT. (2010). Can living in the surroundings of a petrochemical complex be a risk factor for autoimmune thyroid disease? *Environ Res*, Vol.110, No.1, (January 2010), pp. 112-117, ISSN 0013-9351

Dogan M, Acikgoz E, Acikgoz M, Cesur Y, Ariyuca S & Bektas MS. (2011). The frequency of Hashimoto thyroiditis in children and the relationship between urinary iodine level and Hashimoto thyroiditis. *J Pediatr Endocrinol Metab*, Vol.24, No.(1-2), (2011), pp. 75-80, ISSN 2191-0251

Duron F, Dubosclard E, Ballot E & Johanet C (2004). *Encycl Med Chir Endocrinol Nutrition* Thyroidites, 10-008-A-40

Dultz G, Matheis N, Dittmar M, Rohrig B, Bender K & Kahaly GJ. (2009). The protein tyrosine phosphatase non-receptor type 22 C1858T polymorphism is a joint susceptibility locus for immunthyroiditis and autoimmune diabetes. *Thyroid*, Vol.19, No.2, (February 2009), pp. 143-148, ISSN 1050-7256

Elleuch-Bougacha N, Maalej A, Makni H, Bellassouad M, Abid M, Jouida J, Ayed K, Charron D, Tamouza R & Ayadi H. (2001). HLA class I and II polymorphisms in a large multiplex family with AITDs. *Clin Endocrinol (Oxf)*, Vol.55, No.4, (October 2001), pp. 557-558, ISSN 0300-0664

Eschler DC, Hasham A & Tomer Y. (2011). Cutting edge: the etiology of AITDs. *Clin Rev Allergy Immunol*, Vol.41, No.2, (October 2011), pp. 190-197, ISSN 1559-0267

Everett LA, Glaser B, Beck JC, Idol JR, Buchs A, Heyman M, Adawi F, Hazani E, Nassir E, Baxevanis AD, Sheffield VC & Green ED. (1997). Pendred syndrome is caused by mutations in a putative sulphate transporter gene (PDS). *Nat Genet*, Vol.17, No.4, (December 1997), pp. 411-422, ISSN 1061-4036

Fountoulakis S & Tsatsoulis A. (2004). On the pathogenesis of autoimmune thyroid disease: a unifying hypothesis. *Clin Endocrinol (Oxf)*, Vol.60, No.4, (April 2004), pp. 397-409, ISSN 0300-0664

Fountoulakis S, Vartholomatos G, Kolaitis N, Frillingos S, Philippou G & Tsatsoulis A. (2008) Differential expression of Fas system apoptotic molecules in peripheral lymphocytes from patients with Graves'disease and Hashimoto's thyroiditis. *Eur J Endocrinol*, Vol. 156, No. 6, (Jun 2008) pp. 853-9 ISSN 0804-4643

Friedrich N, Schwarz S, Thonack J, John U, Wallaschofski H & Volzke H. (2008). Association between parity and autoimmune thyroiditis in a general female population. *Autoimmunity*, Vol.41, No.2, (March 2008), pp. 174-180, ISSN 1607-842X

Giordano C, Richiusa P, Bagnasco M, Pizzolanti G, Di Blasi F, Sbriglia MS, Mattina A, Pesce G, Montagna P, Capone F, Misiano G,Scorsone A, Pugliese A & Galluzzo A. (2001). Differential regulation of Fas-mediated apoptosis in both thyrocyte and lymphocyte cellular compartments correlates with opposite phenotypic manifestations of autoimmune thyroiddisease. *Thyroid*, Vol. 11, No. 3, (Mar 2001), pp. 233-44, ISSN 1557-9077

Hadj Kacem H, Rebai A, Kaffel N, Masmoudi S, Abid M & Ayadi H. (2003). PDS is a new susceptibility gene to AITDs: association and linkage study. *J Clin Endocrinol Metab*, Vol.88, No.5, (May 2003), pp. 2274-2280, ISSN 1945-7197

Hadj Kacem H, Rebai A, Kaffel N, Abid M & Ayadi H. (2006). Evidence for linkage and association between AITDs and the 18q12-q21 region in a large Tunisian family. *Int J Immunogenet*, Vol.33, No.1, (February 2006), pp. 25-32, ISSN 1744-3121

Hadj-Kacem H, Rebuffat S, Mnif-Feki M, Belguith-Maalej S, Ayadi H & Peraldi-Roux S. (2009). AITDs: genetic susceptibility of thyroid-specific genes and thyroid autoantigens contributions. *Int J Immunogenet*, Vol.36, No.2, (April 2009), pp. 85-96, ISSN 1744-3121

Hall R & Stanbury JB. (1967). Familial studies of autoimmune thyroiditis. *Clin Exp Immunol*, Vol.2(Suppl), (December 1967), pp. 719-725, ISSN 1365-2249

Hawkins BR, Lam KS, Ma JT, Wang C & Yeung RT. (1987). Strong association between HLA DRw9 and Hashimoto's thyroiditis in southern Chinese. *Acta Endocrinol (Copenh)*, Vol.114, No.4, (April 1987), pp. 543-546, ISSN 0001-5598

Hollowell JG, Staehling NW, Flanders WD, Hannon WH, Gunter EW, Spencer CA & Braverman LE. (2002). Serum TSH, T(4), and thyroid antibodies in the United States population (1988 to 1994): National Health and Nutrition Examination Survey (NHANES III). *J Clin Endocrinol Metab*, Vol.87, No.2, (February 2002), pp. 489-499, ISSN 1945-7197

Honda K, Tamai H, Morita T, Kuma K, Nishimura Y & Sasazuki T. (1989). Hashimoto's thyroiditis and HLA in Japanese. *J Clin Endocrinol Metab*, Vol.69, No.6, (December 1989), pp. 1268-1273, ISSN 0021-972X

Huang CM, Wu MC, Wu JY & Tsai FJ. (2002). Association of vitamin D receptor gene BsmI polymorphisms in Chinese patients with systemic lupus erythematosus. *Lupus*, Vol.11, No.1, (January 2002), pp. 31-34, ISSN 0961-2033

Inoue N, Watanabe M, Nanba T, Wada M, Akamizu T & Iwatani Y. (2009). Involvement of functional polymorphisms in the TNFA gene in the pathogenesis of AITDs and production of anti-thyrotropin receptor antibody. *Clin Exp Immunol*, Vol.156, No.2, (May 2009), pp. 199-204, ISSN 1365-2249

Inoue N, Watanabe M, Morita M, Tatusmi K, Hidaka Y, Akamizu T & Iwatani Y. (2011). Association of functional polymorphisms in promoter regions of IL5, IL6 and IL13 genes with development and prognosis of AITDs. *Clin Exp Immunol*, Vol.163, No.3, (March 2011), pp. 318-323, ISSN 1365-2249

Ito C, Watanabe M, Okuda N, Watanabe C & Iwatani Y. (2006). Association between the severity of Hashimoto's disease and the functional +874A/T polymorphism in the interferon-gamma gene. *Endocr* J, Vol.53, No.4, (August 2006), pp. 473-478,ISSN 1348-4540

Jaume JC, Guo J, Pauls DL, Zakarija M, McKenzie JM, Egeland JA, Burek CL, Rose NR, Hoffman WH, Rapoport B & McLachlan SM. (1999). Evidence for genetic transmission of thyroid peroxidase autoantibody epitopic "fingerprints". *J Clin Endocrinol Metab*, Vol.84, No.4, (April 1999),pp. 1424-1431, ISSN 1945-7197

Kaczmarek E, Lacka K, Jarmolowska-Jurczyszyn D, Sidor A & Majewski P. (2011). Changes of B and T lymphocytes and selected apopotosis markers in Hashimoto's thyroiditis. *J Clin Pathol*, Vol.64, No.7, (July 2011), pp. 626-630, ISSN 1472-4146

Kahles H, Ramos-Lopez E, Lange B, Zwermann O, Reincke M & Badenhoop K. (2005). Sex-specific association of PTPN22 1858T with type 1 diabetes but not with Hashimoto's thyroiditis or Addison's disease in the German population. *Eur J Endocrinol*, Vol.153, No.6, (December 2005), pp. 895-899, ISSN 0804-4643

Kammoun-Krichen M, Bougacha-Elleuch N, Makni K, Rebai M, Peraldi-Roux S, Rebai A, Mnif M, Abid M, Jouida J & Ayadi H. (2007). Association analysis of interleukin gene polymorphisms in AITDs in the Tunisian population. *Eur Cytokine Netw*, Vol.18, No.4, (December 2007), pp. 196-200, ISSN 1148-5493

Kammoun-Krichen M, Bougacha-Elleuch N, Makni K, Mnif M, Jouida J, Abid M, Rebai A & Ayadi H. (2008). A potential role of TNFR gene polymorphisms in AITDs in the Tunisian population. *Cytokine*, Vol.43, No.2, (August 2008), pp. 110-113, ISSN 1043-4666

Kelso A. (1998). Cytokines: principles and prospects. *Immunol Cell Biol*, Vol.76, No.4, (August 1998), pp. 300-317, ISSN 0818-9641

Lander E & Kruglyak L. (1995). Genetic dissection of complex traits: guidelines for interpreting and reporting linkage results . *Nat Genet*, Vol.11, No.3, (November 1995), pp. 241-247, ISSN 1061-4036

Lassoued S, Mseddi M, Mnif F, Abid M, Guermazi F, Masmoudi H, El Feki A & Attia H. (2010). A comparative study of the oxidative profile in GD, Hashimoto's thyroiditis, and papillary thyroid cancer. *Biol Trace Elem Res*, Vol.138, No.(1-3), (December 2010), pp. 107-115, ISSN 1559-0720

Liu Z, Wang H, Xiao W, Wang C, Liu G & Hong T. (2010) Thyrocyte interleukin-18 expression is up-regulated by interferon-γ and may contribute tothyroid destruction in Hashimoto's thyroiditis. *Int J Exp Pathol*, Vol.91, No.5, (Oct 2010), pp. 420-5 ISSN 1936-2625

Maalej A, Makni H, Ayadi F, Bellassoued M, Jouida J, Bouguacha N, Abid M & Ayadi H. (2001a). A full genome screening in a large Tunisian family affected with thyroid autoimmune disorders. *Genes Immun*, Vol.2, No.2, (April 2001), pp. 71-75, ISSN 1466-4879

Maalej A, Bougacha N, Rebai A, Bellassouad M, Ayadi-Makni F, Abid M, Jouida J, Makni H & Ayadi H. (2001b). Lack of linkage and association between AITDs and the CTLA-4 gene in a large Tunisian family. *Hum Immunol*, Vol.62, No.11, (November 2001), pp. 1245-1250, ISSN 0198-8859

Maalej A, Rebai A, Ayadi A, Jouida J, Makni H & Ayadi H. (2004). Allelic structure and distribution of 103 STR loci in a Southern Tunisian population. *J Genet*, Vol.83, No.1, (April 2004), pp. 65-71, ISSN 0022-1333

Maalej A, Petit-Teixeira E, Chabchoub G, Hamad MB, Rebai A, Farid NR, Cornelis F & Ayadi H. (2008). Lack of association of VDR gene polymorphisms with thyroid autoimmune disorders: familial and case/control studies. *J Clin Immunol*, Vol.28, No.1, (January 2008), pp. 21-25, ISSN 0271-9142

MacGregor AJ, Snieder H, Schork NJ & Spector TD. (2000). Twins. Novel uses to study complex traits and genetic diseases. *Trends Genet*, Vol.16, No.3, (March 2000), pp. 131-134, ISSN 0168-9525

Martin L. (1945). The hereditary and familial aspects of exophthalmic goitre and nodular goitre. *Q J Med*, Vol.14, (October 1945), pp. 207-219, ISSN 1460-2393

McDermott MF, Ramachandran A, Ogunkolade BW, Aganna E, Curtis D, Boucher BJ, Snehalatha C & Hitman GA. (1997). Allelic variation in the vitamin D receptor influences susceptibility to IDDM in Indian Asians. *Diabetologia*, Vol.40, No.8, (August 1997), pp. 971-975, ISSN 0012-186X

Menconi F, Monti MC, Greenberg DA, Oashi T, Osman R, Davies TF, Ban Y, Jacobson EM, Concepcion ES, Li CW & Tomer Y. (2008). Molecular amino acid signatures in the MHC class II peptide-binding pocket predispose to autoimmune thyroiditis in humans and in mice. *Proc Natl Acad Sci U S A*, Vol.105, No.37, (September 2008), pp. 14034-14039, ISSN 0027-8424

Mitsiades N, Poulaki V, Kotoula V, Mastorakos G, Tseleni-Balafouta S, Koutras DA & Tsokos M. (1998). Fas/Fas ligand up-regulation and Bcl-2 down-regulation may be significant in the pathogenesis of Hashimoto's thyroiditis. *J Clin Endocrinol Metab*, Vol. 83, No.6, (June 1998), pp. 2199-2203, ISSN 1945-7197

Mooij P, de Wit HJ & Drexhage HA. (1993). An excess of dietary iodine accelerates the development of a thyroid-associated lymphoid tissue in autoimmune prone BB rats. *Clin Immunol Immunopathol*, Vol. 69, No.2, (November 1993), pp. 189-198, ISSN 0090-1229

Mori K & Yoshida K. (2010). Viral infection in induction of Hashimoto's thyroiditis: a key player or just a bystander? *Curr Opin Endocrinol Diabetes Obes*, Vol.17, No.5, (October 2010), pp. 418-424, ISSN 1752-2978

Morris GP, Brown NK & Kong YC. (2009). Naturally-existing CD4(+)CD25(+)Foxp3(+) regulatory T cells are required for tolerance to experimental autoimmune thyroiditis induced by either exogenous or endogenous autoantigen. *J Autoimmun*, Vol 33, No. 1, (Aug 2009), pp. 68-76, ISSN 1095-9157

Nanba T, Watanabe M, Akamizu T & Iwatani Y. (2008). The -590CC genotype in the IL4 gene as a strong predictive factor for the development of hypothyroidism in Hashimoto disease. *Clin Chem*, Vol.54, No.3, (March 2008), pp. 621-623

Pani MA, Knapp M, Donner H, Braun J, Baur MP, Usadel KH & Badenhoop K. (2000). Vitamin D receptor allele combinations influence genetic susceptibility to type 1 diabetes in Germans. *Diabetes*, Vol.49, No.3, (March 2000), pp. 504-507, ISSN 1939-327X

Pani MA, Seissler J, Usadel KH & Badenhoop K. (2002). Vitamin D receptor genotype is associated with Addison's disease. *Eur J Endocrinol*, Vol.147, No.5, (November 2002), pp. 635-640, ISSN 0804-4643

Parish NM & Cooke A. (2004). Mechanisms of autoimmune thyroid disease. *Drug Discovery Today Disease Mechanisms*, Vol.1,No.3, (December 2004), pp. 337-344, ISSN 1740-6765

Pauls DL, Zakarija M, McKenzie JM & Egeland JA. (1993). Complex segregation analysis of antibodies to thyroid peroxidase in Old Order Amish families. *Am J Med Genet*, Vol.47, No.3, (September 1993), pp. 375-379, ISSN 0148-7299

Pedersen OM, Aardal NP, Larssen TB, Varhaug JE, Myking O & Vik-Mo H.(2000). The value of ultrasonography in predicting autoimmune thyroid disease. *Thyroid*, Vol 10, No. 3, (Mar 2000), pp 251-9, ISSN 1557-9077

Rekha PL, Ishaq M & Valluri V. (2006). A differential association of interferon-gamma high-producing allele T and low-producing allele A (+874 A/T) with Hashimoto's thyroiditis and GD. *Scand J Immunol*, Vol.64, No.4, (October 2006), pp. 438-443, ISSN 0300-9475

Risch N. (1990). Linkage strategies for genetically complex traits. II. The power of affected relative pairs. *Am J Hum Genet*, Vol.46, No.2, (February 1990), pp. 229-241, ISSN 0002-9297

Sakai K, Shirasawa S, Ishikawa N, Ito K, Tamai H, Kuma K, Akamizu T, Tanimura M, Furugaki K, Yamamoto K & Sasazuki T. (2001). Identification of susceptibility loci for autoimmune thyroid disease to 5q31-q33 and Hashimoto's thyroiditis to 8q23-q24 by multipoint affected sib-pair linkage analysis in Japanese. *Hum Mol Genet*, Vol.10, No.13, (Jun 2001), pp. 1379-1386, ISSN 0964-6906

Scott DA, Wang R, Kreman TM, Sheffield VC & Karniski LP. (1999). The Pendred syndrome gene encodes a chloride-iodide transport protein. *Nat Genet*, Vol.21, No.4, (April 1999), pp. 440-443, ISSN 1061-4036

Shai R, Quismorio FP, Jr., Li L, Kwon OJ, Morrison J, Wallace DJ, Neuwelt CM, Brautbar C, Gauderman WJ & Jacob CO. (1999). Genome-wide screen for systemic lupus erythematosus susceptibility genes in multiplex families. *Hum Mol Genet*, Vol.8, No.4, (April 1999), pp. 639-644, ISSN 0964-6906

Tandon N, Zhang L & Weetman AP. (1991). HLA associations with Hashimoto's thyroiditis. *Clin Endocrinol (Oxf)*, Vol.34, No.5,(May 1991), pp. 383-386, ISSN 0300-0664

Taylor JC, Gough SC, Hunt PJ, Brix TH, Chatterjee K, Connell JM, Franklyn JA, Hegedus L, Robinson BG, Wiersinga WM, Wass JA, Zabaneh D, Mackay I & Weetman AP. (2006). A genome-wide screen in 1119 relative pairs with autoimmune thyroid disease. *J Clin Endocrinol Metab*, Vol.91, No.2, (February 2006), pp. 646-653, ISSN 0021-972X

Teng X, Shan Z, Chen Y, Lai Y, Yu J, Shan L, Bai X, Li Y, Li N, Li Z, Wang S, Xing Q, Xue H, Zhu L, Hou X, Fan C & Teng W. (2011). More than adequate iodine intake may increase subclinical hypothyroidism and autoimmune thyroiditis: a cross-sectional study based on two Chinese communities with different iodine intake levels. *Eur J Endocrinol,* Vol.164, No.6, (Jun 2011), pp. 943-950, ISSN 1479-683X

Tomer Y, Barbesino G, Greenberg DA, Concepcion E & Davies TF. (1999). Mapping the major susceptibility loci for familial Graves' and Hashimoto's diseases: evidence for genetic heterogeneity and gene interactions. *J Clin Endocrinol Metab,* Vol.84, No.12, (December 1999), pp. 4656-4664, ISSN 1945-7197

Tomer Y, Greenberg DA, Concepcion E, Ban Y & Davies TF. (2002). Thyroglobulin is a thyroid specific gene for the familial AITDs. *J Clin Endocrinol Metab,* Vol.87, No.1, (January 2002), pp. 404-407, ISSN 1945-7197

Tomer Y, Ban Y, Concepcion E, Barbesino G, Villanueva R, Greenberg DA & Davies TF. (2003). Common and unique susceptibility loci in Graves and Hashimoto diseases: results of whole-genome screening in a data set of 102 multiplex families. *Am J Hum Genet,* Vol.73, No.4, (October 2003), pp. 736-747,ISSN 0002-9297

Tomer, Y., Menconi, F., Davies, T.F., Barbesino, G., Rocchi, R., Pinchera, A. Concepcion E & Greenberg DA. (2007) Dissecting genetic heterogeneity in autoimmune thyroid diseases by subset analysis. *J of Autoimmun,* vol. 29, (Sep-Nov 2007), pp. 69-77, ISSN 1095-9157

Tomer Y. (2010). Genetic susceptibility to autoimmune thyroid disease: past, present, and future. *Thyroid,* Vol.20, No.7, (July 2010), pp. 715-725, ISSN 1050-7256

Toulis KA, Anastasilakis AD, Tzellos TG, Goulis DG & Kouvelas D. (2010). Selenium supplementation in the treatment of Hashimoto's thyroiditis: a systematic review and a meta-analysis. *Thyroid.,* Vol. 20, No. 10, (Oct 2010), pp. 1163-73, ISSN 1557-9077

Tunbridge WM, Evered DC, Hall R, Appleton D, Brewis M, Clark F, Evans JG, Young E, Bird T & Smith PA. (1977). The spectrum of thyroid disease in a community: the Whickham survey. *Clin Endocrinol (Oxf),* Vol.7, No.6, (December 1977), pp. 481-493, ISSN 0300-0664

Tunbridge WM & Vanderpump MP. (2000). Population screening for autoimmune thyroid disease. *Endocrinol Metab Clin North Am,* Vol.29, No.2, (June 2000), pp. 239-253, v, ISSN 0889-8529

Ueda H, Howson JM, Esposito L, Heward J, Snook H, Chamberlain G, Rainbow DB, Hunter KM, Smith AN, Di Genova G, Herr MH, Dahlman I, Payne F, Smyth D, Lowe C, Twells RC, Howlett S, Healy B, Nutland S, Rance HE, Everett V, Smink LJ, Lam AC,Cordell HJ, Walker NM, Bordin C, Hulme J, Motzo C, Cucca F, Hess JF, Metzker ML, Rogers J, Gregory S, Allahabadia A,Nithiyananthan R, Tuomilehto-Wolf E, Tuomilehto J, Bingley P, Gillespie KM, Undlien DE, Rønningen KS, Guja C, Ionescu-Tîrgovişte C, Savage DA, Maxwell AP, Carson DJ, Patterson CC, Franklyn JA, Clayton DG, Peterson LB, Wicker LS, Todd JA & Gough SC. (2003). Association of the T-cell regulatory gene CTLA4 with susceptibility to autoimmune disease. *Nature,* Vol.423, No.6939, (May 2003), pp. 506-511, ISSN 0028-0836

Vaidya B, Imrie H, Perros P, Young ET, Kelly WF, Carr D, Large DM, Toft AD, Kendall-Taylor P & Pearce SH. (2000). Evidence for a new Graves disease susceptibility locus at chromosome 18q21. *Am J Hum Genet*, Vol.66, No.5, (May 2000), pp. 1710-1714, ISSN 0002-9297

Vanderpump MP, Tunbridge WM, French JM, Appleton D, Bates D, Clark F, Grimley Evans J, Hasan DM, Rodgers H, Tunbridge F, et al. (1995). The incidence of thyroid disorders in the community: a twenty-year follow-up of the Whickham Survey. *Clin Endocrinol (Oxf)*, Vol 43 No. 1, (Jul 1995), pp. 55-68, ISSN 1365-2265

Villanueva R, Greenberg DA, Davies TF & Tomer Y. (2003). Sibling recurrence risk in autoimmune thyroid disease. *Thyroid*, Vol.13, No.8, (August 2003), pp. 761-764, ISSN 1050-7256

Vyse TJ & Todd JA. (1996). Genetic analysis of autoimmune disease. *Cell*, Vol.85, No.3, (May 1996), pp. 311-318

Wang C & Crapo LM. (1997). The epidemiology of thyroid disease and implications for screening. *Endocrinol Metab Clin North Am*, Vol.26, No.1, (March 1997), pp. 189-218, ISSN 0889-8529

Yamada H, Watanabe M, Nanba T, Akamizu T & Iwatani Y. (2008). The +869T/C polymorphism in the transforming growth factor-beta1 gene is associated with the severity and intractability of autoimmune thyroid disease. *Clin Exp Immunol*, Vol. 151, No.3, (March 2008), pp. 379-382, ISSN 1365-2249

Zaletel K, Krhin B, Gaberscek S & Hojker S. (2006). Thyroid autoantibody production is influenced by exon 1 and promoter CTLA-4 polymorphisms in patients with Hashimoto's thyroiditis. *Int J Immunogenet*, Vol.33, No.2, (April 2006), p. 87-91, ISSN 1744-3121

Zaletel K, Krhin B, Gaberscek S, Bicek A, Pajic T & Hojker S. (2010). Association of CT60 cytotoxic T lymphocyte antigen-4 gene polymorphism with thyroid autoantibody production in patients with Hashimoto's and postpartum thyroiditis. *Clin Exp Immunol*, Vol.161, No.1, (July 2010), pp. 41-47, ISSN 1365-2249

Zeitlin AA, Heward JM, Newby PR, Carr-Smith JD, Franklyn JA, Gough SC & Simmonds MJ. (2008). Analysis of HLA class II genes in Hashimoto's thyroiditis reveals differences compared to GD. *Genes Immun*, Vol.9, No.4, (June 2008), pp. 358-363, ISSN 1466-4879

4

Hashimoto's Disease - Involvement of Cytokine Network and Role of Oxidative Stress in the Severity of Hashimoto's Thyroiditis

Julieta Gerenova, Irena Manolova and Veselina Gadjeva
Medical Faculty, Trakia University, Stara Zagora, Bulgaria

1. Introduction

Autoimmune thyroid diseases (AITDs) such as Hashimoto's disease (HD) and Graves'disease (GD) are archetypes of organ-specific autoimmune disease (Davies et al., 1988; Volpe, 1995). Hashimoto's disease (HD), Hashimoto's thyroiditis (HT) or chronic autoimmune lymphocytic thyroiditis was first described by H. Hashimoto in 1912 as struma lymphomatosa (Hashimoto H.,1912). Histological and cytological features of HT include a dense thyroidal accumulation of lymphocytes, plasma cells and occasional multinuclear giant cells. The epithelial cells are enlarged, with a distinctive eosinophilic cytoplasm, owing to increased number of mitochondria. HD is characterized by the presence of thyroid autoantibodies to thyroglobulin (Tg) and to thyroid peroxidase (TPO). The autoantibodies present in this disorder were identified in 1956 by Roitt et al. (Roitt et al., 1956).

HT is the most common underlying cause for hypothyroidism. It has been estimated that about 3–4% of the population suffers from HT. This disorder is most commonly found in middle-aged and elderly females, but it also occurs in other age groups (Canaris et al. 2000). HT is distributed throughout the world without racial and ethnic restriction.

The severity of HT vary among patients. Most patients with HD maintain a lifetime euthyroid state without any medical treatment, whereas others become hypothyroid. The immunological differences that underlie differences in severity remain unclear. Various cytokines may play role in this process; thyroid autoantibodies are independently involved in the severity of HD (Ito et al., 2006). The increased oxidative stress and a deficiency of cellular antioxidative defense in HT patients may be related to the processes of development of hypothyroidism.

In this view, to clarify the role of serum cytokines and antioxidant enzyme activities in different stages of disease we investigated three sub-groups of patients with autoimmune thyroiditis according to the thyroid function: group I —euthyroid subjects; group II—hypothyroid subjects; and group III—subjects treated with Levothyroxine and healthy controls.

2. Genetic and environmental factors

The interaction between internal (genetic) and external (environmental and endogenous) factors is required to initiate Hashimoto's disease. Environmental triggers of HT include high iodine intake, selenium deficiency, pollution, stress, bacterial and viral infections, cytokine therapy (Noel et al., 2002; Tomer & Davies, 1993; Bartalena et al., 2007). Probably puberty, pregnancy and menopause are factors contributing to disease. The role of dietary iodine is well defined in epidemiological studies and in animal models and seems to be the most significant environmental factor to induce thyroiditis. Environmental factors (particularly, iodine intake and infection) could cause insult of the thyrocyte followed by abnormal expression of major histocompatibility complex (MHC) class I and class II molecules, as well as changes to genes or gene products (such as MHC class III and costimulatory molecules) needed for the thyrocyte to become an antigen-presenting cell (APC). In this stage, a modulating role of sequence variants of human leukocyte antigen (HLA) class II molecules could become pivotal in binding and presenting thyroid antigenic peptides derived from Tg, TPO and TSHR (thyroid-stimulating hormone receptor) (Weetman, 2003). Selenium is other micronutrient involved in thyroid hormone metabolism, which exert various effects, while maintaining the cell reduction-oxidation balance (Beckett & Arthur, 2004; Duntas, 2009). Genetic variations in Tg, and probably in TSHR and other thyroid-specific genes, might be responsible for generating an autoimmune response. Genetic factors predominate, accounting for approximately 80% of the likelihood of developing AITDs, whereas at least 20% is due to environmental factors.

3. Pathogenesis

Several antibody and cell-mediated mechanisms contribute to thyroid injury in autoimmune hypothyroidism. In general, in case of Hashimoto's thyroiditis, the expressions of death receptors such as CD95 and death receptor ligands such as CD95L and TRAIL in the thyroid tissue appear to be much higher compared to normal subjects. Also, the expression of positive effectors of apoptosis such as caspase 3 and 8, as well as Bax and Bak appear to be relatively high in thyroiditis samples as compared to controls. This expression pattern clearly supports enhanced apoptosis as the mechanism underlying the loss of thyrocytes in Hashimoto's thyroiditis. There is significant expression of Fas/CD95 and its ligand in the thyrocytes who undergo apoptosis in Hashimoto's thyroiditis. Cytokines appear to play a crucial role in the pathology of the disease by enhancing the expression of caspases and there by sensitizing cells to FAS mediated apoptosis (Weetman, 2004).

3.1 B Cell response

Three principal thyroid autoantigens mentioned above are involved in AITDs. These are TPO, Tg and the TSH receptor. TPO Abs appear involved in the tissue destructive processes associated with the hypothyroidism observed in Hashimoto's and atrophic thyroiditis. The appearance of TPO Abs usually precedes the development of thyroid dysfunction. Some studies suggest that TPO Abs may be cytotoxic to the thyroid (Chiovato et al., 1993; Guo et al., 1997). The pathologic role of Tg Abs remains unclear. TPO Abs and/or Tg Abs are frequently present in the sera of patients with AITDs (Doullay et all., 1991). However, occasionally patients with AITDs have negative thyroid autoantibody test results.

Longitudinal studies suggest that TPO Abs may be a risk factor for future thyroid dysfunction; changes in autoantibody concentrations often reflect a change in disease activity.

TPO is a 110 kD membrane bound hemo-glycoprotein with a large extracellular domain, and a short transmembrane and intracellular domain. TPO is involved in thyroid hormone synthesis at the apical pole of the follicular cell. Several isoforms related to differential splicing of TPO RNA have been described. TPO molecules may also differ with respect to their three-dimensional structure, extent of glycosylation and heme binding. Most of the TPO molecules do not reach the apical membrane and are degraded intracellularly. TPO autoantibodies were initially described as anti-microsomal autoantibodies (AMA) since they were found to react with crude preparations of thyroid cell membranes. The microsomal antigen was later identified as TPO (Czarnocka et al., 1985). TPO Abs is the most sensitive test for detecting autoimmune thyroid disease (Mariotti et al., 1990). TPO Abs are typically the first abnormality to appear in the course of developing hypothyroidism secondary to Hashimoto's thyroiditis. In fact, when TPO Abs are measured by a sensitive immunoassay, over 95% of subjects with Hashimoto's thyroiditis have detectable levels of TPO Abs.

Tg - the prothyroid globulin, is a high molecular weight (660 kDa) soluble glycoprotein made up of two identical subunits. Tg is present with a high degree of heterogeneity due to differences in post-translational modifications (glycosylation, iodination, sulfation etc). During the process of thyroid hormone synthesis and release, Tg is polymerized and degraded. Consequently, the immunologic structure of Tg is extremely complex. The heterogeneity of Tg Abs are restricted in patients with AITDs compared with other thyroid disorders. Tg Abs measurements do not appear to be a useful diagnostic test for AITDs in areas of iodide sufficiency (Ericsson et al., 1985; Nordyk et al., 1993). Tg Abs are found in less than 60% of patients with lymphocytic thyroiditis.

Tg and TPO antibodies occur in very high concentration in patients with Hashimoto's thyroiditis and primary myxedema. Both of the antibodies show partial restriction to the IgG1 and IgG4 subclass. Tg antibodies usually mediate Antibody mediated cytotoxicity (ADCC), where as TPO antibodies form terminal complement complexes within the thyroid gland. Cell mediated injury may be necessary for TPO antibodies to gain access to their antigen and become pathogenic.

Thyroid stimulating antibodies (TS Abs) occurs in 10% to 20% of patients with autoimmune hypothyroidism (AH) but their effects are obscured by TSH-R-blocking antibodies and destructive processes.

Karanikas at al. demonstrate that high TPO Abs titres correlate with increased frequencies of T cells producing cytokines, enhancing cellular cytotoxic immunity, e.g. Interferon Gamma (IFN-γ) and Tumor necrosis factor -alpha (TNF-α), reflecting high disease activity. The role of thyroid autoantibodies in different stage of Hashimoto's disease remains unclear. (Karanikas at al., 2005).

To clarify the prevalence of TPO Abs in different stages in Hashimoto's thyroiditis we measured serum levels of TPO Abs in 128 out-patients with autoimmune thyroiditis from the Department of Internal Medicine, Stara Zagora University Hospital (Bulgaria), with HT and in 52 healthy controls. In all patients diagnosis had been made by enlarged thyroid glands, elevated TPO Abs and/or typical hypoechogenicity of the thyroid in high-resolution sonography. In negative TPO Abs patients fine needle aspiration biopsy (FNAB) was performed and typical cytological features of autoimmune thyroiditis were found. Serum levels of TSH, free thyroxin (fT4) were estimated. Fasting samples of venous blood were collected in the morning between 8.00 and 10.00 h. Serum samples were routinely collected and stored frozen at -20 C until assayed. At the time of sampling, neither of the patients and control subjects had clinical signs or symptoms of intercurrent illness. TPO Abs were measured by ELISA, using commercially available kits (The Binding Site LTD, England). FT4 was measured by competitive immunoassay on the ACS180 (Chiron Diagnostics USA). TSH was measured by a third generation two-site chemiluminometric assay on the ACS180. The reference range was 11.5-22.7 pmol/l for fT4 and 0.35-5.5 μIU/ml for TSH. Patients were divided into tree subgroups according to the thyroid function. Group I (n=40) involved subjects with normal thyroid function (TSH and fT4 within the normal range). Group II (n=17) included patients with hypothyroidism (high levels of TSH and low or normal serum levels of fT4). In group III (n=71) were enrolled subjects with hypothyroidism treated with Levothyroxine (LT4) in a dosage to maintain TSH and fT4 within the normal range. The medication of Levothyroxine (range: 50-200 μg) was given in the fasting state. Fifty two healthy subjects were included as controls. Informed consent was obtained from all participants in the study according to the ethical guidelines of the Helsinki Declaration. The relevant clinical and biochemical data of all of patients studied and controls are summarized in Table 1.

Variables	Controls	HT	Range
N	52	128	
Gender (M/F)	9/43	9/119	
Age (years)	44.6±1.8	47.0±1.2	
TSH (mIU/l)	1.3±0.8 [1]	14.4±4.3 [1]	0.35-5.5
fT4 (pmol/l)	15.8±0.6 [2]	12.8±2.8 [2]	12-22
TPO Abs (U/ml)	12,7±1,9 [3]	528±39,2 [3]	< 150
TPO Abs Neg/Pos(%)	52/0 (0%) [4]	35/93 (73%) [4]	

Statistical significance: 1, 2, 3, 4 : $p<0.05$

Table 1. Clinical features of controls and Hashimoto's thyroiditis patients included in the study (mean±SEM).

Statistical analysis was carried out using the Statistica 5.5 for Windows. The results were reported as means ± SD (SE). Student's *t*-test or non-parametric Mann Whitney U test were used to determine whether differences between means were significant. Correlations between the different parameters were calculated by linear regression analysis. $P \leq 0.05$ was considered statistically significant.

The clinical and biochemical data of subgroups of Hashimoto's thyroiditis patients are presents in Table 2.

Characteristics	Group I	Group II	Group III	Range
N	40	17	71	
Gender (M/F)	0/40	1/16	8/63	
Age (years)	48.8±1.8	47.6±3.5	46.2±1.7	
TSH (mIU/l)	2.4±1.3 [1]	18.6±4.8 [1,2]	3.7±2.6 [2]	0.35-5.5
fT4 (pmol/l)	14.6±2.2 [3]	10.3±3.1 [3,4]	17.1±4.4 [4]	12-22
TPO Abs (U/ml)	397±57 [5,6]	691±95 [5]	574±58 [6]	<150
TPO Abs Neg/Pos(%)	16/24 (60%)[7]	1/16 (94%)[7]	18/53 (75%)	

Statistical significance: 1, 2, 3, 4, 5, 6, 7 : $p<0.05$

Table 2. Baseline characteristics and TPO Abs levels in Hashimoto's thyroiditis patients – euthyroid group (Group I), hypothyroid group (Group II) and group of patients treated with Levothyroxine (Group III) (mean±SEM).

We found statistical significant differences of serum TPO Abs levels in sub-groups of patients with autoimmune thyroiditis compared to controls. Concentrations of TPO Abs in euthyroid group (397±57 U/ml) are lower in comparison with both hypothyroid group (691±95 U/ml) and group of patients treated with levothyroxine (574±58 U/ml) (p=0.02; p=0.03 respectively). After treatment with thyroid hormones serum levels of TPO Abs declined without reached statistical significance. We found significantly higher TPO Abs (+) patients in hypothyroid group in comparison with euthyroid Hashimoto's group (x2 =6.63, p=0.01). Ito at al. also found significantly higher titers of TPO Abs in HT patients with overt hypothyroidism than in those with euthyroidism (Ito at al., 2006). The same study showed the significant association of IFN-γ gene polymorphisms with the severity of autoimmune thyroid diseases (Ito et al., 2006). In work of Schmidt et al. serum TPO Abs levels also declined on HT patients, but after a mean 50 months of treatment with levothyroxine (Schmidt et al., 2008). We may conclude that patients with euthyroid HT differ immunologically from patients with hypothyroid HT.

3.2 T Cell response

3.2.1 Cytokines and Th1/Th2 balance

Cytokines are small glycoprotein chemical structures that act in paracrine and endocrine fashion as soluble signals between cells and play a pivotal role in the immune response. They are the hormonal messengers responsible for most of the biological effects in the immune system, such as cell-mediated immunity and allergic type responses. T lymphocytes are a major source of cytokines. A wide array of cytokines including interleukin (IL)-2, IFN-γ, TNF-α, IL-4, IL-6, IL-10, IL-12, IL-13 and IL-15 are produced by the lymphocytes with some variation between patients (Nilsson et al., 1998). There are two main subsets of T lymphocytes, distinguished by the presence of cell surface molecules known as CD4+ and cytotoxic T cells (CD8+). T lymphocytes expressing CD4+ are also known as helper T cells, and these are regarded as being the most prolific cytokine producers. CD4+ T helper lymphocytes play a key role in the pathogenesis of inflammatory and autoimmune diseases via the production of distinctive sets of cytokines (Druet et al., 1996). On the basis of their pattern of cytokine synthesis, CD4+ Th (helper) cells were originally classified into Th1 and Th2 lymphocytes, which are involved in cellular and humoral immune responses, respectively (Tato et al., 2006). The cytokines produced are known as Th1-type cytokines and Th2-type cytokines. Type 1 helper T cells are characterized by the production of pro-inflammatory cytokines like IFN-γ, IL-2, IL-12, IL-15, IL-18 and TNF-beta. Th1 cells are involved in cell-mediated immunity. The cytokines produced by Th1 cells stimulate the phagocytosis and destruction of microbial pathogens. Type 2 helper T cells are characterized by the production of IL-4, IL-5, IL-6, IL-9, IL-10, and IL-13. Th2 cells are thought to play a role in allergy responses and facilitate humoral immune responses. Cytokines like IL-4 generally stimulate the production of antibodies. Improved understanding of Th1 and Th2 differentiation will improve our overall understanding of the immune system. Th1 and Th2 lymphocyte subpopulations are with different in some cases even contradictory functions (Ajjan et al., 1996; Sterzl 1999). A third subset of CD4+ cells (Th3 lymphocytes) mainly synthesize transforming growth factor - beta (TGF-β) and are considered as regulatory cells (Shevach, 2000).

Disturbed mechanism of innate immunity, resulting from macrophage activation through innate immunity receptors may be the basis of pathologically high levels of cytokine production and activation (Boraschi D. & Dinarello C.A., 2006). Classical macrophage activation in response to microbial products has long been recognised and gives rise to potent effector macrophages (M1), which kill microorganisms and tumour cells and produce proinflammatory cytokines and chemokines (including IL-12, TNF-α, IL-1, IL-6, IL-8). More recently, it has been shown that anti-inflammatory molecules, such as glucocorticoid hormones, IL-4, IL-13 and IL-10, are more than simple inhibitors of macrophage activation, in that they induce a distinct activation pathway (alternatively activated macrophages) (Gordon, 2003; Mosser, 2003). Alternative macrophage activation with IL-4 and IL-13 induces M2 macrophages, which can regulate inflammatory responses and adaptive Th1 immunity (Mantovani et al., 2002; Mantovani et al., 2004). Classically and alternatively activated (polarised) macrophages have been referred to as M1 and M2, in analogy with the Th1/Th2 dichotomy in T cell responses. M1 or M2 polarised macrophages differ in terms of receptor expression, cytokine and chemokine production, and effector function. Differential cytokine production characterises polarised macrophages. The M1 phenotype includes IL-12 and TNF-α, while M2 macrophages typically produce IL-10, the IL-1 receptor antagonist (IL-1Ra) and the type II IL-1 receptor (IL-1RII). Differential production of chemokines, which attract Th1 *versus* Th2 or T regulatory cells, integrates M1 and M2 macrophages in circuits of amplification and regulation of polarised T cell responses. The microenvironment thus influences macrophage activation and their subsequent functions. In this light, genetic and environmental conditions that promote M1/Th1 polarisation and inhibit M2/Th2 regulatory activity may contribute to the establishment of a chronic inflammatory condition. This may develop into autoimmunity following triggering events (e.g., an infection or trauma) that would induce an autoimmune adaptive response, through mechanisms of molecular mimicry.

IL-12 is a proinflammatory cytokine mainly produced by activated macrophages, dendritic cells, and granulocytes (Hsieh et al., 1993; Macatonia et al., 1993; Heufler et al., 1996). It acts upon T, B, and natural killer (NK) lymphocytes, although it is best known for inducing the differentiation of CD4+ T lymphocytes from a Th0 to a Th1 phenotype (Trinchieri, 1993). IL-12 is a heterodimer (p70) composed of a p40 subunit that is expressed predominantly on antigen-presenting cells and a p35 subunit that is present constitutively in numerous cells. Both subunits, have to be secreted by the same cell for production of a bioactive molecule. IL-12 binds to a specific plasma membrane receptor, ultimately resulting in transcription of the genes involved in prototypic Th1 responses, such as IFN-γ. In light of its ability to stimulate Th1 responses, IL-12 has been invoked as a key cytokine in the pathogenesis of organ-specific autoimmune diseases, which are often mediated by cellular immunity (Trinchieri, 2003).

IL-18 is related to the IL-1 family in terms of its structure, receptor family and signal transduction pathways (Fantuzzi & Dinarello, 1999). The production of bioactive IL-18 is a multistep process involving synthesis of the precursor, synthesis and activation of the cleaving enzyme caspase-1, maturation and extracellular transport (Dinarello, 1999; Gracie et al., 2003). Mainly produced by macrophages and APC (Okamura H et al. 1995), IL-18 acts in synergy with IL-12 for Th1 differentiation (Kohno et al.,1997; Robinson et al., 1997; Micallef et al., 1996). It also exerts pro-inflammatory properties by inducing the production of IL-1beta, TNF-α, chemokines, nitric oxide and prostaglandins (Puren et al., 1998; Olee et al., 1999). The pleiotropic activities of IL-18 suggest an important role of this cytokine in the triggering and polarization of the immune response (Liew FY., 2003). Activated macrophages and Kupffer cells were first described to produce high levels of IL-18 (Okamura H. et al., 1995). IL-18 is also produced by dendritic and Langerhans cells (Brossart et al., 1998) and APC represent the major source of IL-18 production (Akita et al., 1997). Like IL-1beta, IL-18 exerts proinflammatory properties, but this cytokine is also related to IL-12 in view of its capacity to induce the production of Th1 cytokines and to enhance cell-mediated immune cytotoxicity. Indeed, enhanced production and activity of IL-18 appears to be at a fundamental level in autoimmune pathologies.

IFN-γ, also called immune or type II interferon is a pleiotropic cytokine involved in the regulation of nearly all phases of immune and inflammatory responses, including the activation, growth and differentiation of T-cells, B-cells, macrophages, NK cells and other cell types such as endothelial cells and fibroblasts. It enhances MHC expression on antigen-presenting and IFN--γ production is characteristic of Th1 differentiation (Romagnani, 1997). IFN-γ enhances the cytotoxic activity of T cells, macrophages and natural killer cells and thus has antiproliferative effects. It also increases the production of antibodies in response to antigens administered simultaneously with alpha-interferon, possible by enhancing the antigen-presenting function of macrophages (Mitcham, 2005). IFN-γ is produced by Th0-cells, activated Th1-cells (CD4+) and cytotoxic T cells (CD8+), and by NK cells. Practically any antigen can cause the secretion of IFN-γ in one or other way, and it is enhanced by IL-2 and IL-12 which induce the NK-cells, and Th cells to form IFN- γ. B-lymphocytes need IL-1 to produce IFN-γ. During its secretion, IFN-γ influences on the secreting cells as well as on the cells around through IFN- γ - receptors. The first necessary step in the functioning of the IFN-γ pathway is its interaction with receptors located on the surface of the cells. IFN-γ stimulates the expression of class I and class II MHC molecules and co-stimulatory molecules on antigen presenting cells; promotes the differentiation of naive helper T cells into Th1 cells; activates polymorphonuclear leukocytes (PMN) and cytotoxic T cells and increases the cytotoxicity of NK cells and suppresses humoral immunity.

IL-6 is a multi-functional cytokine, produced by lymphoid and non-lymphoid cells of the body, having regulatory effects on the immune and the hemopoietic system and causing an acute-phase reaction (Heinrich et al., 1990). IL-6 together with IL-2, TNF-α and other cytokines is an essential part of the accessory signal which is needed for the activation and the proliferation of antigen-stimulated T-lymphocytes. Interleukin-6 is especially important in the early stages of T-cell differentiation. In this phase, it reinforces the effect of IL-2 and promotes the differentiation of CD4 cells into T helper 2 cells (Janeway et al., 2001). It controls the growth and proliferation of early progenitor cells in the thymus and bone marrow and is later important in both T-cell and NK cell activation (Lee et al.; 1989). The molecular form of IL-6 responsible for T-cell activation is released by monocytes. It augments the early events of activation. (Heinrich et al., 1990; Van Snick, 1990) IL-6 also functions as the required second signal in both antigen- or mitogen-activated T-cells. (Clark & Shu, 1990) This protein holds a very important role in the life of NK cells. IL-6 provides support for continued development throughout the life of a natural killer cell (Van Snick, 1990). Interleukin-6 is very important in the stimulation of differentiation and proliferation of B-cells. Its most noted effect is found in the induction of permanent differentiation of B-cells into plasma cells, antibody producing cells (Nawata et al., 1989). IL-6 enhances the release of antibodies by acting as a growth factor for already differentiated plasma cells. It stimulates mostly the release of IgG and IgA antibodies from these cells. IL-6 induces increased production of antibodies in B-cells (Nawata et al., 1989).

IL-10 is a small protein known as a cytokine that functions as an important regulator of the immune system. Although IL-10 is known to have many different roles in the immune system, its two major activities include inhibition of cytokine production by macrophages and inhibition of the accessory functions of macrophages during T cell activation (Abbas et al., 1994). The effects of these actions cause IL-10 to play mainly an anti-inflammatory role in the immune system IL-10 is mainly produced by the Th2 subset of CD4$^+$ helper cells. However, it is also produced by some activated B cells, some Th1 cells (in humans), activated macrophages, and some other cells. Kinetics studies demonstrate that IL-10 is synthesized later than other immunoregulatory cytokines by activated T cells or monocytes. This data may reveal the regulatory role of IL-10 in later phases of the immune response (Delves et al., 1998). Studies have shown IL-10 to be an immunosuppressive agent that inhibits the synthesis of several monocyte and Th1 cell-derived cytokines (IL-1, -2, -6, -8, -12, TNF-beta, INF-γ). Moreover IL-10 has been demonstrated to down-regulate class II MHC expression thereby inhibiting the antigen-presenting capacity of monocytes. Like other cytokines interleukin-10 has many effects upon the functions of cells such as lymphocytes, monocytes, natural killer cells, and dendritic cells. Specifically, IL-10 is a cytokine that regulates immune-mediated inflammation. It appears to have two major functions: (1) to inhibit cytokine (i.e., TNF, IL-1, chemokine, and IL-12) production by macrophages and (2) to inhibit the accessory functions of macrophages in T cell activation. IL-10 accomplishes the latter function through the reduced expression of MHC class II molecules and certain co-stimulators (e.g., B7). The cumulative effect of these functions acts to inhibit T cell-mediated immune inflammation. IL-10 also has stimulatory actions on B cells and may function as a switching factor for the production of IgG4 in humans (homologous to IgG1 in mice) (Delves et al., 1998)

TNF- α is a pleiotropic inflammatory cytokine. This cytokine possesses both growth stimulating properties and growth inhibitory processes, and it appears to have self regulatory properties as well. TNF-α is produced by neutrophils, macrophages, activated T- and B-lymphocytes, NK-cells, lymphokine-activated killer cell, astrocytes, endothelial cells, smooth and muscle cells. TNF-α has been implicated in the mediation of a number of diseases including septic shock syndrome, cachexia, AIDS and in pathogenesis of certain autoimmune diseases. TNF-α production may play a key kinetic role by amplifying release of cytokines IL-1α, IL-1β, and IL-6 and thereby affecting the severity of a response (Amiot et al., 1997). TNF-α participates in both inflammatory disorders of inflammatory and non inflammatory origin (Strieter al., 1993). TNF-α is an acute phase protein which initiates a cascade of cytokines and increases vascular permeability, thereby recruiting macrophage and neutrophils to a site of infection.

IL-15 shares many activities exerted by IL-2 including the stimulation and expansion of T cells thymocytes, B cells and natural killer cells owing to the fact that the receptors for IL-2 and IL-15 share the same β and γ subunits. At least in murine models, IL-15 unlike IL-2 fails to significantly activate the apoptotic pathways when stimulating T cells as well as other responding lineages, suggesting that IL-15 promotes the establishment of long-term memory T cells. IL-15 is produced by a variety of tissues, including skeletal muscle, kidney, placenta, hematopoietic stromal cells etc. IL-15 is expressed by a wide range of human tissues and cell lines, including skeletal muscle, placenta, and epithelial cell cultures (Tagaya et al., 1996). This cytokine induces T and B cell proliferation and it is essential for cell survival and for maintenance of long-lived memory cells (Perera et al., 1999; Oh et al., 2008). IL-15 is known to have noninflammatory actions because it can be detected in normal muscle tissue, where it is thought to have an anabolic activity and can modulate adipose tissue deposition (Quinn et al., 2009).

TGF-$ß_1$ belong to a family of multifunctional polypeptides and is produced by a wide variety of lymphoid and nonlymphoid cells. The TGF-ßs are involved in a variety of different biological processes, including tumorigenesis, fibrosis, hemopoiesis, and immunoregulation (Prud'homme & Piccirillo, 2000; Grande, 1997). Lymphoid cells mostly produce TGF-$ß_1$, an isoform that is also found in large amounts in bones and platelets and in the serum (Letterio & Roberts 1998). The activation of TGF-$ß_1$ may be mediated by macrophages in inflammatory sites (Wallick et al., 1990). Regarding the immunoregulating role of TGF-$ß_1$, this is an immunosuppressive cytokine, as it inhibits T and B cell proliferation, natural killer cell cytotoxic activity, and the generation of T cell cytotoxicity (Rook et al., 1986; Lee et al. 1987). Furthermore, TGF-$ß_1$ is able to inhibit both T helper type 1 and T helper type 2 cytokine production and decreases the interferon- γ -induced expression of HLA class II antigens (Czarniecki et al., 1988).

3.2.2 Cytokines and the thyroid

Both CD4+ and CD8+ T-Cells occur in thyroid lymphocytic infiltrate with a preponderance of CD4+ cells. There is an increase in activated T Cells expressing markers like HLA-DR. Thyroid cells express MHC class-II molecules as well as other immunologically important molecules and behaves as an APC. Expression of ICAM-1, LFA-3 and MHC class I molecules by thyrocytes is enhanced by IL-1, TNF-α and IFN-γ (Weetman, 2004). This response increases the ability of cytotoxic T cells to mediate lysis. Thyroid cell destruction is mediated by Fas dependent mechanisms (Weetman, 2004; Wu et al., 1994). Cytokines and other toxic molecules such as nitric oxide and reactive oxygen metabolites probably also contribute directly to cell mediated tissue injury (Weetman, 2011). (Fig. 1)

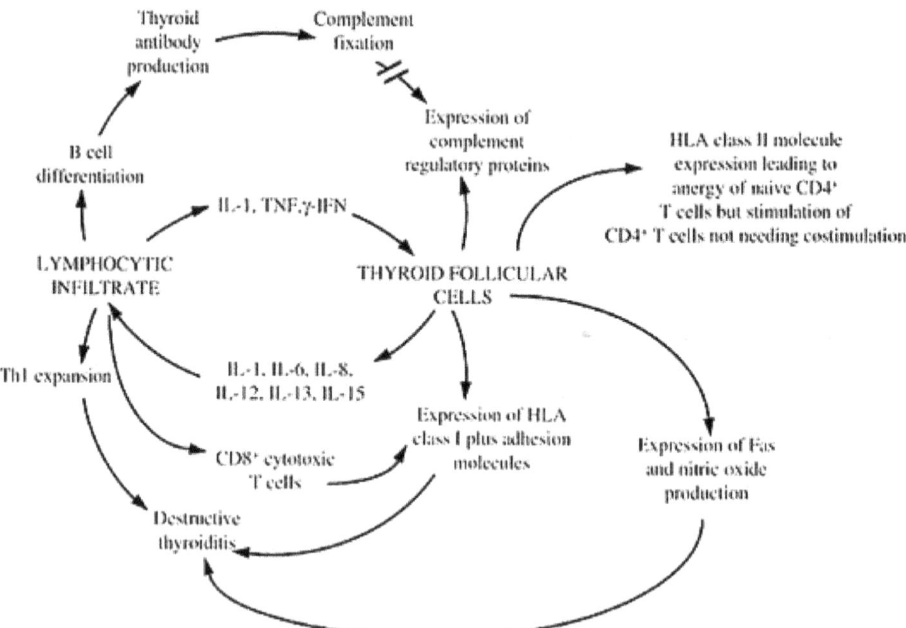

Fig. 1. Interaction between thyroid cells and the immune system via cytokines.

Humoral immunity exacerbates cell-mediated damage in a secondary fashion, both by direct complement fixations (TPO antibodies) and by ADCC (Chiovato et al., 1993). Complement attack initiated via the classic or alternative pathway, impairs the metabolic function of thyroid cells and induces them to secrete IL-1, IL-6, reactive oxygen metabolites and prostaglandin. All of these enhance the autoimmune response.

As well as T and B cell, dendritic cells and monocyte/ macrophages accumulate in the thyroid. Presumably they play a major role as APC and capable of providing co-stimulatory signals. Thyroid cell-derived monocyte chemoattractant-I, produced after TNF-α, IFN-γ, or IL-1 stimulation, is likely to be responsible for the accumulation of monocytes, which are important source of cytokines (Simons, 1998). Many cytokines are now known to be produced by thyroid cells especially after stimulation with IL-1, including IL-1, IL-6, IL-8, IL-12, IL-13 and IL-15 (Weetman et al. 1990; Weetman et al. 1992; Ajjan et al. 1997).

Gene expression of IL-1, IL-2, IL-4, IL-6, IL-8, IL-10, IL-12, IL-13, IL-14, IL-15, IL-16, IFN-γ, TNF-α and a number of chemokines have been shown in both GD and HT tissue samples

(Ajjan et al. 1996; Azmi et al. 1997; Ashhab et al., 1999). Generally, a mixed Th1 and Th2 pattern has been found in the samples analysed, although some studies, using quantitative techniques, have shown a Th1 response in HT and a Th2 response in GD (Heuer et all. 1996). However, the analysis of mRNA can be misleading, as gene expression does not necessarily correlate with protein production. To address this issue, immunohistochemical methods have been applied which demonstrated cytokine protein production by a variety of cells in AITDs tissue in vivo. IFN-γ was found in infiltrating lymphocytes, IL-1 in endothelial cells, whereas IL-1, IL-6 and TNF-α were produced by thyroid follicular cells (TFC) (Ajjan et al. 1996).

Cytokine production by TFC in vitro can be stimulated by IL-1, IFN-γ and TNF-α, and this may be important in increasing the size and the activity of the infiltrate in vivo. Cytokines enhance the expression of adhesion molecules on TFC and can stimulate nitric oxide and prostaglandin production by these cells, which may further have a role in localising and augmenting the inflammatory reaction (Ajjan et al. 1996).

MHC class I expression is upregulated on TFC by IFN-γ and TNF-α treatment in vitro, which may play a role in tissue destruction through T-cell-mediated cytotoxicity (Ajjan et all. 1996). IFN-γ also enhances MHC class II expression on TFC in vitro, which may have a role in enhancing the proliferation of non-B-7-dependent T cells, but may also have a protective role as detailed below.

Apoptosis seems to play a role in AITDs, in particular HT (Palazzo et al. 2000). Cytokines can upregulate proapoptotic genes and downregulate antiapoptotic genes on TFC predosposing these cells to apoptosis.

TFC are resistant to complement-mediated cell lysis, an effect mediated in part by the expression of several protective proteins, which can be upregulated by cytokines (Ajjan et al. 1996). IFN-γ and TNF-α treatment of TFC in vitro renders these cells resistant to cell-mediated cytotoxicity, whereas TGF-β_1 inhibits T cell proliferation and thyroid autoantigen recognition (Ajjan et al. 1996).

IL-1 and IL-6 enhance TFC proliferation in culture but can also have inhibitory effects if cells are stimulated with TSH, emphasising the complex interaction of these molecules in vivo. IFN-γ and TNF-α inhibit TFC growth and proliferation, without affecting cell viability (Ajjan et al. 1996). TPO gene expression and Tg production are decreased by cytokine treatment of TFC in vitro, which may affect iodine organification in vivo (Rasmussen et all. 1994). IFN-γ can also downregulate TSHR gene expression (Nishikawa et al., 1993).

Levels of IL-5 are increased in GD and HT sera (Hidaka et all., 1998), whereas IL-6, IL-8 and IL-12 concentration is increased in GD sera compared with controls (Tamaru et al., 1999; Salvi et al., 2000). Increased serum levels of IFN-γ, IL-4, IL-6, IL-10 and TNF-α were found in GD compared with controls indicating a mixed Th1/Th2 response in this disease (Al-Humaidi, 2000). In recent study Sieminska at al. found increased production of IL-6 in postmenopausal women with Hashimoto's thyroiditis (Sieminska et al., 2010). On balance, the concept of a predominance of a Th1 and Th2 response, in HT and GD respectively, is almost certainly an over-simplification as features of cell-mediated and humoral immunity can be found in both diseases. Some authors considered HT as Th1 disease (Phenekos et al., 2004; Colin et al., 2004), others found a mixed Th1 and Th2 pattern (Heuer et al., 1996;

Weetman A.P, 2004). Th1-associated cytokines have antagonistic and counterregulatory effects on the functions of Th2 type cells and vice versa (Mosmann & Sad, 1996; Elenkov & Chrousos, 1999). Cytokines can modulate Th1/Th2 cell differentiation via chromatin remodeling of Th cell loci (Murphy & Reiner, 2002, Morinobi et al., 2004; Spilianakis & Flavell, 2004).

The role of cytokines in different stages of Hashimoto's thyroiditis is not well established and their participation in processes leading to hypothyroidism remains contradictory. Relatively few studies are available on the role of IL-12 and IL-18 in autoimmune lymphocytic thyroiditis, either in patients with Hashimoto's thyroiditis or in mice. IL-15 mRNA was detected in the majority of thyroid tissue samples from patients with multinodular goiter, GD, and HT (Ajjan et al. 1996). Furthermore the expression of IL-15 was increased after stimulation of TFC cells with TSH, IL-1 or IFN-γ, suggesting that these cells are a source of IL-15 in the thyroid.

To provide the involvement of Th1 and Th2 lymphocyte subpopulations and to clarify the role of some cytokines in different stages of Hashimoto's disease we investigated 128 out-patients from the Department of Internal Medicine, Stara Zagora University Hospital (Bulgaria), with autoimmune thyroiditis. Fifty two healthy subjects were included as controls. In all patients diagnosis had been made by enlarged thyroid glands, elevated TPO Abs and/or typical hypoechogenicity of the thyroid in high-resolution sonography. In negative TPO Abs patients FNAB was performed and typical cytological features of autoimmune thyroiditis were found. Serum levels of TSH, free thyroxin (fT4) were estimated. Fasting samples of venous blood were collected in the morning between 8.00 and 10.00 h. Serum samples were routinely collected and stored frozen at -20 C until assayed. At the time of sampling, neither of the patients and control subjects had clinical signs or symptoms of intercurrent illness. Concentrations of IL-12, IL-18, IFN-γ, IL-10, IL-6, TNF-α, IL-15 and TGF- $ß_1$ in the serum samples of patients and controls were evaluated by ELISA, using commercially available kits (R&D Systems, Minneapolis, USA). Patients were divided into tree subgroups according to the thyroid function. Group I (n=40) involved subjects with normal thyroid function (TSH and fT4 within the normal range). Group II (n=17) included patients with hypothyroidism (high levels of TSH and low or normal serum levels of fT4). In group III (n=71) were enrolled subjects with hypothyroidism treated with Levothyroxine (LT4) in a dosage to maintain TSH and fT4 within the normal range. The medication of Levothyroxine (range: 50-200 μg) was given in the fasting state. Informed consent was obtained from all participants in the study according to the ethical guidelines of the Helsinki Declaration.

The relevant clinical and biochemical data of all of patients studied and controls are summarized in Table 1. and Table 2.

The results obtained for cytokine levels in blood serum are shown in Table 3.

IL-18 was significantly higher in all HT patients (p=0.02) and both group II (p=0.03) and group III (p=0.01) in comparison with controls. The mean serum IL-12 levels in patients with HT were significantly higher than those in control subjects (p=0.014). (Fig.2) The serum IL-12 levels were also higher in sub-groups in patients, statistically significant in group I and group III (p=0.015 and p=0.036 respectively) in comparison with controls. (Fig.3) Concentrations of IL-10 in sub-groups of patients - I and II tended to be lower in comparison with controls. IL-15 was significantly lower in group II in comparison with controls ($p<0.05$). Serum concentrations of TGF- ß$_1$ were not statistically different in sub-groups of patients and controls, but in all sub-groups of HT patients levels tended to be lower than in controls.

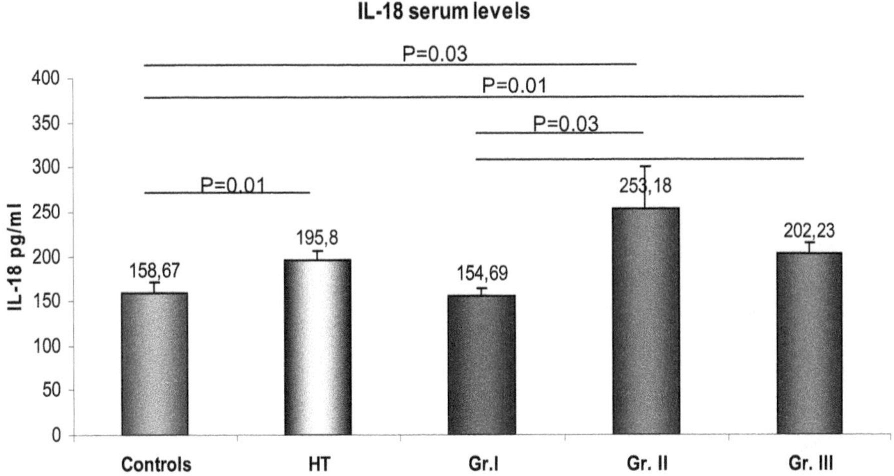

Fig. 2. IL-18 serum levels in controls, in all patients with Hashimoto's thyroiditis (HT), in euthyroid group (Gr. I), hypothyroid group (Gr. II) and group of patients treated with Levothyroxine (Gr. III). Data are presented as mean ± SEM.

The relevant clinical and biochemical data of all of patients studied and controls are summarized in Table 1. and Table 2. The results obtained for cytokine levels in blood serum are shown in Table 3.

Variables	Controls	HT	Group I	Group II	Group III
IL-10	0.77 ± 0.23	1.34±0.89	0.41±0.17	0.51±0.23	1.85±1.38
IL-15	2.06±0.24 [1]	1.48±0.11	1.67±0.21 [2]	0.62±0.40 [1,2]	1.56±0.12
IL-18	158.67±13.14 [3,4,5]	195.80±10.64 [4]	154.69±9.84 [6,7]	253.18±46.51[3,6]	202.23±13.26 [5,7]
TGF-β_1	25874,1±2894	18742±737	18967±1151	19830±2516	18305±1011
TNF-α	10.99±0.60	10.27±0.45	10.54±0.53	11.18±0.97	9.35±0.85
IL-12	67.99±9.85 [8,9,10]	93.48±7.05 [8]	103.73±14.409 [9]	83.41±14.0	90.48±8.19 [10]
IFN-γ	1.79±0.11 [11]	1.61±0.72	1.68±0.12	1.56±0.29 [11]	1.58±0.09
IL-6	1.47±0.29	2.22±0.36	1.79±0.50	3.96±1.30	1.71±0.29

Statistical significance: 1, 2, 3, 4, 5, 6, 7, 8, 9, 10, 11: $p<0.05$

Table 3. Cytokine concentrations (pg/ml) in all Hashimoto's thyroiditis patients and in particular groups of patients: euthyroid group (Group I), hypothyroid group (Group II) and group of patients treated with Levothyroxine (Group III) and controls (mean±SEM).

To further analyze the balance of immune regulation (Th1/Th2 balance) in individuals, the ratio between IL-12 and IL-6 was calculated. In comparison to control subjects, a clear bias towards Th1-dominated immune reactivity was found in group I - euthyroid Hashimoto's patients ($p=0.018$).

We found statistically significant lower serum levels of TGF-$ß_1$ in TPO Abs (+) patients (17802±876 pg/ml) in comparison with TPO Abs (-) patients (21200±1291 pg/ml) ($p=0.018$, Mann Whitney U test).

An advantage of investigating serum cytokine levels in ATD is the ability to analyse cytokine profile early in the disease process, when the immune response is presumably more specific. However, serum cytokine levels may not reflect the intrathyroidal cytokine profile as levels of some cytokines may be very low in the periphery (falling below the detection sensitivity of the assay), despite high intrathyroidal concentrations.

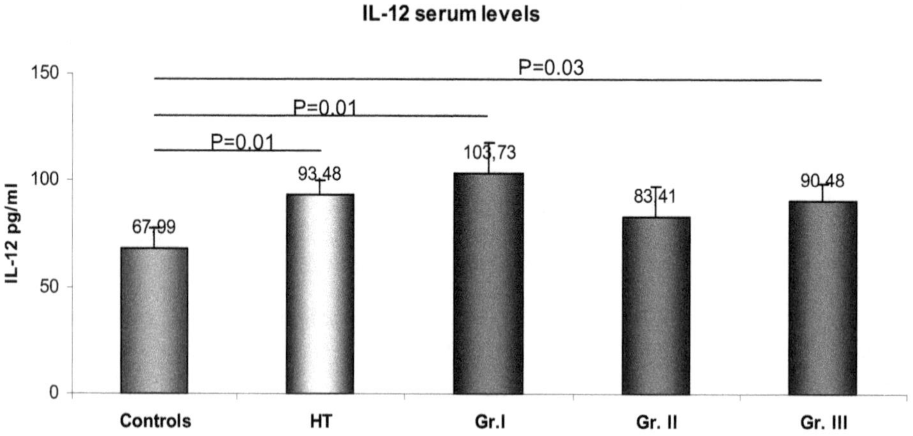

Fig. 3. IL-12 serum levels in controls, in all patients with Hashimoto's thyroiditis (HT), in euthyroid group (Gr. I), hypothyroid group (Gr. II) and group of patients treated with Levothyroxine (Gr. III). Data are presented as mean ± SEM.

Our results demonstrate that serum IL-12 levels were increased in all sub-groups in patients independently of functional state of the disease. The ratio between IL-12 and IL-6 demonstrate a clear bias towards Th1-dominated immune reactivity in group of euthyroid Hashimoto's patients in comparison to control subjects. In our previous work we found significantly increased serum levels of IL-12 in patients suffering from both GD and HT, which suggests that IL-12 might affect the immune response in both GD and HT (Halacheva et al., 2005). The results shown in the existing research carried out so far on IL-12 serum levels in GD and HT are contradictory. Phenekos et al. have shown that IL-12 serum concentrations were significantly higher than those in normal controls in HT patients but were not increased in patients suffering from GD (Phenekos et al., 2004). During iodine-induced autoimmune (lymphocytic) thyroiditis in NOD mouse IL-12 is produced in the thyroid gland early and throughout the course of the disease (Bonita et al., 2003). Kimura at al. have shown that the local production of IL-12 in the thyroid enhances the expression of sodium-iodide symporter and inhibits thyroid hormonogenesis downstream of the organification, thus inducing primary hypothyroidism; and the disease promoting effect of IL-12 was independent of of interferon-γ (Kimura et al., 2005). On the basis of our results and data from experimental mouse models we may conclude that the effect of IL-12 on the initiation and regulation of immune responses and also on thyroid function is crucial in Hashimoto's thyroiditis.

We found that serum levels of IL-18 were significantly higher in HT; particularly in patients with severe disease and no change significantly after treatment with Levothyroxine in comparison with controls. Concentrations of IL-10 in sub-groups of patients tended to be lower in comparison with controls. Phenekos et al. demonstrated significantly increased IL-18 serum levels in HT patients than those in normal controls and in patients suffering from GD and toxic nodular goiter (Phenekos et al., 2004). IL-18 expression was increased in the thyroid tissues of HT compared with control thyroid tissues in canine model and in humans (Choi et al., 2006, Liu et al., 2010). IL-18 acts in synergy with IL-12 for Th1 differentiation induce the production of Th1 cytokines and inhance cell-mediated cytotoxicity (Lebel-Binay et al., 2000).; Increased serum levels of IL-18 particularly in patients with severe disease and no change significantly after treatment with Levothyroxine suggest an altered immunological status in severe hypothyroid stage of the disease and during Levothyroxine replacement remained unchanged. Mazziotti et al. found different expression of IL-4 in CD4+ in hypothyroid and euthyroid patients with HT (Mazziotti et al., 2003). Taking together our and these results suggest a different immunological status for euthyroid and hypothyroid HT patients and the interaction between IL-12 and IL-18 may be related to development of thyroid destruction.

Our results indicate lower serum levels of IL-15 in hypothyroid HT patients. Treatment with Levothyroxine increases serum levels of IL-15. In study of Ajjan at al. IL-15 was detected in all HT samples, and the expression was increased after stimulation of thyroid follicular cells with TSH, but all patients had been treated with Levothyroxine before surgery (Ajjan et al., 1997). IL-15 expression has been detected in numerous tissues, many of which are not sites of immune responses (Fehniger & Caligiuri, 2008). Accordingly we may suppose that decreased serum levels of IL-15 in hypothyroid HT may be related to the process of thyroid apoptosis and hypometabolism of all tissues.

TGF-$ß_1$ regulate proliferation of follicule cells of the thyroid in many experiments *in vitro*. It has been proved that TGF- $ß_1$ is an immunosuppressive cytokine, as it inhibits T and B cell proliferation, natural killer cell cytotoxic activity, and the generation of T cell cytotoxicity (Prud'homme & Piccirillo, 2000). In our work serum levels of TGF-$ß_1$ are not statistically different in sub-groups of patients compared to controls, but in all HT patients they tended to be lower in comparison with controls. Our findings of significantly lower serum levels of TGF-$ß_1$ in TPO Abs (+) patients than TPO Abs (-) suggest that TGF-$ß_1$ may contribute to the severity of autoimmune thyroiditis. Akinci et al. found lower levels of TGF- $ß_1$ in hypothyroid HT patients when compared with control cases and their levels remained unchanged after Levothyroxine replacement (Akinci et al., 2008). Vural at al. also measured decreased plasma TGF-$ß_1$ concentrations in HT patients in comparison with controls (Vural at al., 2009). On the basis of our and these data we suppose that autoimmunity may have been triggered as a result of decreased immunosuppressive effect induced by depressed TGF- $ß_1$ levels in patients with HT.

We may summarize that Th1 pattern of immune response characteristic of cellular immunity is dominant in HT and sub-groups of patients have a different immunological status which contribute to development of hypothyroidism.

3.3 Oxidative stress and antioxidant protection in Hashimoto's thyroiditis

3.3.1 Generation of reactive oxygen metabolites and antioxidant enzymes

Molecular oxygen gives rise to dangerous reactive metabolites upon reduction to water (Fridovich, 1978). The term "free radical" covers any atom or molecule that contains one or more unpaired electrons (Halliwell 1991). Some of the reactive oxygen species (ROS) are free radicals, such as superoxide, nitric oxide and hydroxyl radical, whereas hydrogen peroxide (H2O2) is reactive and important, but not a free radical. Therefore, it is appropriate to speak of reactive oxygen species. ROS are continuously formed in the mitochondrial respiratory chain, via the cyclo-oxygenase pathway and by cellular enzymes, such as xanthine oxidase, NADPH oxidase and cytochrome P450 oxidase (Gadjeva et al., 2000). The main intracellular source of ROS is mitochondria.

A typical feature of free radical reactions is that they proceed as chain reactions, amplifying the damage of the initial event. ROS cause cell injury by reacting with proteins, lipids, and DNA (De Zwart et al., 1999), but they are also an essential part of normal cellular physiology, such as signal transduction. Oxidative reactions occur in living organisms under physiological conditions. ROS and free radicals are essential for numerous metabolic processes. Under physiological conditions, there is a balance between the production and detoxification of ROS. However, any internal or external pathological factor may disrupt this balance, leading to conditions referred to as oxidative stress. Reactive oxygen species - O2-, OH-, H_2O_2 and NO when being in excess cause oxidative damage to molecules. Indeed, oxidative stress plays a significant role in the pathogenesis of several diseases. Excess H_2O_2 has been reported to induce oxidative damage to membrane lipids, proteins and DNA that may result in cell death by necrosis or apoptosis. The levels of lipid peroxidation products (malondialdehyde - MDA) in plasma are widely used in practice as an indicator of free radical damages.

Detoxification of ROS is one of the prerequisites of aerobic life, and hence an elaborate antioxidant system has evolved. Antioxidants are agents that scavenge ROS, prevent their formation, or repair the damage they cause (De Zwart et al., 1999). This complex system consists of antioxidant enzymes (superoxide dismutases, catalase, glutathione peroxidase) and other substrates. Of the antioxidant enzymes superoxide dismutases (SOD) catalyse the conversion of two superoxide molecules to hydrogen peroxide and oxygen, and hydrogen peroxide is mainly eliminated by catalase (CAT) and glutathione peroxidase (GPX).

SOD is an endogenously produced intracellular enzyme present in essentially every cell in the body. Cellular SOD is actually represented by a group of metalloenzymes with various prosthetic groups. The prevalent enzyme is cupro-zinc (CuZn) SOD, which is a stable dimeric protein.

Catalase is a protein enzyme present in most aerobic cells in animal tissues. Catalase is present in all body organs being especially, concentrated in the liver and erythrocytes. The brain, heart, skeletal muscle contains only low amounts.

Glutathione peroxidase is a selenium-dependent enzyme, which decomposes H_2O_2 and various hydro- and lipid peroxides. (Kinnula et al. 1995). The classical form of GPX is cellular and dispersed throughout the cytoplasm, but GPX activity is also found in mitochondria. GPX is considered more important in physiologic conditions (reviewed by Kinnula et al., 1995). Selenium is essential for the protein synthesis and enzymatic activity of GPX.

SOD is considered fundamental in the process of eliminating ROS by reducing (adding an electron to) superoxide to form H_2O_2. Catalase and the selenium-dependent glutathione peroxidase are responsible for reducing H_2O_2 to H_2O. Catalase and glutathione peroxidase seek out hydrogen peroxide and convert it to water and diatomic oxygen. An increase in the production of SOD without a subsequent elevation of catalase or glutathione peroxidase leads to the accumulation of hydrogen peroxide, which gets converted into the hydroxyl radical.

The respective enzymes that interact with superoxide and H_2O_2 are tightly regulated through a feedback system. Excessive superoxide inhibits glutathione peroxidase and catalase to modulate the equation from H_2O_2 to H_2O. Likewise, increased H_2O_2 slowly inactivates CuZn-SOD. Meanwhile, catalases and glutathione peroxidase, by reducing H_2O_2, conserve SOD; and SOD, by reducing superoxide, conserves catalases and glutathione peroxidase. Through this feedback system, steady low levels of SOD, glutathione peroxidase, and catalase, as well as superoxide and H_2O_2 are maintained, which keeps the entire system in a fully functioning state (Fig.4). (Gadjeva et al., 2000; Al-Gubory K et al.; 2010).

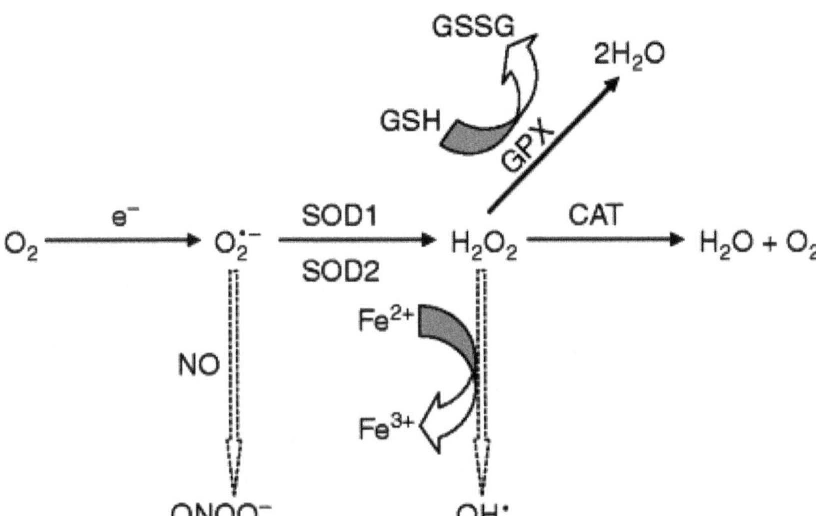

Fig. 4. Schematic representation of the pathways producing reactive oxygen species (ROS) and key cellular antioxidant enzymatic systems controlling ROS production.

3.3.2 Oxidative stress and antioxidant protection in Hashimoto's thyroiditis

In the thyroid hydrogene peroxide is necessary for thyroid hormonogenesis acting at different steps of the process. Excess H_2O_2 has been reported to induce oxidative damage to membrane lipids, proteins and DNA that may result in cell death by necrosis or apoptosis. The levels of lipid peroxidation products (malondialdehyde - MDA) in plasma are widely used in practice as an indicator of free radical damages. To prevent the damages caused by the ROS, multiple defense systems, collectively called antioxidants, are present in human serum, erythrocytes as well in the tissues. The presence of following antioxidative enzymes in the thyroid gland has been documented: superoxide dismutase, catalase and glutathione peroxidase. GPX and TR (thioredoxin reductase) are selenoenzymes capable of modifying cell function by acting as antioxidants.

In the thyroid, ROS and free radicals are constantly formed and participate in physiological and pathological processes in the gland. For example, H_2O_2 is necessary for thyroid hormonogenesis (Nunez & Pommier, 1982; Fayadat et al., 1999). But an *in vitro* experimental study H_2O_2 has been found to influence the process of cell death (Riou et al., 1998).

Cells have developed a comprehensive set of antioxidant defense mechanisms to limit the action of ROS. SOD catalyse the conversion of two superoxide molecules to H_2O_2 and oxygen. CAT and GPX mainly eliminate H_2O_2, as primary participants in the most important antioxidant enzyme pathways. The involvement of hyperthyroidism due to Graves' disease in lipid peroxidation and antioxidant enzyme activities has been studied (Komosinska-Vassev et al., 2000; Gerenova & Gadjeva, 1996). The papers concerninig the influence of hypothyroidism have shown that this condition results in complex effects such as the augmentation of SOD and GPX activities and significant decrease of the CAT activity in rat liver mitochondria in experimental work (Das & Chainy, 2001) and augmentation of oxidative stress and disturbance of antioxidant defense in humans (Erdamar et al.,2008). The complex regulation of ROS generation and free radical-scavenging systems activity in patients with Hashimoto's thyroiditis in different stages of disease activity has not been studied. The study of Hashimoto's thyroiditis is plagued by the difficulties in examining a disease that progresses over long periods of time (Davies & Amino, 1993; Dayan & Daniels, 1996).

In our previous study we investigated the possible induction of oxidative stress and changes in antioxidant enzyme activities in Hashimoto's thyroiditis and compared these parameters in different subgroups of patients (Gerenova & Gadjeva, 2007). For this purpose seventy-one patients with autoimmune thyroiditis and 30 healthy controls were studied. Patients were divided into tree subgroups according to the thyroid function: group I - euthyroid subjects; group II - hypothyroid subjects; group III - subjects with hypothyroidism treated with Levothyroxine (LT4) to maintain TSH and fT4 winthin the normal range. The levels of of lipid peroxidation products - MDA in the plasma, and the antioxidant defences such as SOD, CAT and GPX activities in erythrocytes were measured.

Between June 2003 and April 2005 seventy-one out-patients (4 males, 67 females, of mean age 45.9±13.1 years) from the Department of Internal Medicine, Stara Zagora University

Hospital (Bulgaria) with Hashimoto's thyroiditis were recruited and investigated in prospective study. From 74 patients selected, 71 agreed to participate in the study. In all patients diagnosis had been made by enlarged thyroid glands, elevated TPO Abs and/or Tg Abs as well as typical hypoechogenicity of the thyroid in high-resolution sonography. Serum levels of TSH, free thyroxin (fT4) and lipid profile [total cholesterol (TC), triglyceride (TGs), LDL- and HDL- cholesterol (LDL-C and HDL-C)] were estimated. Patients were divided into tree subgroups according to the thyroid function. Group I (n=19) involved subjects with normal thyroid function (TSH and fT4 within the normal range). Group II (n=20) included patients with hypothyroidism (high levels of TSH and low or normal serum levels of fT4). In group III (n=32) were enrolled subjects with hypothyroidism treated with Levothyroxine (LT4) in a dosage to maintain TSH and fT4 within the normal range. The medication of Levothyroxine was given in the fasting state, mean Levothyroxine doses were 83.2±27.7 μg daily (range: 50-200 μg).

Blood samples, obtained from 30 healthy individuals (4 males, 26 females, of mean age 43.8 ± 12.3 years) who had no family history of autoimmune disease were used as controls. To eliminate the factors, that might affect parameters of oxidative stress, we excluded from Hashimoto's thyroiditis patients and healthy controls, all smoking and alcohol drinking subjects, as well as individuals suffering from acute or chronic diseases. Informed consent was obtained from all participants in the study according to the ethical guidelines of the Helsinki Declaration. Fasting samples of venous blood were collected in the morning between 8.00 and 10.00 h. FT4 was measured by competitive immunoassay on the ACS180 (Chiron Diagnostics USA). TSH was measured by a third generation two-site chemiluminometric assay on the ACS180. The reference range was 11.5-22.7 pmol/l for FT4 and 0.35-5.5 μIU/ml for TSH. Serum TC, HDL-C and TG concentrations were determined enzymatically in the routine laboratory by automated procedures (Roche). Serum LDL-C was calculated according to the Friedewald formula.

Blood for determining the parameters of oxidative stress was collected in tubes containing ethylendiamine-tetraacetic acid (EDTA), centrifuged at 3000 rpm for 15 min and plasma was carefully separated. The erythrocyte pellets were washed three times with saline, and 0.5 ml of the cell suspension was diluted with 2 ml cold water to lyse the erythrocytes. To 0.2 ml lysat 1.8 ml water and ethanol/chloroform (3:5/v:v) were then added to precipitate hemoglobin. The tubes were shaken vigorously for 5 min. The supernatant was used for determination of enzyme activity.

Total amount of lipid peroxidation products in the plasma of healthy volunteers and patients was estimated using the thiobarbituric acid (TBA) method, which measures the malondialdehyde (MDA) reactive products (Plaser et al., 1996). The results were expressed as μM/l. Superoxide dismutase activity was determined as described by Sun et al., (Sun at al., 1988) with minor modifications. The results were expressed as U/gHb. Catalase activity in the erythrocyte lysats was assessed by the method described by Beers and Sizer (Beers & Sizer, 1952). The hemoglobin concentration of lysate was determined by the cyanmethemoglobin method (Mahoney et al., 1993). Glutathione peroxidase activity was measured by the method of Paglia et al (Paglia et al., 1967). Activity was given in units per g hemoglobin (U/g Hb).

Characteristics	Group I	Group II	Group III
N	N=19	N=20	N=32
Age (yr)	46.1±14.9	41.8±14.5	48.4±10.7
Sex F/M	17/2	1/19	1/31
BMI (kg/m^2)	27.6±3.2	28.4±5.9	28.8±5.8
TSH basal (mIU/l)	2.3±1.2 *	16.0±4.9 * #	3.9±4.8 #
Free T4 (pmol/l)	14.8±1.3 *	10.6±2.4 *#	16±2.4#
Total cholesterol (mmol/l)	6.0±1.1	6.3±1.3	5.6±0.8
LDL-C (mmol/l)	4.0±1.0	3.8±1.1	3.5±0.6
HDL-C (mmol/l)	1.4±0.5	1.6±0.3	1.4±0.3
Triglycerides (mmol/l)	1.6±0.6	1.6±0.9	1.4±1.1

* $p<0.05$; # $p<0.05$ are statistically significant (Student's t-test)

Table 4. Baseline characteristics of Hashimoto's thyroiditis patients - euthyroid group (Group I), hypothyroid group (Group II) and group of patients treated with Levothyroxine (Group III). The results are expressed as mean ± S.D

Statistical analysis was carried out using the Statistica 5.5 for Windows. The results were reported as means ± SD (SE). Student's *t*-test was used to determine whether differences between means were significant. Correlations between the different parameters were calculated by linear regression analysis. $P \leq 0.05$ was considered statistically significant. Clinical and biochemical data of subgroups of Hashimoto's thyroiditis patients are presented in Table 4. In hypothyroid Hashimoto's patients cholesterol levels tended to be higher compared to euthyroid patients and patients treated with LT4. Results of studied parameters of oxidative stress in controls and Hashimoto's patients are listed in Table 5.

There were no significant changes of plasma levels of MDA between the groups of patients (group I - 1.68±0.08; group II - 1.90±0.13; group III – 1.71±0.07 μmol/l; respectively) as well as between the patients and the controls (1.70±0.06 μmol/l). Only plasma levels of MDA in hypothyroid Hashimoto's patients (group II) tended to be higher. No significant differences in SOD activity in erythrocytes were observed between the groups of patients (group I - 2377±262; group II - 2602±190; group III – 2308±267 U/gHb; respectively) and the controls

(2597±156 U/gHb. Our results showed that CAT activity was significantly lower in hypothyroid patients (group II) in comparison with controls (16016±3875 vs 26855±2272 U/gHb, p=0.01) and in coparison with subjects treated with LT4 (group III) (16016±3875 vs 29250±3939 U/gHb, p=0.02). Erythrocyte CAT activity of patients in euthyroid stage (group I) was also found significantly decreased compared to the controls (18733±3188 vs 26855±2272 U/gHb, p=0.04). Activity of GPX in erythrocytes in hypothyroidism (group II) was higher compared to control group (8.3±0.6 vs. 6.4±0.4 U/gHb, p=0.02). In euthyroid Hashimoto's patients (group I) and in patients treated with LT4 (group III), the activity of GPX was found significantly decreased in comparison with hypothyroid patients (5.7±1.1 vs 8.3±0.6 and 5.2±1.1 vs 8.3±0.6 U/gHb; p=0.05, p=0.047, respectively). GPX activity in both groups I and III, also tended to be lower in comparison with controls, but not significantly (Fig. 5).

Groups Parameters	**Controls**	**Group I**	**Group II**	**Group III**
N	30	19	20	32
MDA (μmol/l)	1.70 ± 0.06	1.68 ± 0.08	1.90 ± 0.13	1.71 ± 0.07
SOD (U/gHb)	2597 ± 156	2377 ± 262	2602 ± 190	2308 ± 267
CAT (U/gHb)	26855 ± 2272 [a b]	18773 ± 3188 [b]	16016 ± 3875 [a c]	29250 ± 3939[c]
GPX (U/gHb)	6.4 ± 0.4 [a]	5.70 ± 1.1 [c]	8.3 ± 0.6 [a b c]	5.2 ± 1.1 [b]

The results are expressed as mean ± S.E.

Student's *t-test* was used to compute the statistical significance of values

[a]CAT $_p$<0.05; [b]CAT $_p$ <0.05; [c]CAT$_p$ < 0.05

[a]GPX: $_p$<0.05; [b]GPX $_p$ <0.05; [c]GPX $_p$ < 0.05

Table 5. Levels of lipid peroxidation products – malondialdehyde (MDA) (μmol/l) in the plasma and the activities of antioxidative enzymes superoxide dismutase (SOD) (U/gHb), catalase (CAT) (U/gHb), and glutathione peroxidase (GPX) (U/gHb) in erythrocytes of control group and Hashimoto's thyroiditis patients – euthyroid group (Group I), hypothyroid group (Group II) and group of patients treated with Levothyroxine (Group III).

Significant negative linear correlation was found between activities of GPX and CAT in control group (r=- 0.57, p<0.05). However, no correlation was noted between activities of GPX and CAT in patient's groups. Significant negative correlation was also observed between serum levels of TSH and CAT activity (r= -0.40, p<0.05) in both groups euthyroid (group I) and hypothyroid (group II) Hashimoto's patients.

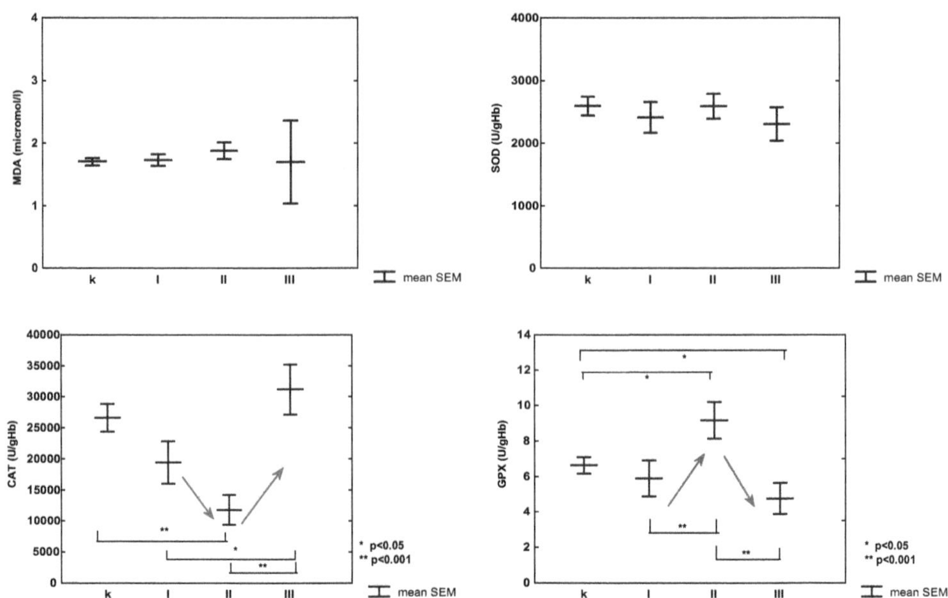

Fig. 5. Comparison of MDA levels in plasma and the activities of antioxidative enzymes superoxide dismutase (SOD) (U/gHb), catalase (CAT) (U/gHb), and glutathione peroxidase (GPX) (U/gHb) in erythrocytes of control group and Hashimoto's thyroiditis patients - euthyroid group (I), hypothyroid group (II) and group of patients treated with Levothyroxine (III). The results are expressed as mean ± S.E.

The thyroid function is normal in a great number of patients with Hashimoto's thyroiditis. Some of them, however, may progress to hypothyroidism over time. Although the highest titers of TPO antibodies are found in hypothyroid patients with Hashimoto's thyroiditis, they can also be found in euthyroid patients, that is, the correlation of titers with thyroid functional status is contradictory (Amino et al., 1976, Aksoy et al., 2005; Ito et al., 2006). Pathogenitic role of TPO Abs is not clearly established, but they are recognized as marker of aitoimmune thyroid diseases and the presence of TPO Abs indicates that, the processes of thyroid destruction started many years, before establishment of thyroid hypofunction (Kraiem, 1998). Thyroid cells undergoing apoptosis occur with high level of frequency in thyroids from patients with Hashimoto's thyroiditis (Kotani et al., 1995; Okayasu et al., 1995; Tanimoto et al., 1995). Many of the apoptotic cells in these glands are detected in areas of disrupted follicles in proximity to infiltrating lymphoid cells (Kotani et al., 1995; Hammond et al., 1997). This suggests that the thyroid destruction in this disease occurs through thyroid cell apoptosis.

In hypothyroid Hashimoto's patients both the level of MDA tended to be higher as well as the cholesterol levels compared to euthyroid patients and patients treated with LT4. This might lead to the development and progression of atherosclerosis and possibly contribute to enhanced atherosclerosis risk in this group.

Our data showed a lack of significant changes in activities of SOD in all groups of Hashimoto's patients compared to controls, but in contrast, the results concerninig GPX and

CAT activities differed significantly in studied groups. At high concentrations ROS have been reported to induce oxidative damage to membrane lipids, proteins and DNA, and that might result in cell death by necrosis or apoptosis (Gamaley & Klyubin, 1999; Hampton & Orrenius, 1997). Both GPX and CAT are major defense against harmful side effect of ROS in cells and in cultured thyrocytes both have a high capacity to degrade exogenious H_2O_2 (Björkman & Ekholm, 1995). Specifically, the observations indicate that GPX is involved in the degradation of fairly low H_2O_2 levels (100 μmol/l) whereas CAT is required to degrade H_2O_2 at mmol/l concentrations. In thyroid tissue GPX is active in the cytosol and conceivably degrade H_2O_2 produced at the apical plasma membrane as soon as it enters the cell. CAT on the other hand, is mainly enclosed in the peroxisomes and therefore not directly accessible at the side of H_2O_2 production. It is thus possible that the impaired GPX and CAT activities may lead to H_2O_2-induced apoptosis to thyroid cells in Hashimoto's thyroiditis patients.

Our study clearly demonstrates lower activities on both enzymes - CAT and GPX in euthyroid Hashimoto's patients. In hypothyroid stage, GPX production increased probably through hyperstimulation of TSH receptor by TSH (Beckett & Arthur, 2005), but CAT activity remained reduced. Significant negative linear correlation was found between activities of GPX and CAT in control group, but no correlation was noted between activities of GPX and CAT in patient's groups. In *in vitro* study Demelash et al. found that impaired capacity of GPX to degrade H_2O_2 in cultured thyroid pig cells aggravates the apoptic response (Demelash et al., 2004). This data and our results suggest the possibility that reduced GPX and CAT activities in euthyroid Hashimoto's patients might participate in the initiation of the autoimmune process and might lead to H_2O_2-induced damage of thyroid cells related to cytosolic oxidative stress. The compensatory increased activity of GPX in hypothyroid stage of disease is not sufficient to protect the thyrocytes from harmful effects of excess H_2O_2.

After restoring euthyroidism with LT4 medication MDA reached levels close to control group and CAT activity increased while GPX again tended to be lower. Under *in vitro* conditions thyroid hormones triidothyronine and thyroxine revealed the capacity to scavenge free radicals (Aziol et al., 2001). Erdamar et al. demonstrate an increased generation of reactive oxygen species and impairment of the antioxidant system in patients with hypothyroidism due to Hashimoto's thyroiditis.; after restoring euthyroidism the values normalize (Erdamar et al.,2008). These findings indicate that thyroid hormones have a strong impact on oxidative stress and the antioxidant system. Our results demonstrate that treatment with LT4 in Hashimoto's patients is useful, but insufficient to normalize all of parameters of oxidative stress. Aksoy et al. found significant decrease of TPO Abs and Tg Abs in euthyroid Hashimoto's thyroiditis after prophylactic thyroid hormone replacement, but increase of CD8+ cell counts (Askoy et al., 2005). We may suppose that thyroid hormones in small doses may be used in some groups of euthyroid Hashimoto's thyroiditis patients e.g. with subtle brain dysfunction or depression in view of their antioxidant properties.

Selenium supplementation produced a significant decline in TPO Abs in hypothyroid Hashimoto's patients (Gärtner et al., 2002; Duntas et al., 2003). In experimental study selenium increases cellular levels of GPX and CAT (Alvarado al., 2006). Our results indicate a deficiency of cellular antioxidative defense in Hashimoto's thyroiditis patients in all stages of disease and the observed imbalance may be connected to the processes of thyroid cell apoptosis. We may speculate that the supplementation with antioxidants including selenium, from an early stage of the disease, in addition to thyroid hormone replacement may have positive benefit in Hashimoto's disease's treatment.

4. Conclusion

In the past decade, significant progress has been made in our understanding of the genetic and environmental triggers contributing to HD. Meanwhile, HT is also a heterogeneous disorder exhibiting various clinicopathological presentations and outcomes. The thyroid autoantibodies, cytokines and antioxidative cellular enzymes are involved in the severity of Hashimoto's thyroiditis and they may be influenced by ethnic differences and environmental factors. The determination of cytokines in peripheral blood provides information about the involvement of cytokine network in the severity of Hashimotos's thyroiditis and variations in their concentrations may be connected with different clinical course of disease in patients. Our results have shown that IL-12 and IL-18 play an influential role in inflammatory response; in the induction and perpetuation of chronic inflammation in autoimmune thyroiditis. These findigs suggest that antagonists to these cytokines may have a potential therapeutic role against Hashimoto's thyroiditis. We found a deficiency of cellular antioxidative defense in Hashimoto's thyroiditis patients in all stages of disease and the observed imbalance may be connected to the processes of thyroid cell apoptosis. Levothyroxine treatment and the supplementation with antioxidants mainly with selenium restore the imbalance, but what is needed is a new type of antioxidant, such as a CAT/GPX mimetic, that works continuously and may be a powerful new approach for correction of Hashimoto's thyroiditis-induced oxidative stress. Further studies are necessary to establish the exact mechanism of autoantibodies, cytokines and antioxidant enzymes interaction influencing the severity of Hashimoto's thyroiditis.

5. Acknowledgements

This work was partially supported by Grant for Scientific research project 3/2009 of The Medical Faculty, Trakia University, Stara Zagora from Ministry of Education, Science and Sports Bulgaria.

6. References

Abbas A.; Lichtman A. & Pober J. (1994) *Cellular and Molecular Immunology*. 2nd Ed. Philadelphia: W.B. Saunders Company.

Ajjan R.A; Watson P.F & Weetman A.P. (1996) Cytokines and thyroid function. *Advances in Neuroimmunology,*Vol. 6, pp 359-386.

Ajjan R.A; Watson P.F & Weetman A.P. (1997) Detection of IL-12, IL-13 and IL-15 messenger ribonucleic acid in the thyroid of patients with autoimmune thyroid disease. *J Clin Endocrinol Metab* Vol. 82, No. 2, pp. 666-669.

Akinci B.; Comiekci A.; Yener S.; Bayraktar F.; Demir T.; Azcan M.A.; Yuksel F &Yesil S. (2008) Hashimoto's thyroiditis, but not treatment of hypothyroidism, is associated with altered TGF-beta 1 levels. *Arch Med Res*, Vol. 39, No 4, pp. 397-401.

Akita K.; Ohtsuki T.; Nukada Y.; Tanimoto T.; Namba M.; Okura T.; Takakura-Yamamoto R.; Torigoe K.; Gu Y.; Su M. S. S. *et al.* (1997). Involvement of caspase-1 and caspase-3 in the production and processing of mature human interleukin-18 in monocytic THP.1 cells. *J. Biol. Chem.* Vol. 272, pp 26595-26603.

Aksoy DY, Kerimoglu U, Okur H.; Canpinar H.; Karaagauglu E,; Yetin S. Kansu E. & Gedik O. (2005) Effects of prophylactic thyroid hormone replacement in euthyroid Hashimoto's thyroiditis. *Endocr J*, Vol. 52, No 3, pp 337-343.

Al-Gubory K.; Garrel K.; Delatouche L.; Heyman Y. & Chavatte-Palmer P. (2010) Antioxidant adaptive responses of extraembryonic tissues from cloned and non-cloned bovine conceptuses to oxidative stress during early pregnancy. *Reproduction*, Vol. 140, pp 175–181 www.reproduction-online.org

Al-Humaidi MA. Serum cytokine levels in Graves' disease. (2000) *Saudi Med J* Vol. 7, pp. 639-644.

Alvarado C.; Alvarez P.; Jimenez L. & De la Fuente M. (2006) Oxidative stress in leukocytes from young prematurely aging mice is reversed by supplementation with biscuits rich in antioxidants. *Dev Comp Immunol;*, Vol. 30, No 12, 1168-1180.

Amiot F.; Fitting C.; Tracey K.; Cavaillon J.M. & Dautry F. (1997). Lipopolysaccharide-Induced Cytokine Cascade and Lethality in LT-α/TNF-α Deficient Mice. *Molecular Medicine.* Vol. 12, No 3, pp 864-875.

Amino N.; Hagan SR.; Yamada N. & Refetoff H.S. (1976) Measurement of circulating thyroid microsomal antibodies by the tanned red cell haemagglutination technique: its usefulness in the diagnosis of autoimmune thyroid disease. *Clin Endocrinol*, Vol. 5, 115-125.

Ashhab Y.; Dominguez O.; Sospedra M.; Roura-Mir C.; Lucas-Martin A. & Pujol-Borrell R. (1999) A one-tube polymerase chain reaction protocol demonstrates CC chemokine overexpression in Graves' disease glands. *J Clin Endocrinol Metab* Vol. 84, pp. 2873-2882.

Azmi N.; Ajjan R.A.; Findlay C.; Watson P.F. & Weetman A.P. (1997) The detection of IL-14, IL-16 and IL-17 mRNA in the thyroid of patients with autoimmune thyroid disease. *J Endocrinol*, Vol. 155 (supp), p74.

Bartalena L.; Tanda M.L.; Piantanida E.; Lai A.; Compri E. & Lombardi V. (2007) Environment and thyroid autoimmunity; In Wiersinga W.M.; Drexhage H.A.; Weetman A.P et all. (eds.): *The Thyroid and autoimmunity*: Merck European Thyroid SymposiumNoordwijk 2006, June 15-18. Stuttgart, Thieme, 2007, pp 60-73.

Beckett G.J. & Arthur J.R.(2005) Selenium and endocrine systems. *J. Endocrinol.*,Vol.184, pp 455-465.

Beers R. & Sizer T. (1952) Spectrophotometric method for measuring the breakdown of hydrogen peroxide by catalase. *J Biol Chem*, Vol. 195, pp 133-138.

Björkman U. & Ekholm R. (1995) Hydrogen peroxide degradation and glutathione peroxidase activity in cultures of thyroid cells. *Mol Cell Endocrinol*, Vol. 111, pp 99-107.

Bonita R.E.; Rose N.R.; Rasooly L.; Caturegli P.& Burek C.L. (2003). Kinetics of mononuclear cell infiltration and cytokine expression in iodine-induced thyroiditis in the NOD-H2h4 mouse. *Exp. Mol. Pathol.* Vol. 74, pp 1-12.

Boraschi D. & Dinarello C.A. (2006) IL-18 in autoimmunity: review. *Eur. Cytokine Netw.*, Vol. 17, No 4, pp 224-252

Brossart P.; Grunebach F.; Stuhler G.; Reichardt V. L.; Mohle R.; Kanz L. & Brugger W. (1998). Generation of functional human dendritic cells from adherent peripheral blood monocytes by CD40 ligation in the absence of granulocyte-macrophage colony-stimulating factor. *Blood* Vol. 92 pp 4238-4247.

Cadet J.; Delatour T.; Douki T.; Gasparutto D.; Pouget J.P.; Ravanat J.L.; & Sauviago S. (1999) Hydroxyl radicals and DNA base damage. *Mutat Res*, Vol. 424, pp 9-21.

Canaris G.J.; Manowitz N.R. Mayor G.M. & Ridgway E.C. (2000) The Colorado thyroid disease prevalence studies. *Arch. Int. Med.* 160, 526-534.

Chiovato L.; Bassi P.; Santini F.; Mammoli C.; Lapi P.; Carayon P. & Pinchera A. (1993) Antibodies producing complement-mediated thyroid cytotoxicity in patients with atrophic or goitrous autoimmune thyroiditis. *J. Clin. Endocrinol. Metab.* Vol. 77, pp. 1700-1705.

Choi E.; Shin I.; Bhang D.; Lee D.; Bae B.; Kang M.; Kim D.; Hwang M.; Lee C. & Youn H. (2006) Hormonal changes and cytokine mRNA expression in peripheral blood mononuclear cells during the development of canine autoimmune thyroiditis. *Clin Exp Immunol*, Vol. 146, No 1, pp 101-108.

Clark EA & Shu G.(1990) Association between IL-6 and CD40 signaling. IL-6 induces phosphorylation of CD40 receptors. *J Immunol.* Vol. 145, No 5, pp 1400-14066

Colin I.M.; Isaac J.; Dupret P.; Ledant T. & Hautcourt J.L. (2004) Functional lymphocyte subset assessment of the Th1/Th2 profile in patients with autoimmune thyroiditis by flowcytometric analysis of peripheral lymphocytes. *J Biol Regul Homeost Agents*, Vol.18, No 1, pp. 72-76.

Czarniecki C.W.; Chiu H.H.; Wong G.H.; McCabe S.M. & Palladino M.A. (1988) Transforming growth factor-ß1 modulates the expression of class II histocompatibility antigens on human cells. *J Immunol*, Vol.140 pp. 4217–4223.

Czarnocka B.; Ruf J.; Ferrand M.; Carayon P.& Lissitzky S.. (1985) Purification of the human thyroid peroxidase and its identification as the microsomal antigen involved in autoimmune thyroid diseases. *FEBS Letts* Vol. 190, pp 147-151.

Das K. & Chainy G.B. (2001) Modulation of rat liver mitochondrial antioxidant defense system by thyroid hormone. *Biochim. Biophys. Acta*; Vol 27, pp 1-13.

Davies T.F. & Amino N. (1993) A new classification for human autoimmune thyroid disease. *Thyroid*, Vol. 3 pp 331-333.

Davies T.F.; Martin A. & Graves P.N. (1988) Human autoimmune thyroid diseases: cellular and molecular aspects. *Bailliere's Clin Endocrinol Metab*, Vol. 2, pp 911-939.

Dayan C.M. & Daniels G.H. (1996) Chronic autoimmune thyroiditis. *N Engl J Med*, Vol. 335, pp 99-107.

Delves P, Roitt I (eds). 1998. *Encyclopedia of Immunology.* 2nd Ed. San Diego: Academic Press.

Demelash A.; Kalsson J-O.; Nilsson M.. & Björkman U.S. (2004) Selenium has a protective role in caspase-3-dependent apoptosis induced by H2O2 in primary cultured pig thyrocytes. *Eur J Endocrinol*; Vol. 150, pp 841-849.

De Zwart L.L.; Meerman J.H. Commendeur J.N. & Vermulen N.P. (1999) Biomarkrs of free radical damageapplications in experimental animals and in humans. *Free Radical Biology & Medicine*, vol. 26, No 1-2, pp 202-226.

Dinarello CA. Interleukin-18. (1999) *Methods, Vol.* 19, pp 121-132.

Doullay F.; Ruf J.; Codaccioni J.L. & Carayon P. (1991) Prevalence of autoantibodies to thyroperoxidase in patients with various thyroid and autoimmune diseases. *Autoimmunity* Vol. 9, pp 237- 244.

Druet P.; Sheela R. & Pelletier L. (1996) Th1 and Th2 cells in autoimmunity. *Chem Immunol*, Vol. 63, pp 138-170.

Duntas L.H.; Mantzou E.; & Koutras D.A. (2003) Effects of a six month treatment with selenomethionine in patients with autoimmune thyroiditis. *Eur J Endocrinol*, Vol. 148, pp 389-393

Duntas L.H. (2009). Selenium and inflammation: underlying anti-inflammatory mechanism. *Horm Metab Res*. Vol. 41, pp 443-447.

Elenkov l.J. & Chrousos G.P. (1999). Stress hormones, Th1/Th2 patterns, pro/anti-inflammatory cytokines and susceptibility to disease. *TEM*. Vol.10, No 9, 359-367.

Erdamar H.; Demirci H.; Yaman H.; Erbil MK.; Yakar T.; Sancak B.; Elbeg S; Biberoğlu G & Yetkin I.(2008) The effect of hypothyroidism, hyperthyroidism, and their treatment on parameters of oxidative stress and antioxidant status. *Clin Chem Lab Med.*, Vol. 46, No7, 1004-1010

Ericsson U.B.; Christensen S.B. & Thorell J.I. (1985) A high prevalence of thyroglobulin autoantibodies in adults with and without thyroid disease as measured with a sensitive solid-phase immunosorbent radioassay. *Clin Immunol Immunopathol*, Vol. 37, pp 154-162.

Fantuzzi G. & Dinarello C. A. (1999). Interleukin-18 and interleukin-1 beta: two cytokine substrates for ICE (caspase-1). (Review) *J. Clin. Immunol.*Vol. 19, pp 1-11.

Fayadat L. ; Niccoli-Sire P. ; Lanet J. & Franc J-L. (1999) Role of heme in intracellular trafficking of thyroperoxidase and involvement of H_2O_2 generated at the apical surface of thyroid cells in autocatalytic covalent heme binding. *J Biol Chem*, Vol. 274 pp 10533-10558.

Fehniger T.A & Caligiuri A. Interleukin 15: biology and relevance to human disease (2001) 97, *Blood* Vol. 97, No 1, pp. 14-32.

Fridovich I. (1978) Oxygen free radicals and tissue damage: chairman's introduction. *Ciba Found Symp*. Jun 6-8; Vol. 65, pp 1-4.

Gadjeva V.; Vlajkova T.; Popova S.; Hristakieva E.; Ivanova V.; Goicheva P. & Hritozov D. (2000) Reactive oxygen species, antioxidant enzymes and human diseases. *Bulgarian medicine*, Vol. 8, No 5, pp 21-24.

Gamaley I.A. & Klyubin I.V. (1999) Roles of reactive oxygen species: signaling and regulation of cellular functions. *Intern Rev Cytol*, Vol. 188, pp 203-255.

Gärtner R.; Gasnier BCH.; Dietrich W.; Krebs B. & Angstwurm MWA (2002). Selenium supplementation in patients with autoimmune thyroiditis decrease thyroid peroxidase antibodies concentrations. *J Clin Endocrinol Metab*, Vol. 87, pp 1687-1691.

Gerenova J. & Gadjeva V. (2006) Influence of methimazole treatment on parameters of oxidative stress in patients with Graves' disease. *Comp Clin Pathol*, Vol. 15, pp 49-54.

Gerenova J. & Gadjeva V. (2007) Oxidative stress and antioxidant enzyme activities in patients with Hashimoto' thyroiditis. *Comp Clin Pathol*, Vol. 16, pp 259-264.

Gordon S. (2003) Alternative activation of macrophages. *Nat Rev Immunol*, Vol. 3, pp 23-35.

Gracie JA, Robertson SE, McInnes IB. Interleukin-18 (2003) *J Leukoc Biol*, Vol. 73, pp 213-224.

Grande J.P. (1997) Role of transforming growth factor-ß in tissue injury and repair. *Proc Soc Exp Biol Med*, Vol. 214, pp 27–40

Guo J.; Jaume J.C; Rapoport B. & McLachlan S.M. (1997) Recombinant thyroid peroxidase-specific Fab converted to immunoglobulin G (IgG) molecules: evidence for thyroid cell damage by IgG1, but not IgG4, autoantibodies. *J Clin Endocrinol Metab*, Vol. 82, pp 925-931.

Halacheva K., Gerenova J. & Dimova S. (2005) Increased levels of serum interleukin 12 in patients with autoimmune thyroid diseases. *Clinical Application of Immunology*, Vol.3, No 21, pp 480-484.

Halliwell B. (1991) Reactive oxygen species in living systems: source, biochemistry, and role in human disease. *Am J Med.*, Vol. 91, pp 14-22

Hammond L.J.; Lowdell M.W.; Cerrano P.G.; Goode A.W.; Bottazzo G.F. & Mirakian R. (1997) Analysis of apoptosis in relation to tissue destruction associated with Hashimoto's autoimmune thyroiditis. *J Pathol*; Vol. 182, pp 138-144.

Hampton M.B. & Orrenius S. (1997) Dual regulation of caspase activity by hydrogen peroxide: implications for apoptosis. *FEBS Lett*, Vol. 414, pp 552-556.

Hashimoto H. (1912) Zur Kenntniss der lymphomatosen Veranderung der Schilddruse (Struma lymphomatosa). *Arch Klin Chir*; Vol. 97, pp 219-248.

Heinrich P.; Castell J.; & Audust T. (1990) Interleukin-6 and the acute phase response *Biochem. J.* Vol. 265, pp 621-636

Heuer M.; Aust G.; Ode-Hakim S. & Scherbaum W.A.(1996) Different cytokine mRNA profile in Graves' disease, Hashimoto's thyroiditis, and non-autoimmune thyroid disorders determined by quantitative reverse transcriptase polymerase chain reaction (RT-PCR). 6, *Thyroid*, Vol. 6, No 2, pp. 97-105.

Heufler C.; Koch F.; Stanzl U.; Topar G.; Wysocka M.; Trinchieri G.; Enk A.; Steinman R.M.; Romani N. & Schuler G. (1996) Interleukin-12 is produced by dendritic cells and mediates T helper 1 development as well as interferon- production by T helper 1 cells. *Eur J Immunol* Vol. 26, pp 659–668

Hidaka Y.; Okumura M.; Shimaoka Y.; Takeoka K.; Tada H. & Amino N. (1998) Increased serum concentration of interleukin-5 in patients with Graves' disease and Hashimoto's thyroiditis. *Thyroid* Vol. 8, pp. 235-239

Hsieh C.S.; Macatonia S.E.; Tripp C.S.; Wolf S.F.; O'Garra A. & Murphy K.M. (1993) Development of TH1 CD4+ T cells through IL-12 produced by Listeria-induced macrophages. *Science* Vol. 260 pp 547–549.

Ito C.; Watanabe M.; Okuda N.; Watanabe C. & Iwatani Y. (2006) Association between the severity of Hashimoto's disease and the functional +874 A/T polymorphism in the interferon-γ gene. *Endocrine journal*, Vol. 53, No 4, pp. 473-478.

Janeway C.; Travers J.; Mark Walport M.; & Shlomchik M.(2001) The Immune System in Health and Disease *Immunobiology*, 5th edition New York: Garland Science.

Karanikas G.; Schuetz M.; Wahl K.; Paul M.; Kontur S.; Pietschmann P.; Kletter K.; Dudczak R. & Willheim M. (2005) Relation of anti-TPO autoantibody titre and T-lymphocyte cytokine production patterns in Hashimoto's thyroiditis *Clinical Endocrinology,* Vol. 63 No 2, pp 191–196.

Kinnula V.L.; Pietarinen P.; Aalto K.; Virtanen I. & Raivio K.O. (1995) Mitochondrial superoxide dismutase induction does not protect epithelial cells during oxidant exposure in vitro. *Am J Physiol.* Vol. 268, pp 71-77.

Kohno K.; Kataoka J.; Ohtsuki T.; Suemoto Y.; Okamoto I.; Usui M.; Ikeda M. & Kurimoto M. (1997). IFN-gamma-inducing factor (IGIF) is a costimulatory factor on the activation of Th1 but not Th2 cells and exerts its effect independently of IL-12. *J. Immunol.* Vol. 158, pp 1541-1550.

Komosinska-Vassev K.; Olczyk K.; Kucharz E.J.; Marcisz C.; Winsz-Szczotka K. & Kotulska A. (2000) Free radical activity and antioxidant defense mechanisms in patients with hyperthyroidism due to Graves' disease during therapy. *Clin Chim Acta,* Vol. 300, pp 107-117.

Kotani T.; Aratake Y.; Hirai K.; Fukazawa Y.; Sato H. & Ohtaki S. (1995) Apoptosis in thyroid tissue from patients with Hashimoto's thyroiditis. *Autoimmunity,* Vol. 20, pp 231-236.

Kraiem Z. (1998) The measurement of antithyroid autoantibodies in the diagnosis and management of thyroid autoimmune disease. *Clin Rev Allergy Immunol,* Vol. 16, 219-225.

Kimura H.; Tzou S.C.; Rocchi R.; Kimura M.; Suzuki K.; Parlow A.F.; Rose N.R.; & Caturegli P. (2005) Interleukin (IL)-12-driven primary hypothyroidism: the contrasting roles of two Th1 cytokines (IL-12 and interferon -γ). *Endocrinology,* Vol. 146, No 8, pp 3642-3651.

Lebel -Binay S.; Berger A.; Zinzindohoue F.; Cugnenc P-H.; Thiounn N.; Fridman W.H & Pages F. (2000) Inetrleukin-18: biological properties and clinical implications. *European Cytokine Network,* Vol. 11, No 1, pp. 15-26.

Lee G.L.; Ellingsworth L.R.; Gillis S.; Wall R. & Kincade P.W. (1987) ß Transforming growth factors are potential regulators of B lymphopoiesis. *J Exp Med,* Vol. 166, pp 1290–1299

Letterio J.J. & Roberts A.B. (1998) Regulation of immune responses by TGF-ß. *Annu Rev Immunol* Vol. 16, pp 137–161

Liew F.Y. (2003) The role of innate cytokines in inflammatory response. *Immunol. Lett.,* Vol. 85, No 2, pp 131-134.

Lee F, Chiu CP, Wideman J, Hodgkin P, Hudak S, Troutt L, Ng T, Moulds C, Coffman R, Zlotnik A, et al. (1989) Interleukin-6. A multifunctional regulator of growth and differentiation. *Ann N Y Acad Sci.,* Vol. 557 pp 215-228

Liu Z.; Wang H.; Xiao W.; Wang C.; Liu G. & Hong T. (2010) Thyrocyte interleukin-18 expression is up-regulated by interferon-γ and may contribute to thyroid distruction in Hashimoto's thyroiditis. *Int J Exp Pathol,* Vol 91, No 5, pp 420-425.

Macatonia S.E.; Hsieh C.S.; Murphy K.M. & O'Garra A. (1993) Dendritic cells and macrophages are required for Th1 development of CD4+ T cells from ß TCR transgenic mice: IL-12 substitution for macrophages to stimulate IFN- production is IFN--dependent. *Int Immunol* Vol. 5, pp 1119–1128

Mahoney J.J.; Vreman H.; Stevenson D.K. & Van Kessel A.L. (1993) Measurement of carboxyhemoglobin and total hemoglobin by five specialized spectrophotometers (CO-oximeters) in comparison with reference methods. *Clin Chem,* Vol 39, pp 1693-1700.

Mantovani A, Sozzani S, Locati M, Allavena P, Sica A. (2002) Macrophage polarization: tumor-associated macrophages as a paradigm for polarized M2 mononuclear phagocytes. *Trends Immunol, Vol.* 23, pp 549-555.

Mantovani A, Sica A, Sozzani S, Allavena P, Vecchi A, Locati M. (2004)The chemokine system in diverse forms of macrophage activation and polarization. *Trends Immunol, Vol.* 25, pp 677-686.

Mariotti S.; Caturegli P.; Piccolo P.; Barbesino G. & Pinchera A. (1990) Antithyroid peroxidase autoantibodies in thyroid diseases. J *Clin Endocrinol Metab* Vol. 71, pp 661-669.

Mazziotti G.; Sorvillo F.; Naclerio C.; Farzati A.; Cioffi M.; Perna R.; Valentini G.; Farzati B.; Amato G.; & Carella C. (2003) Type-1 response in peripheral CD4+ ana CD8+ T cells from patients with Hashimoto's thyroiditis. *Eur J Endocr,* Vol. 148, pp. 383-388.

Micallef M. J.; Ohtsuki T.; Kohno K.; Tanabe F.; Ushio S.; Namba M.; Tanimoto T.; Torigoe K.; Fujii M.; Ikeda M. *et al.* (1996). Interferon-gamma-inducing factor enhances T helper 1 cytokine production by stimulated human T cells: synergism with interleukin-12 for interferon-gamma production. *Eur. J. Immunol.* Vol. 26, pp 1647-1651.

Mitcham C, Ed. (2005) *Encyclopedia of Science, Technology, and Ethics.* Detroit: Macmillan Reference. 2378 pp. 4 vols.

Morinobi A.; Kanno Y.& O'Shea J.J. (2004) Discrete role for histone acetylation in human T helper 1 cell – specific gene expression. *J. Biol. Chem.* Vol. 279, pp 49640-49646

Mosmann T. R. & Sad S. (1996) The expanding universe of T-cell subsets: Th1, Th2 and more. *Immunol. Today,* Vol.17, pp 138-146.

Mosser DM. (2003) The many faces of macrophage activation. *J Leukoc Biol,* Vol. 73, pp 209-212.

Murphy K.M. & Reiner S.L. (2002) The lineage decisions of helper T cells. *Nat. Rev. Immunol.* Vol.2, pp 933-944.

Nawata Y, Eugui EM, Lee SW & Allison AC. (1989) IL-6 is the principal factor produced by synovia of patients with rheumatoid arthritis that induces B-lymphocytes to secrete immunoglobulins. *Ann N Y Acad Sci.,* Vol. 557, pp 230-238.

Nishikawa T.; Yamashita S.; Namba H.; Usa T.; Tominaga T.; Kimura H.; Izumi M. & Nagataki S. Interferon-g inhibition of human thyrotropin receptor gene expression. (1993) *J Clin Endocrinol Metab* Vol. 77, pp. 1084-1089.

Nilsson M.; Husmark J.; Bjokman U. & Ericson L.E. (1998) Cytokines and thyroid epithelial integrity: Interleukin-1 a induces dissociation of the junctional complex and paracellular leakage in filter-cultured human hydrolytes. *J. Clin. Endocrinol. Metab.* Vol. 83, pp 945-952.

Noel R.R.; Raphael B. & Burek C.L. (2002) Iodine: an environmental trigger of thyroiditis. *Autoimmun. Rev.*, Vol. 1; No 1-2, pp 97-103.

Nordyke R.A.; Gilbert F.I.; Miyamoto L.A. & Fleury K.A. (1993) The superiority of antimicrosomal over antithyroglobulin antibodies for detecting Hashimoto's thyroiditis. *Arch Intern Med*, Vol.153, pp 862-865.

Nunez J. & Pommier J. (1982) Formation of thyroid hormones. *Vitam Horm*, Vol. 39, pp 175-229.

Oh S.; Perera L.P.; Terabe M.; Ni L.; Waldmann T.A. & Berzofsky J.A. (2008) IL-15 as a mediator of CD4+ help for CD8+ T cell longevity and avoidance of TRAIL-mediated apoptosis. *Proc. Natl Acad Sci U S A* Vol. 105, No 13, pp 5201-5206.

Okamura H.; Nagata K.; Komatsu T.; Tanimoto T.; Nukata Y.; Tanabe F.; Akita K.; Torigoe K.; Okura T.; Fukuda S, *et al.* (1995). A novel costimulatory factor for gamma interferon induction found in the livers of mice causes endotoxic shock. *Infect. Immun.* Vol. 63, pp 3966-3972.

Olee T.; Hashimoto S.; Quach J. & Lotz M. (1999). IL-18 is produced by articular chondrocytes and induces proinflammatory and catabolic responses. *J. Immunol.* Vol. 162, pp 1096-1100.

Okamura H.; Tsutsi H.; Komatsu T.; Yutsudo M.; Hakura A.; Tanimoto T.; Torigoe K.; Okura T.; Nukada Y.; Hattori K. *et al.* (1995). Cloning of a new cytokine that induces IFN-gamma production by T cells. *Nature* Vol. 378, pp 88-91.

Okayasu I.; Saegusa M.; Fujiwara M.; Hara Y. & Rose N.R. (1995) Enhanced cellular proliferative activity and cell death in chronic thyroiditis and thyroid papillary carcinoma. *J Cancer Res Clin Oncol*, Vol. 121, pp 746-752.

Oziol L.; Faure P.; Vergely C.; Rochette L.; Artur Y. & Chomard P. (2001) In vitro free radical scavenging capacity of thyroid hormones and structural analogues. *J Endocrinol*, Vol. 170, pp 197-206.

Paglia D.E. & Valentine W.N. (1967) Studies on the quantitative and qualitative characterization of erythrocyte glutathione peroxidase. *J Lab Clin Med*, Vol 70, pp 158-170.

Palazzo F.F.; Hammond L.J.; Goode A.W. & Mirakian R. (2000) Death of the autoimmune thyrocyte: is it pushed or does it jump? *Thyroid* Vol. 10, pp. 561-572.

Perera L.P.; Goldman C.K. & Waldmann T.A. (1999) Il-15 induces the expression of chemokines and their receptors in T lymphocytes. *J Immunol*, Vol. 162, No 5, pp 2606-2612.

Phenekos C.; Vryonidou A.; Gritzapis A.D.; Baxevanis C.N, Goula M. & Papamichail M. Th1 and Th2 serum cytokine profile characterize patients with Hashimoto's thyroiditis (Th1) and Graves' disease (Th2). (2004) *Neuroimmunomodulation*, Vol. 11, No 4, 209-213.

Plaser Z.A.; Cushman L.L. & Jonson B.C. (1966) Estimation of product of lipid peroxidation (Malonyl Dialdehyde) in biochemical systems. *Anal Biochem*; Vol. 16, pp 359-364.

Prud'homme G.J. & Piccirillo C.A. The inhibitory effects of transforming growth factor-beta-1 (TGF-b1) in autoimmune diseases. (2000), *J Autoimmunity*, Vol. 14, No 1, pp. 23-42.

Puren A. J.; Razeghi P.; Fantuzzi G. & Dinarello C. A. (1998). Interleukin-18 enhances lipopolysaccharide-induced interferon-gamma production in human whole blood cultures. *J. Infect. Dis.* Vol. 178, pp 1830-1834.

Quinn L.S.; Anderson B.G.; Strait-Boday L.; Stroud A.M. & Argiles J.M. (2009). Oversecretion of interleukin-15 from skeletal muscle reduces adiposity. *Am J Physiol Endocrinol Metab, Vol.* 296, No 1, pp 191-202.

Rasmussen A.K.; Kayser L.; Rasmussen U.F. & Bendtzen K. (1994) Influence of tumour necrosis factor-b and interferon-g, separately and added together with interleukin-1b, on the function of cultured human thyroid cells. *J Endocrinol* Vol. 143, pp. 359-365.

Rhee SG. (1999) Redox signaling: hydrogen peroxide as intracellular messenger. *Exp Mol Med,* Vol. 31, pp 53-59.

Riou C.; Remy C.; Rabilloud R.; Rousset B. & Fonlupt P. (1998) H_2O_2 induces apoptoses of pig thyrocytes in culture. *J Endocrinol,* Vol. 156, pp 315-322.

Robinson D.; Shibuya K.; Mui A.; Zonin F.; Murphy E.; Sana T.; Hartley S. B.; Menon S.; Kastelein R.; Bazan F. & O'Garra A. (1997). IGIF does not drive Th1 development but synergizes with IL-12 for interferon-gamma production and activates IRAK and NFkappaB. *Immunity* Vol 7, pp 571-581.

Roitt I.M.; Doniach D.; Campbell P.N. & Hudson R.V. (1956). Auto-antibodies in Hashimoto's disease (lymphadenoid goitre). *Lancet;* Vol. 2, pp 820-821.

Romagnani S. The Th1/Th2 paradigm (1997) *Immunol Today,* Vol. 18, No 6, pp. 263-266.

Rook A.H.; Kehrl J.H.; Wakefield L.M.; Roberts A.B.; Sporn M.B.; Burlington D.B.; Lane H.C. & Fauci A.S. (1986) Effects of transforming growth factor ß on the functions of natural killer cells: depressed cytolytic activity and blunting of interferon responsiveness. *J Immunol* Vol. 136, pp 3916–3920

Sadani G.R. & Nadkarni G.D. (1996) Role of tissue antioxidant defense in thyroid cancers. *Cancer Lett,* Vol. 109, pp 231-235.

Salvi M.; Pedrazzoni M.; Girasoli G.; Giuliani N.; Minelli R.; Wall JR. & Roti E. (2000) Serum concentrations of proinflammatory cytokines in Graves' disease: effect of treatment on thyroid function, ophthalmopathy and cigarette smoking. *Eur J Endocrinol* Vol .143, pp. 197-202.

Schmidt M.; Voell M.; Rahiff I.; Dietlein M.; Kobe C.; Faust M. & Schicha H. (2008) Long-term follow-up of antithyroid peroxidase antibodies in patients with chronic autoimmune thyroiditis (Hashomoto's thyroiditis) treated with levothyroxine. *Thyroid,* Vol.18, No 7, 755-760.

Shevach E.M. (2000) Suppressor T cells:rebirth, function and homeostasis. *Curr Biol,* Vol. 10, pp R572-R5.

Sieminska L., Wojciechowska C.; Kos-Kudla B.; Marek B.; Kajdaniuk D.; Nowak M.; Glogowska-Szelag J.; Foltyn W & Strzelczyk J. (2010) Serum concentrations of leptin, adiponectin,, and interleukin 6 in postmenopausal women wiyh Hashimoto's thyroiditis. *Endokrynol Pol* Vol. 61, No1, pp. 112-116.

Simons P.J.; Delemarre F.G.A. & Drexhage H.A.(1998) Antignen-presenting dendritic cells as regulators of the growth of hydrolytes: A role of interleukin-1b and interleukin-6. *Endocrinology.*Vol. 139, pp. 148-156.

Spilianakis C.G. & Flavell R.A. (2004) Long-range intrachromosomal interactions in the T helper type 2 cytokine locus. *Nat. Immunol*, Vol. 5, pp 1017-1027.

Sterzl I: Cytokines - structure and function (1999) I, *Allergie*, Vol. I, No 2, pp. 82-90.

Strieter R., Kunkel S. & Bone R. (1993). Role of Tumor Necrosis Factor-Alpha in Disease States and Inflammation. *Critical Care Medicine*. Vol. 21 (10 Supplement) pp 447-463.

Sugawara M.; Kita T.; Lee E.D.; Takamatsu J.; Hagen J.A.; Kuma K. & Medeiros - Neto G.A. (1998) Deficiency of thyroid superoxide dismutase in endemic goiter tissue. *J Clin Endocrinol Metab*, Vol. 67, pp 1156-1161.

Sun Y.; Oberley L.W. & Li Y. (1988) A simple method for clinical assay of superoxide dismutase. *Clin Chem*; 34: 497-500.

Tagaya Y.; Bamford R.; DeFilippis A. & Waldmann T. (1996) IL-15: A pleiotropic Cytokine with diverse receptor/signaling pathways whose expression is controlled at multiple levels. *Immunity*, Vol.4, pp 329-336.

Tanimoto C.; Hirakawa S.; Kawasaki H.; Hayakawa N. & Ota Z. (1995) Apoptosis in thyroid diseases: a histochemical study. *Endocr J*, Vol. 42, pp 193-201.

Tato CM.; Laurence A. & O'Shea J.J. (2006) Helper Tcell differentiation enters a new era: le roi est mort; vive le roi! *J Exp Med*, Vol. 203, pp 809-812.

Tomer Y. & Davies T.F. (1993). Infection, thyroid disease and autoimmunity. *Endocrine Rewiews*, Vol.14, No 1, pp 107-120.

Trinchieri G (1993) Interleukin-12 and its role in the generation of TH1 cells. *Immunol Today* Vol. 14, pp 335–338

Trinchieri G (2003) Interleukin-12 and the regulation of innate resistance and adaptive immunity. *Nat Rev Immunol* Vol. 3, pp 133–146.

Van Snick J. (1990) Interleukin-6: An Overview *Annual Review of Immunology*, Vol. 8, pp 253-278

Volpe R. (1995) Human autoimmune thyroid disease: recent advances. In: *Thyroid Autoimmunity* (Eds. D.C. Rayner and B.R. Champion). R.G. Landes Company, Texas, pp 199-230.

Vural P.; Degirmencioglu S.; Erden S. & Gelincik A. (2009) The relationship between transforming growth factor – beta 1, vascular endothelial growth factor, nitric oxide and Hashimoto's thyroiditis. *Int. Immunopharmacol.*, Vol.9. No2, 212-215.

Wallick S.C.; Figari I.S.; Morris R.E.; Levinson A.D. & Palladino M.A. (1990) Immunoregulatory role of transforming growth factor ß (TGF-ß) in development of killer cells: comparison of active and latent TGF-ß1. J *Exp Med* , Vol. 172, pp 1777-1784

Weetman A.P. (2003) Autoimmune thyroid disease: propagation and progression. *Eur J Endocrinol*, Vol. 148, pp 1-9.

Weetman A.P. (2004) Cellular immune responses in autoimmune thyroid diseases. *Clin Endocrinol*, Vol. 61, pp. 405-413.

Weetmann A.P. (2011) Autoimmune thyroid disease; in *Oxford Textbook of Endocrinology and Diabetes on line* 2nd Edition, Eds. Wass J. & Stewart, Oxford Univeristy Press; oted.oxfordmedicine.com

Weetman A.P.; Bright-Thomas R. & Freeman M. (1990) Regulation of interleukin-6 release by human thyrocytes. *J Endocrinol*, Vol. 127, pp. 357–361.

Weetman A.P.; Bennett G.L. & Wong WLT. (1992) Thyroid follicular cells produce interleukin-8. *J. Clin. Endocrinol. Metab.* Vol. 75, pp. 328–330.

Wu Z.; Podack E.R.& McKenzie J.M. (1994) Perforin expression by thyroid infiltrating T cells in autoimmune thyroid disease. *Clin. Exp. Immunol.* Vol. 98, pp. 470-477.

5

Hashimoto's Thyroiditis

Arvin Parvathaneni, Daniel Fischman and Pramil Cheriyath
Pinnacle Health System-Harrisburg Hospital
Harrisburg, Pennsylvania,
USA

1. Introduction

Hashimoto's thyroiditis is a common autoimmune disorder, which causes significant morbidity. Its pathophysiological hallmark is lymphocytic infiltration of thyroid follicles resulting in autoimmune glandular destruction. Various studies have successfully outlined the genetic and environmental factors responsible for the causation of the disease. In this chapter we will discuss our current understanding of these factors and delineate how Hashimoto's thyroiditis serves as a paradigm not just for disease of the thyroid gland, but also for autoimmune disease in the human body. Our focus is on the varying presentations of the disease and the relationship between Hashimoto's thyroiditis and other autoimmune diseases frequently associated with it. The etiological factors and the pathophysiological changes which lead to the development of disease are discussed. Common diagnostic modalities are described, and the need for correlation between the various available diagnostic tests is explained. Various treatment strategies and the appropriate choice for different forms of presentation are discussed. Hashimoto's encephalopathy, a rare complication, will be addressed separately as its unusual presentation often results in misdiagnosis of the underlying pathology.

2. Background

Hashimoto's thyroiditis was first described in 1912 by Dr. Hakuru Hashimoto. Based on the histological findings, Hashimoto originally used the term "Struma Lymphomatosa." Over the years, this disease has been called by several names including lymphocytic thyroiditis, autoimmune thyroiditis, chronic thyroiditis, and lymph adenoid goiter. The debate about the relationship between Hashimoto's thyroiditis and Graves' disease has been ongoing for many decades as they differ in clinical and immunological presentation. However, Hashimoto's thyroiditis and Graves' disease, which depict the two extremes of the clinical spectrum, are now included in a common entity called autoimmune thyroid disease. It is now believed that they share a common autoimmune pathology and are believed to be triggered by multiple genetic and environmental factors. Hashimoto's thyroiditis was initially perceived as an uncommon disease and most cases were incidentally diagnosed through histopathological examination of the thyroid gland after thyroidectomy. The advent of newer diagnostic modalities with increased diagnostic sensitivity made it possible to unveil more cases of Hashimoto's thyroiditis. With the increasing number of cases, the association of Hashimoto's thyroiditis with other autoimmune diseases is being studied extensively. Type 1 diabetes, multiple sclerosis, rheumatoid arthritis, celiac disease, vitiligo, and chronic urticaria have all been reported to be frequently associated with Hashimoto's thyroiditis.

3. Incidence and distribution of the disease

Hashimoto's thyroiditis is about 15-20 times more common in women than in men and frequently involves people between the ages of 30 and 50 years of age. Determining the exact incidence and prevalence rates for Hashimoto's thyroiditis has been difficult due to variable expression of this disease. Some studies estimate that the current prevalence rate in the United States ranges between 0.3%-1.2% (Staii et al., 2010). Other studies estimate the prevalence among the general population to be approximately 2% (Wang et al., 1997). When attempts have been made to characterize the prevalence prospectively, with the aid of organized programs of ultrasound guided biopsy, the prevalence described has been at least 5%. It should be noted that studies employing the diagnostic modality of ultrasound guided biopsy have recorded prevalence rates higher than studies using other investigative modalities (Staii et al., 2010). The National Health and Nutrition Evaluation Study-3 (NHANES-3) study has shown the prevalence of subclinical and clinical hypothyroidism to be 4.6% and 0.3%, respectively, in the United States (Hollowell et al., 2002). The Whickham survey, an epidemiological study conducted in the United States, has revealed the prevalence of hypothyroidism to be 1.5% in females and less than 0.1% in males (Tunbridge et al., 1997). During the past few decades there has been a reported increase in the incidence of Hashimoto's thyroiditis, which could be attributed to newer diagnostic modalities such as needle biopsies and serological tests, and their increased sensitivity when compared to the older methods. (McConahey et al., 1962). Studies about age-specific incidence rates of Hashimoto's thyroiditis indicate the existence of a random distribution in both men and women and have shown an initial lag in the first few years of their life followed by a constant rate after this (Volpe et al., 1973). A few studies have suggested a slight increase in the prevalence of autoimmune thyroiditis in adolescent girls following use of iodized food products ingested to prevent iodine deficiency (Zois et al., 2003).

4. Etiology

The etiology of Hashimoto's thyroiditis is considered to be multifactorial, involving the interplay of various environmental and genetic factors. Studies conducted on the genetic associations of Hashimoto's thyroiditis have shown that the human leukocyte antigen (HLA) region, which plays a major role in other autoimmune disorders, is associated with development of Hashimoto's thyroiditis (Fisher, G.F., 2000). The association of Hashimoto's thyroiditis with various other autoimmune diseases has further reinforced the probable involvement of genetic factors in the etiology. The major histocompatability complex (MHC), cytotoxic T-lymphocyte association (CTLA-4) and the human leukocyte antigen (HLA) are the genetic factors which are purported to play a major role in the pathogenesis. The selection of thyroid cells in the thymus and presentation of antigens in the periphery are modulated by, the human MHC analog, HLA. The sensitivity and specificity of the affinity to bind the peptides and recognize T-cells is determined largely by the genetic polymorphisms exhibited by the MHC molecule. The possible polymorphisms within the MHC molecules play a pivotal role in the predisposition to autoimmune disease (Gebe et al., 2002). The association between the genetics of Hashimoto's thyroiditis and HLA gene loci has been investigated by serotyping the HLA, and deoxyribonucleic acid (DNA) typing the sequence- specific oligonucleotides. Different subsets of HLA genes have been found to show varying degree of associations with Hashimoto's thyroiditis in different races. The HLA class 1 and class 2 genes both showed association with Hashimoto's thyroiditis in Asian populations, while only HLA class 1 demonstrated the association in Caucasians. (Wu et al., 1994). No significant associations have been found between Hashimoto's thyroiditis and HLA class 3 or non-HLA genes of the HLA region (Hunt et al., 2001). An association between CTLA-4 and Hashimoto's thyroiditis has been noted in significant number of cases (Einarsdottir et al., 2003). CTLA-4 plays a vital role in upholding immunological self tolerance in the body and its down regulation is believed to be the initiating step for the pathogenesis of Hashimoto's thyroiditis as well as other autoimmune disorders such as Graves' disease (Chistiakov & Turakulov, 2003).

In addition to the genetic factors numerous external factors also play a vital role in the etiology of the disease, preferentially affecting genetically predisposed individuals. The common environmental factors which act as triggers to initiate the insult on thyroid tissue include infections, cytokine therapy, selenium and iodine intake. Epidemiological studies and animal models have shown that among the factors that initiate the process, iodine appears to be the most significant (Boukis et al., 1983). Some studies have established smoking as an important risk factor for the causation of hypothyroidism in patients with Hashimoto's thyroiditis (Fukata et al., 1996).

5. Pathogenesis

The pathogenesis of Hashimoto's thyroiditis is a complex multistep process which involves various genetic, environmental and immunological factors (Figure 1). In a nut shell, loss of immune tolerance to normal thyroid cells leads to production of antibodies directed against thyroid tissue, which causes the destruction of the thyroid gland. The initial inflammatory changes in the disease process are triggered when genetically predisposed individuals are exposed to the above mentioned environmental factors. The major histocompatability complex (MHC) class 2 antigen presenting cells, which include dendritic cells and macrophages, invade the thyroid gland after the initial inflammatory process. These cells present the autoantigen components of the thyroid gland to the immune system for processing. Among the myriad of potential auto-antigens, thyroglobulin, the main protein produced in thyroid tissue, is believed to play a central role in the pathogenesis of this disease (Champion et al., 1991). The thyroglobulin protein has been reported to have approximately 40 different types of epitopes, which play a vital role in the pathogenesis of the disease (Male et al., 1985). In contrast to the epitope recognition pattern of normal individuals, the epitope recognition pattern of the antibodies in autoimmune thyroid disease is altered triggering immune and inflammatory processes (Dietrich et al., 1991). Thyroid peroxidase, an enzyme that catalyzes the oxidation of iodine, also plays a significant role as an autoantigen in the disease pathogenesis. Moreover, 180 different types of thyroid peroxidase antibodies have been identified, thus far. Studies have confirmed that even though antibodies against thyrotropin receptor and sodium iodide symporter have been detected in patients with autoimmune thyroid disease, they do not play a significant role in the pathogenesis of this condition.

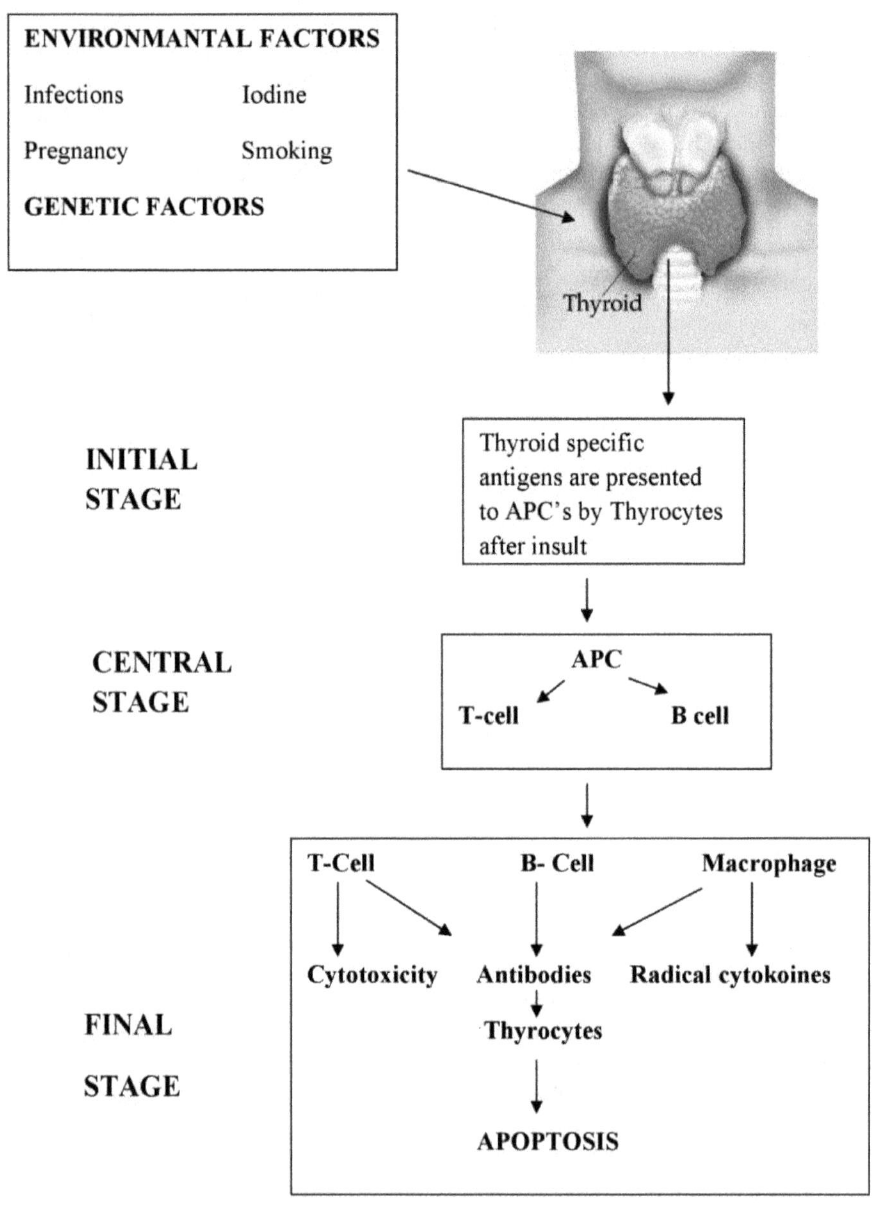

Legend: APC = Antigen Presenting Cell

Fig. 1. A schematic presentation of etiopathogenesis of Hashimoto's thyroiditis. (Casselman, W, G., 1996).

The major step in the pathogenesis is the formation of autoreactive cells directed against the thyroid gland, which could result from defects in central tolerance or defects in the peripheral tolerance. Loss of immune tolerance has been associated with genetically determined immune defects or with the lack of regulatory T-cells which impose the suppressive function (Martin, 1992). This is followed by formation, clonal expansion, and maturation of self-reactive T-lymphocytes and B-lymphocytes in the draining lymph nodes. This step is then followed by a central phase of autoimmunity, characterized by uncontrolled production of self-reactive cells and autoantibodies in response to the presented antigens. This process initially occurs in the lymph nodes but as the disease progresses the production process shifts to the thyroid gland where the development of lymphoid tissue follows. The stimulated B-lymphocytes produce antithyroglobulin (TGAB) and antithyroid peroxidase (ATPO) antibodies which are directed against thyroid cells. The autoreactive T-cells, which are produced in the disease process, infiltrate the thyroid gland and mediate destruction through cytotoxicity with the aid of CD+8 cells. The macrophages which are stimulated in this process produce numerous cytokines which, along with antibodies, initiate the process of tissue destruction via apoptosis.

As a final step in the process, caspases, which are self-activated through proteolytic cleavage, induce enzymes which are directly involved in the destruction of thyroid gland. In a normal thyroid gland, the production of new cells and the destruction of old cells are tightly regulated so that a constant proportion of functioning cells is always present. During the course of the disease, the control over destruction of cells in the thyroid gland is lost. Genetic susceptibility is one of the factors that plays a vital role in deregulation of the regular destructive mechanisms in the thyroid gland. Several other triggers which have an influence on the expression of Bcl-2, the apoptosis inhibitor, or Fasl membrane ligand also are crucial in the initiation of the apoptosis process (Giordano et al., 2001). Thyroid cells in tissue affected with Hashimoto's thyroiditis, when compared to normal thyroid cells, are capable of producing more Fasl proteins leading to an increased tempo of apoptosis (Limachi & Basso, 2002). The severity of the disease and the clinical outcome are determined by the rate at which apoptosis occurs in the thyroid gland. Expression of these proteins has direct correlation to the severity of the disease and as the rate of apoptosis increases, the mass of hormonally-active thyroid tissue decreases resulting in diminished production of thyroid hormones and more significant disease manifestations.

6. Signs and symptoms

Thyroid hormone is capable of influencing the function of every cell in the body. The basic function of thyroid hormone is to increase the basal metabolic rate of the body. The symptoms of Hashimoto's thyroiditis are predominantly due to decreased production of thyroid hormone, which occurs as a result of destruction of thyroid tissue, ultimately leading to decreased metabolism. Indeed, most symptoms are not manifested in the early stages of the disease; as the disease advances and the degree of hypothyroidism increases, the symptoms become more evident. The decreased production of thyroid hormone adversely affects various major organ systems. Dysfunction of the cardiovascular system is manifested as bradycardia, while nervous system dysfunction manifests as slowed speech and delayed reflexes. Gastrointestinal symptoms include constipation, increased bile reflux and ascites. When the metabolic rate drops to a critical level, a life threatening emergency called myxedema coma occurs. Myxedema is usually characterized by hypothermia, hypoglycemia, altered sensorium and severe bradycardia. In severely hypothyroid Individuals, triggers such as stress, infection, surgery and traumatic injuries may also predispose to the development of myxedema.

In contrast to hypothyroid patients, patients in a euthyroid state do not experience any symptoms or exhibit any signs of the disease, and in most cases the diagnosis is incidental. Moreover, some individuals may not present with any clinical features except an enlarged thyroid gland and the diagnosis is made by investigating the goiter. The goiter, by itself, can cause cosmetic disfigurement in its initial stages and as its size increases, it can lead to pressure symptoms including pain in the neck, dysphagia, and dyspnea in some cases. Furthermore, a rapid growth in the goiter is sometimes noted, which should arouse suspicion for a tumor. Tumors of the thyroid gland, which sometimes arise in the background of Hashimoto's thyroiditis, usually manifest as solitary or multiple nodules typically discovered incidentally during a regular physical examination. In addition to the previously noted symptoms, accumulation of the matrix proteins, such as metalloproteases, might lead to swelling of the extremities and face. Though extremely rare in children, Hashimoto's thyroiditis can lead to detrimental effects on growth and physical maturation. Moreover, short stature and mental retardation are the features which are most commonly observed in children suffering from Hashimoto's thyroiditis.

In addition to the symptoms of hypothyroidism, people suffering from Hashimoto's thyroiditis sometimes experience symptoms due to other autoimmune diseases. Muscle pain is present in 25.5% of patients with Hashimoto's thyroiditis. Rheumatic manifestations in autoiummune thyroiditis are reported to be ten times more frequent when compared to nonautoimmune thyroiditis. (Becker et al., 1963). Furthermore, the initial presentation sometimes can be very subtle. For instance, occasionally, irritatability, depression, confusion, and fatigue have been reported as initial complaints in patients later diagnosed with Hashimoto's thyroiditis (Hall et al., 1982). Unfortunately, in many instances these cases were misdiagnosed as psychiatric disorders before being correctly diagnosed as due to thyroid hormone deficiency.

7. Clinical course of the disease

Hashimoto's thyroiditis has a highly variable clinical presentation; patients may either be hypothyroid, euthyroid or hyperthyroid. About 20% of the patients exhibit signs and symptoms of mild hypothyroidism at the initial presentation. However, the severity of the symptoms increases with the progression of the disease (Gordin et al., 1974). This increase in the severity of symptoms is attributed to gradual destruction of the thyroid gland. Furthermore, as the hypothyroidism worsens, the patient is at increased risk of developing myxedema coma as a result of complete thyroid atrophy (Buchanan & Harden, 1965). A goiter, usually with gradual enlargement of the gland, may be the sole presentation in some instances. (Tunbridge et al., 1977). The other features which are usually associated with Hashimoto's thyroiditis are not exhibited along with the goiter.

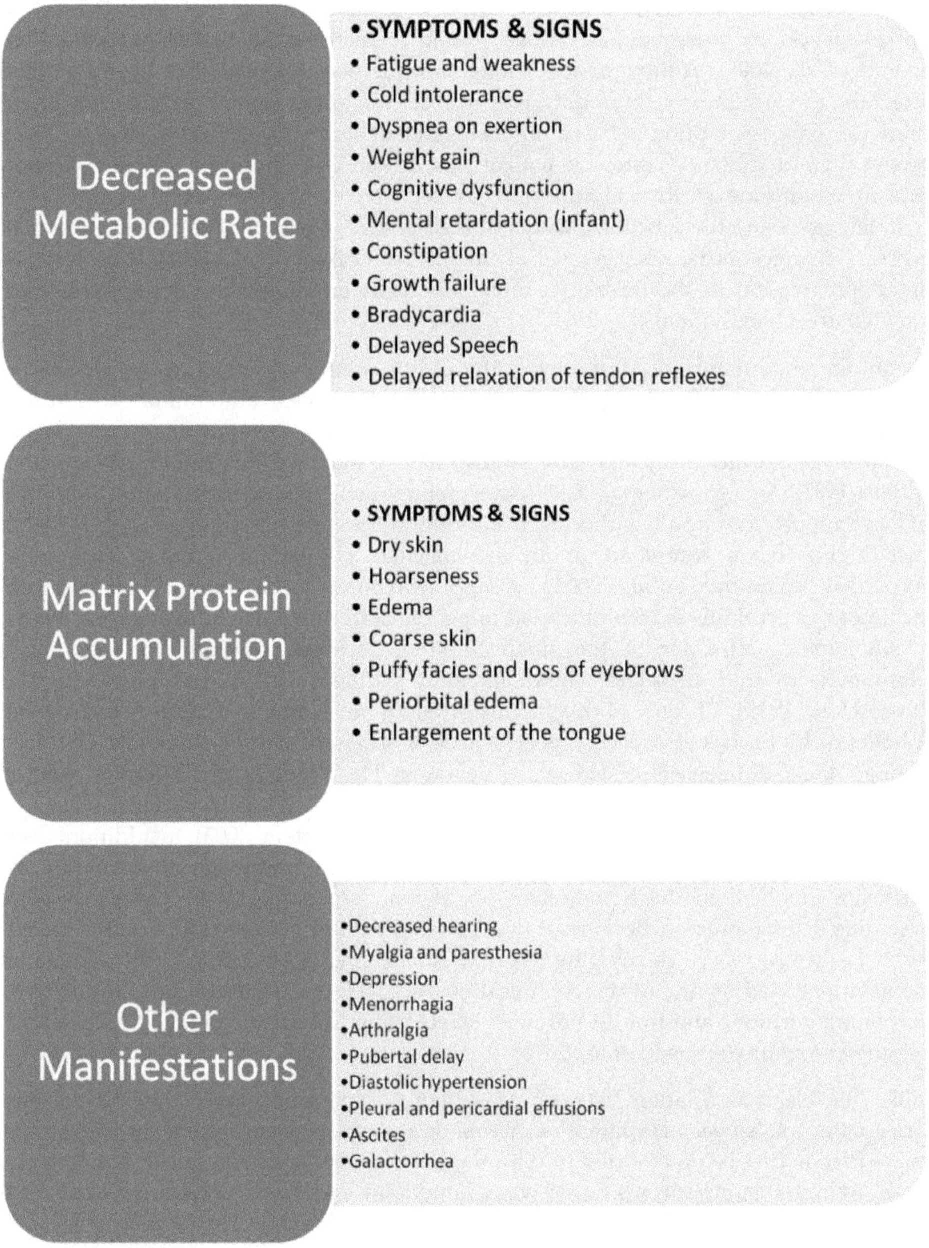

Fig. 2. Symptoms and signs of hypothyroidism based on specific pathophysiology

Some patients are initially euthyroid and are at risk of developing hypothyroidism as the disease progresses. The concomitant presence of a goiter along with elevated thyroid antibody levels, at presentation, has been found to increase the risk of hypothyroidism (Radetti et al., 2006). Although, for a long time, it was believed that hypothyroidism secondary to Hashimoto's thyroiditis was irreversible, some recent studies have proved otherwise. This assumption is based on observational studies which revealed a decline in titers of thyroid antibodies after the patient was treated with thyroid hormone. Therefore, frequent monitoring of thyroid function has been recommended which would help in accurately assessing the functional status of the thyroid and enable the physician to make necessary changes in the management of the disease (Takasu et al., 1992). Identifying the clinical progression of the disease is important in determining the nature of treatment provided to each individual.

The autoimmune nature of Hashimoto's thyroiditis predisposes patients to concomitant development of additional autoimmune diseases. One such autoimmune disorder is systemic lupus erythematosus. This particular association was reported as early as 1957 (Wilkinson & Sacker, 1957) and later studies have confirmed this finding (Weetman & Walport 1987; Pyne & Isenberg, 2002). An increased incidence of Hashimoto's thyroiditis has been reported in adults suffering from vitiligo; the risk has been assessed to be 2.5 times higher when compared to an age-matched population without Hashimoto's thyroiditis (Kakourou et al., 2005). As per Kakourou et al, annual screening for Hashimoto's thyroiditis is recommended in people suffering with vitiligo. Celiac disease, an autoimmune disorder of the small intestine, is more common in people with autoimmune thyroid disorders when compared to those with other thyroid disorders (Cuoco et al., 1999). Chronic idiopathic urticaria, an autoimmune disorder characterized by bouts of hives, has also been reported to be associated with Hashimoto's thyroiditis although the pathogenesis of chronic urticaria in Hashimoto's thyroiditis is not well understood. Furthermore, chronic idiopathic urticaria has also been reported in euthyroid patients who are seropositive for antithyroid antibodies (Rottem, 2003). In addition, the C-cells in the thyroid gland, which are responsible for the production of calcitonin, and which are involved in the homeostasis of calcium, are damaged by the Hashimoto's thyroiditis disease process. Because of this, patients with Hashimoto's thyroiditis patients have an inherent risk of developing hypocalcemia (Lima et al., 1998). Dyslipedemia has also been reported as one of the complications of Hashimoto's thyroiditis, with thyroid stimulating hormone and free T4 hormone levels being inversely correlated with severity of lipid abnormality (Tagami et al., 2010).

Unlike the clear association between Hashimoto's thyroiditis and other autoimmune diseases, the link between Hashimoto's thyroiditis and cancer is not well delineated. Despite the association first being reported in 1951, the link still remains obscure and is a subject of debate. In investigating various tumor types, lymphoma and papillary carcinoma of thyroid (PTC) are most commonly associated with Hashimoto's thyroiditis. The incidence of thyroid carcinoma in people with Hashimoto's thyroiditis has been reported to be as high as 36.4% (Pino Rivero et al., 2004). Although a chimeric gene rearrangement has been proposed as the molecular basis for the development of thyroid carcinoma in the presence of Hashimoto's thyroiditis, recent studies have not supported this supposition. Interestingly, no such rearrangements were detected in patients diagnosed with papillary thyroid cancer in the background of Hashimoto's thyroiditis, while in patients diagnosed first with PTC, the prevalence of these rearrangements was found to be 33% (Nikiforova et al., 2002). Unlike with production of chimeric gene products, the tumor protein P63 is believed to play a vital role in the development of PTC in patients with previously established Hashimoto's thyroiditis. Moreover, supporting evidence can be inferred from the absence of these proteins in thyroid tissue devoid of PTC or Hashimoto's thyroiditis (Unger et al., 2003). Similar to PTC, B-cell lymphoma of the thyroid gland has been found to be associated with Hashimoto's thyroiditis. The histological features of this specific lymphoma have been found to be similar to those of mucosa associated lymphoid tumors (Hygek & Isaacson, 1988).

8. Diagnosis

Assessing the metabolic status of the patient and identifying the type of lesion present are of vital importance in making an accurate diagnosis of Hashimoto's thyroiditis. The first step is to assess the thyroid hormone status, which reflects glandular function. Although the presence of goiter alone, without associated hyperthyroid symptoms, is suggestive of Hashimoto's thyroiditis, the presence of a goiter in a hypothyroid patient is considered to be strongly indicative of Hashimoto's thyroiditis. Triiodothyronine (T3), tetraiodothyronine (T4) and thyroid stimulating hormone (TSH) levels are the commonly employed lab studies used to assess the level of function of the thyroid gland. Among these parameters, TSH has been reported to be the most sensitive marker of hypothyroidism. Even after the diagnosis is established, frequent monitoring of TSH is done to assess the response to treatment and progression of the disease. After the assessment of patient's thyroid function status, the focus shifts to indentifying the presence of antithyroid antibodies. It should be noted that while the presence of antithyroid peroxidase (ATPO) and antithyroglobulin (TGAB) antibodies are both positively correlated with Hashiomoto's thyroiditis, the correlation is slightly higher for TGAB than ATPO. (Kasagi et al., 1996). Even in the absence of hypothyroid symptoms, the presence of antithyroid antibodies would indicate underlying lymphocytic infiltration of the gland, and be indicative of autoimmune disease (Yoshida et al., 1978). In an attempt increase the certainty of the diagnosis, antimicrosomal antibodies have been found to afford greater diagnostic accuracy when compared to antithyroglobulin antibodies. However, for those cases in which Hashimoto's thyroiditis is suspected clinically but antibody titers are not elevated, fine needle aspiration (FNA) and cytological examination continue to play a defining role in establishing the diagnosis (Baker et al., 1982; Kumar et al., 2002; Takashi et al., 2008).

In delineating key cytological findings, extent of lymphocytic infiltration and the presence of Hurthle cells has been found to be directly proportional to the severity of the disease. Also, as the disease progresses, colloid in the thyroid gland is destroyed and the spaces between follicular cells shrink, altering the microscopic appearance of FNA biopsy specimens. In further elaboration on how microscopic appearance correlates with disease severity, extent of involved tissue has been found to be directly proportional to severity of the disease. Despite the diagnostic sensitivity and accuracy of cytological analysis, in some instances, the presence of numerous hyperplastic follicular cells may lead to a false diagnosis of follicular carcinoma. Alternatively, the diagnosis of some neoplasms, like Hurthle cell tumor, could be misdiagnosed as Hashimoto's thyroiditis due to the presence of a large number of Hurthle cells (MacDonald & Yazdi, 1999). In addition to the above investigations, accurate diagnosis must also incorporate clinical correlation.

Radioactive iodine uptake (RAIU) is another modality which is commonly employed in diagnosing thyroid disorders. The role of RAIU in the diagnosis of Hashimoto's thyroiditis has been debated for many years (Cohen et al., 1965). A potentially less obtrusive study which may be performed to discern thyroid pathology is an ultrasound. Ultrasonography provides information regarding anatomic characteristics of the gland and identifies any major changes in the gland. Ultrasonography can be helpful in discerning Hashimoto's thyroiditis in goiters of unknown etiology and can identify the cause of functional impairment as well as the necessity for treatment (Sostre & Reyes, 1991).

The physical characteristics of the thyroid gland, serum TSH levels, serum antithyroid antiglobulin titer, radioactive iodine uptake of the gland, and the response to the perchlorate discharge test are widely used in making an accurate diagnosis of the disease. Indeed, the clinician can feel reasonably confident in their diagnosis of Hashimoto's thyroiditis if at least two of the above mentioned tests support the diagnosis (Fisher et al., 1975). Some recent studies have subclassified Hashimoto's thyroiditis as IgG-4 thyroiditis and nonIgG-4 thyroiditis. This distinction may be important in that IgG-4 thyroiditis has been associated with severe lymphoplasmacytic infiltration, marked fibrosis, and lymphoid follicle formation in contrast to nonIgG-4 thyroiditis, which exhibits more mild histopathological changes (Li., 2009). Thus, this classification might be helpful in assessing the severity of the disease and could be used in determining the most appropriate treatment options for patients.

Furthermore the disease process must be differentiated from some commonly occurring thyroid disorders such as nontoxic nodular goiter and Graves' disease. The presence of a multinodular goiter with gross nodularity is usually considered to be evidence against the diagnosis of Hashimoto's thyroiditis but it cannot be ruled out based on this finding (Takashi et al., 2008). Unlike Hashimoto's thyroiditis, multinodular goiter is usually characterized by euthyroid status and absence of antithyroid antibodies. Hashimoto's thyroiditis and multinodular goiter commonly coexist in patients thus, FNA is commonly employed to differentiate these two entities. Tumor of thyroid gland is another entity which has to be differentiated from Hashimotos' thyroiditis. Rapid growth of the gland and persistent pain usually arouses suspicion of tumor. The confirmatory diagnosis of tumor is usually performed with the aid of FNA. Thyroid lymphoma may develop in some cases of Hashimoto's thyroiditis. Some studies have indicated that using reverse transcriptase polymerase chain reaction might be helpful in differentiating thyroid lymphoma and Hashimoto's thyroiditis (Takano et al., 2000). Furthermore, although Hashimoto's thyroiditis typically presents with hypothyroid symptoms, patients may occasionally present with hyperthyroidism and thyrotoxicosis. This necessitates the differentiation of Hashimoto's thyroiditis from Graves' disease, in cases associated with symptoms of excess thyroid hormone.

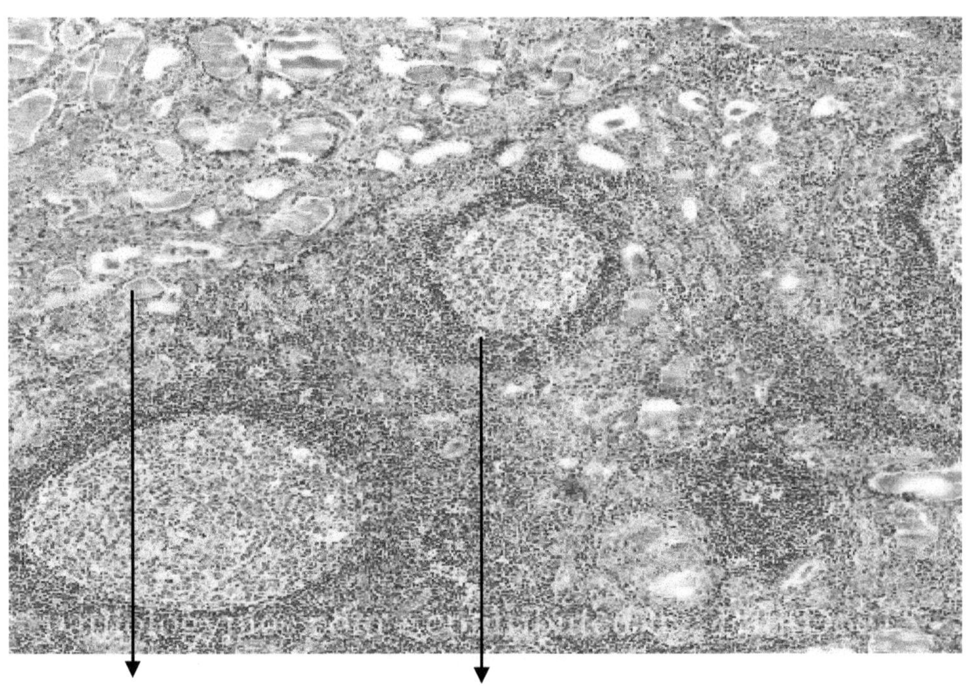

Fig. 3. Histological section thyroid gland affected with Hashimoto's Disease (Datto & Youens, 2007).

9. Treatment

Options in the treatment of Hashimoto's thyroiditis include medical therapy and surgical resection of the gland. The appropriate choice depends on disease presentation and extent of gland involvement. In some instances, patients may present without symptoms, and may not require immediate intervention. (Vickery & Hamlin, 1961). However, continuing debate surrounds whether prophylactic replacement of thyroid hormone has therapeutic benefit in euthyroid-appearing patients with Hashimoto's thyroiditis (Chiovato et al., 1986). Recently, studies have shown that prophylactic treatment in euthyroid patients can slow the progression of the disease and significantly reduce levels of antithyroid antibodies; however, the long-term benefits of this approach have not yet been confirmed (Padberg etal 2004). Furthermore, ultrasound studies have shown that thyroid size diminishes in response to thyroid hormone replacement, even in euthryoid patients (Hegedus et al., 1991). Moreover, reversibility in the progression of the disease appears to be quicker and more pronounced in younger patients than in more mature patients. This difference may be attributable to the extent of glandular involvement and increased degree of fibrosis in older populations, making reversibility of the underlying pathology less feasible.

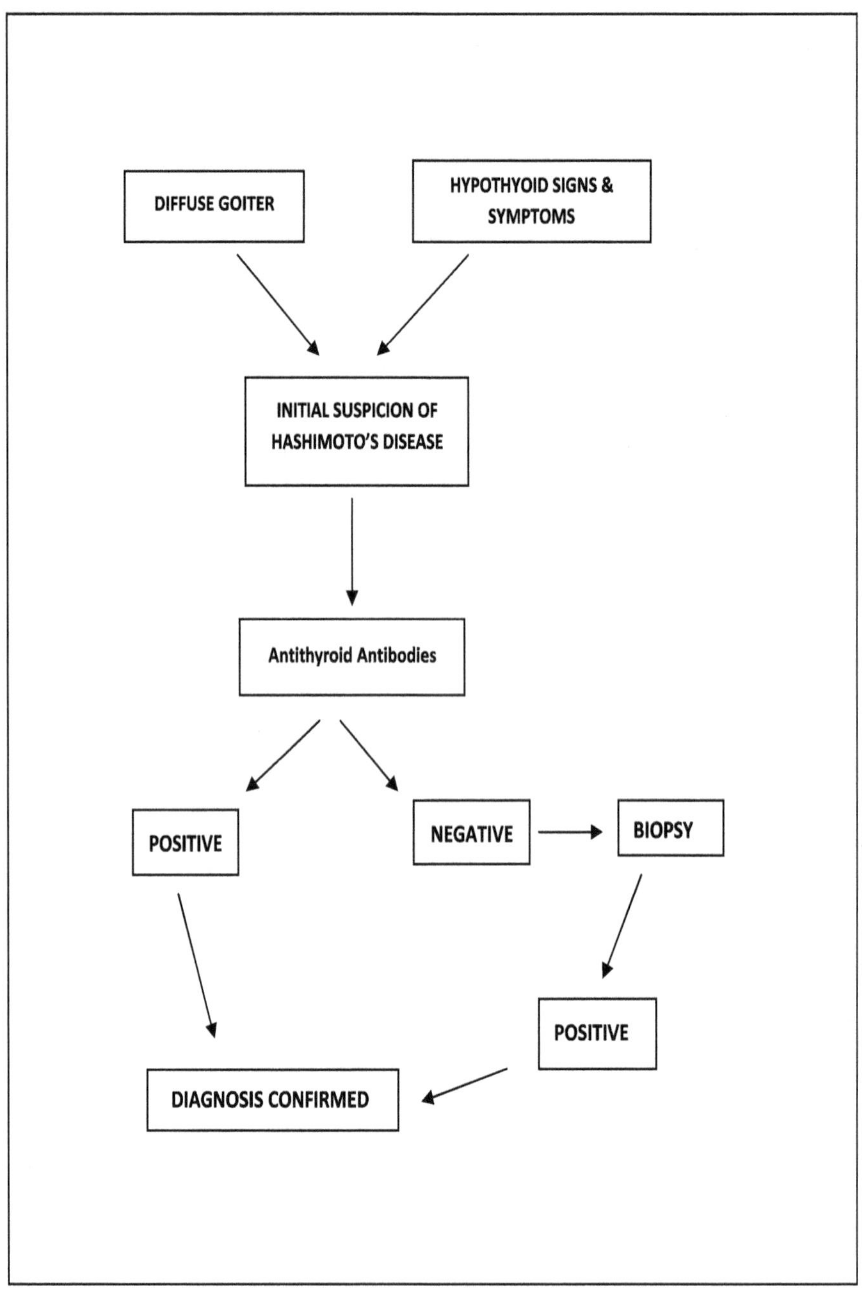

Fig. 4. Flow diagram representing the diagnosis of Hashimoto's thyroiditis

After assessment of the functional status of thyroid gland, thyroid hormone replacement therapy is instituted in all Hashimoto's thyroiditis patients with documented hypothyroidism. Thyroid hormone replacement is also indicated in the presence of a goiter, if the goiter is small in size and is causing minimal pressure symptoms or disfigurement. The initial dosage of the thyroid hormone is determined based upon the patient's body mass, cardiovascular condition, concomitant co-morbid conditions and pregnancy status. The daily dosing in healthy young individuals is usually calculated as 1.7 micrograms/Kilogram of body weight per day which typically ranges between 75-125 micrograms per day. Most hypothyroid patients suffering with Hashimoto's thyroiditis will need lifelong replacement of thyroid hormone. External supplementation of thyroid hormone will not only correct the metabolic status of the person but it is also postulated to modify the course of the disease. Long term follow up of patients treated with thyroxine has shown reduced antithyroid peroxidase antibodies after a mean time of 50 months, with a small number of patients being reported as seronegative (Schmidt et al., 2008). Moreover, about 20% of patients suffering from Hashimoto's thyroiditis-related hypothyroidism recovered normal thyroid function when challenged with thyroid releasing hormone (TRH). In addition, a few studies have shown that if patients recover normal thyroid gland function, they might remain euthyroid, despite not taking hormone therapy, for a mean period of approximately 8 years (Takasu et al., 1990).

In contrast to hormone replacement therapy, nutritional therapies, which focus on modifying the body's immune response and resultant destruction of thyroid tissue, continue to be an area of keen interest. Selenium, a trace element which plays an important role in modifying inflammatory and immune responses in the body, has been proposed to have disease-modifying properties in Hashimoto's thyroiditis. The rationale for using this nutrient stems from the discovery that the enzymes iodothyronine deiodinase, glutathione peroxidase and thioredoxin reductase, which maintain thyroid gland homeostasis, are selenium dependant. One study investigating the effect of selenium supplementation on Hashimoto's thyroiditis found significant reduction in the levels of antithyroid peroxidase (ATPO) following 6 months of therapy. Further decline in antibody levels was observed when the therapy was continued, with antibody levels increasing after therapy was terminated. (Mazokapakis et al., 2007).

In some cases, pharmacotherapy and hormone replacement might not be sufficient to treat the symptoms of Hashimoto's thyroiditis and surgical therapy is required. Surgical therapy is indicated in patients suffering from severe, painful goiter or experiencing pressure symptoms resulting from tracheal encroachment, which include dysphasia or dyspnea. In an attempt to create guidelines for thyroid resection, the following factors have been found to play a major role in determining when to pursue surgical resection (Thomas & Rutledge, 1981):

1. Dominant mass unresponsive to thyroxine therapy
2. Increase in the size of the mass despite thyroxine therapy
3. History or physical examination findings suggestive of malignancy
4. Indeterminate findings on cutting needle biopsy

A small group of patients, with Hashimoto's thyroiditis, present with pain and tenderness rather than a goiter or hypothyroidism. Thyroidectomy has been proven to be effective in these patients as treatment with thyroid hormone replacement or corticosteroids will not alleviate their symptoms (Kon & Degroot, 2003). Painful Hashimoto's thyroiditis is an atypical variant characterized by recurrent attacks of fever and thyroid pain in the presence of antithyroid antibodies. These cases do not respond to the regular anti-inflammatory agents, which have been found to be effective in controlling pain associated with other forms of thyroiditis. In assessing the risk/benefit trade-off of thyroid resection, the complication risk involved in performing thyroidectomy in patients with Hashimoto's thyroiditis is reported to be very low, but the presence of unsuspected coexisting malignancies is common (Shih et al., 2008). Moreover, prophylactic removal of a nodular thyroid gland is done in selected cases to prevent the development of thyroid cancer, which would be typically diagnosed at a later stage. It should be noted that the effectiveness of this approach has been widely debated and remains a point of research interest. In cases with documented thyroid cancer, removal of the gland followed by radiotherapy or chemotherapy, depending on the type of tumor, is the definitive therapy. The presence of tumors coexistent with Hashimoto's thyroiditis does not alter surgical management when compared to cases of Hashimoto's thyroiditis uncomplicated by neoplasm (Singh et al., 1999). Surgical removal of the thyroid gland has been tried with variable success in cases of Hashimoto's thyroiditis associated with chronic urticaria, when anti-allergic and corticosteroid therapies have proven ineffective. Briefly summarized; thyroid hormone status, pressure symptoms associated with an enlarged gland, and presence of associated symptoms or other autoimmune disorders should be considered in making an accurate treatment choice.

10. Hashimoto's encephalopathy

Hashimoto's encephalopathy or encephalitis is a rare neuroendocrine entity and is described as an autoimmune encephalopathy, which occurs in patients diagnosed with Hashimoto's thyroiditis. Similar to Hashimoto's thyroiditis, it can affect individuals of all age groups, and is more common in women than in men. Hashimoto's encephalopathy is frequently misdiagnosed since symptoms at presentation are predominantly neurological. Some cases have been reported where patients presented with Hashimoto's encephalopathy long before there was any clinical suspicion for Hashimoto's thyroiditis (Peschen-Rosin et al., 1999). Hashimoto's encephalopathy was first described in 1961, in a 48 year-old man who was hypothyroid and who experienced recurring episodes of encephalopathy and stroke-like symptoms (Brain et al., 1966). Some authors prefer using the term corticosteroid-responsive encephalopathy rather than Hashimoto's encephalopathy as the pathogenesis of this condition is still a topic of widespread conjecture (Fatourechi, 2005). The estimated prevalence of this condition is 2.1/100,000 (Ferracci & Giani, 2003). The actual prevalence of the disease could be much higher since many cases of Hashimoto's encephalopathy are presumed to remain undiagnosed. Studies attempting to describe the pathophysiological mechanisms behind this condition have suggested the possible role of autoimmune processes. Similar to Hashimoto's thyroiditis, patients with Hashimoto's encephalopathy have high levels of antithyroid antibodies and respond to immunosuppressive therapy, supporting the involvement of an autoimmune mechanism in its pathogenesis (Schiess & Pardo, 2008). An underlying immune mechanism is further supported by autopsy studies which revealed histopathological changes such as lymphocyte infiltration of the leptomeninges, and gliosis of cortical gray matter, basal ganglia, thalamus and hippocampus, which are reminiscent of autoimmune injury to other organs of the body (Duffey & Yee, 2003). The presentation of Hashimoto's encephalopathy can be either acute or subacute, and is characterized by a relapsing-remitting or progressive course of seizures, tremors, ataxia, myoclonus, psychosis, and stroke-like neurological findings. The literature indicates that the initial clinical presentation can be classified either as a vasculitic type, with predominantly stroke-like symptoms and mild cognitive impairment, or a diffuse progressive type with predominant cognitive impairment (Kothbauer-Marggreiter et al., 1996). In contrast to disease prevalence findings in adults, very few instances of Hashimoto's encephalopathy have been reported in the pediatric age group. Pediatric Hashimoto's encephalopathy is characterized by seizures, hallucinations, and confusion, and suspicion should arise when a progressive decline in school performance is observed (Vasconcellos et al., 1998).

The diagnosis of Hashimoto's encephalopathy continues to be a diagnosis of exclusion. Serum titers of antithyroid antibodies will be elevated and cerebrospinal fluid analysis will show increased protein levels. Other possible causes of encephalopathy including infections, metabolic and electrolyte derangements, toxic ingestions, vascular abnormalities, and neoplastic or paraneoplastic syndromes must be ruled out before a Hashimoto's encephalopathy diagnosis is made. Electroencephalogram and imaging studies in patients with suspected Hashimoto's encephalopathy typically exhibit nonspecific changes, in the absence of infection, tumor, or stroke (Marshall & Doyle, 2006). The antibody titers in Hashimoto's encephalopathy are not suggestive of the severity or the type of clinical presentation. Early diagnosis and prompt intervention are of critical importance in effectively treating this condition, and significantly reducing its morbidity and mortality. The first line of treatment is usually corticosteroids, and in cases where steroids are contraindicated, other immunosuppressive agents have been employed with good efficacy. In steroid unresponsive cases, administration of plasmapheresis has been shown effective in controlling symptoms (Nagpal & Pande, 2004). Periodic intravenous exchange may also be used for steroid non-responders, but no superiority has been established when compared to plasmapheresis. The duration of the treatment is highly variable, however approximately 90% of the cases will remain in remission after treatment.

11. Conclusion

In this chapter, we have discussed the epidemiology, presumed pathogenesis, diagnosis and treatment of Hashimoto's thyroiditis. We have also discussed potential complications including other autoimmune diseases and neoplasms. In many ways, Hashimoto's thyroiditis serves as a paradigm for autoimmune disease throughout the body. Our understanding of how a genetic predisposition can be modified by environmental exposure is expanding. Our grasp of how aggressive immune suppression can alter disease course is growing. As with many subjects in medicine, with knowledge comes more questioning of what we know. Just as in other disease states, we must eagerly seek out both the questions and the answers.

12. Acknowledgements

The authors acknowledge Helen Houpt, MSLS for her editorial assistance in the production of this manuscript.

13. References

Baker, B, A., Gharib, H., Markowitz, H. (1983). Correlation of Thyroid Antibodies and Cytologic Features in Suspected Autoimmune Thyroid Disease. *The American Journal of Medicine*, Vol. 74, No. 6, (June, 1983), pp. (941-944), doi: 10.1016/0002-9343(83)90786-6.

Becker, K, L., Ferguson, R, H., Mc cohaney, W, M. (1963). The Connective Tissue Diseases and Symptoms Associated with Hashimoto's Thyroiditis. *The New England Journal of Medicine*, Vol. 263, (February, 1963), pp. (277-280).

Boukis, M, A., Koutras, D, A., Souvatzoglou, A., Evangepolau, K., Vrontakis, M., Moulapoulaos, S, D. (1983). Thyroid Hormone and Immunologic Studies in Endemic Goiter. *The Journal of Clinical and Endocrinology and Metabolism*, Vol, 57, (1983), pp. (859-862).

Brain, L., Jellinek, E, H., Ball, K. (1966). Hashimoto's disease and encephalopathy. *Lancet*, Vol. 2, (1966), pp (512–514).

Buchanan, W, W., Harden, R, M. (1965). Primary Hypothyroidism and Hashimoto's Thyroiditis. *Archives of Internal Medicine*, Vol. 115, No. 4, (April, 1965), pp. (411-417).

Casselman, W, G. (1996). Thyroid, In: Index of Medical Word origins, (1996), Available from: <Hashimoto's Thyroiditistp://www.billcasselman.com/dictionary_of_medical_der ivations/dmd_nine.Hashimoto's Thyroiditism>.

Champion, B, R., Page, K, R., Parish, N., Rayner, D, C., Dawe, K., Biswas-Hughes, G., Cooke, A., Geysen, M., Roitt, I, M. (1991). Identification of a Thyroxine-Containing Self-Epitope of Thyroglobulin Which Triggers Thyroid Auto reactive T Cells. *The Journal of Experimental Medicine*, Vol. 174, (August, 1991), pp. (363-370), ISSN 0022-1007/91/08/0363/08.

Chistiakov, D.A., Turakulov, R.I. (2003). CTLA4 and its role in autoimmunr thyroid disease. *Journal of Molecular Endocrinology*, Vol. 31, (August, 2003), pp. (21-36), doi: 10.1677/jme.0.0310021.

Chiovato, L., Marcocci, C., Mariotti, S., Mori, A., Pinchera, A. (1986). L-thyroxine therapy induces a fall of thyroid microsomal and thyroglobulin antibodies in idiopathic myxedema and in hypothyroid, but not in euthyroid Hashimoto's thyroiditis. *Journal of Endocrinological Investigation*, Vol. 9, No. 4, (August, 1986), pp. (299-305).

Cohen R,J., Stansifer P,D., Barrett, O. (1965). Radioactive Iodine Uptake In Hashimoto's Thyroiditis. *Archives of Internal Medicine*, Vol. 116, (July, 1965), pp. (111-112), PubMed PMID: 14338941.

Cuoco, L., Certo, M., Jorizzo, R, A., De Vitis, I., Tursi,, A., Papa, A., De Marinis, L., Fedeli, P., Fedeli, G., Gasbarrini, G. (1999). Prevalence and Early Diagnosis of Celiac Disease in Autoimmune Thyroid Disorders. *Italian Journal of Gastroenterology and Hepatology*, Vol. 31, No. 4, (May, 1999), pp. (283-287).

Datto, M., Youens, K. (2007). Hashimotos Thyroiditis, In: *Pathology Pics,* February, 2008, Available from <www.pathologypics.com/pictview.aspx?id=291>.

Dietrich, G., Piechaszuk, M., Pau, B., Kassatchkine, M, D. (1991). Evidence for a Restricted Idiotypic and Epitope Specificity of Anti-thyroglobulin Auto antibodies in Patients with Autoimmune Thyroiditis. *European Journal of Immunology,* Vol. 21, No. 3, (March, 1991), pp. (811-814), doi: 10.1002/eji.1830210340.

MacDonald, L., Yazdi, H, M. (1999). Fine Needle Aspiration Cytology of Hashimoto's Thyroiditis: Sources of Diagnostic Error. *Acta Cytologica,* Vol. 43, No. 3, (June, 1999), pp. (400-406).

Dufey, P., Yee, S., Reid, I, N., Bridges, L, R. (2003). Hashimoto's Encephalopathy: Postmortem Findings after Fatal Status Epilepticus. *Neurology,* Vol. 61, No. 8, (October, 2003), pp. (1124-1126), doi: 10.1212/01.WNL.0000090462.62087.

Einarsdottir, E., Soderstrom, I., Lofgren-Burstrom, A., Haraldsson, S., Nilsson-Ardnor, S., Penha-Goncalves, C., Lind, L., Holmgren, G., Holmberg, M., Asplund, K., Holmberg, D. (2003). The CTLA-4 Region as a General Autoimmunity Factor: An Extended Pedigree Provides Evidence for Synergy with the HLA locus in the Etiology of Type 1 Diabetes Mellitus, Hashimoto's Thyroiditis and Grave's Disease. *European Journal of Human Genetics,* Vol. 11, (2003), pp. (81-84).

Fatourechi, V. (2005). Hashimoto's Encephalopathy: Myth or Reality? An Endocrinologists Perspective. *Best Practice and Research Clinical Endocrinology and Metabolism,* Vol. 9, No. 1, (2005), pp. (53-66), doi: 10.1016/j.beem.2004.11.006.

Fisher, D.A., Oddie, T.H., Johnson, D.E., Nelson, J.C (1975). The Diagnosis Of Hashimoto's Thyroiditis. *The Journal of Clinical Endocrinology and Metabolism,* Vol. 40, No.5, (May, 1975), pp. (795-801), doi:10.1210/jcem-40-5-795.

Fischer, G, F. (2000). Molecular Genetics of HLA. *Vox Sanguinis,* Vol. 78, No. 10, (2000), pp. (261-264), ISSN 0042-9007.

Ferracci, F., Bertiato, G., Moretto, G. (2004). Hashimoto's encephalopathy Epidemiological Data and Pathogenetic Considerations. *Journal of the Neurological Sciences,* Vol. 217, No. 2, (February, 2004), pp. (165-168). PubMed PMID:14706219

Fukata, s., Kuma, K., Sugawara, M. (1996). Relationship Between Cigarette Smoking and Hypothyroidism in Patients with Hashimoto's Thyroiditis. *Journal of Endocrinological Investigation,* Vol. 19, No. 9, (1996), pp. (607-612), ISSN 0391-4097.

Gebe, J, A., Swanson, E., Kwok, W, W. (2002). HLA Class II Peptide-Binding and Autoimmunity. *Tissue Antigens,* Vol. 59, No. 2, (February, 2002), pp. (78-87).

Giordano, C., Richiusa, P., Bagnasco, M., Pizzolanti, G., Di Blasi, F., Sbriglia, M, S., Mattina, A., Pesce, G., Montagna, P., Capone, F., Misiano, G., Scorsone, A., Pugilese, A., Galluzzo, A. (2001). Differential Regulation of Fas-Mediated Apoptosis in Both Thyrocyte and Lymphocyte Cellular Compartments Correlates with Opposite Phenocytic Manifestations of Autoimmune Thyroid Disease. *Thyroid,* Vol. 11, No. 3, (March, 2001), pp. (233-244), doi: 10.1089/105072501750159615.

Gordin, A., Saarinen, P., Pelkonen, A., Lamberg, B. (1974). Serum Thyroglobulin and the Response to Thyrotropin Releasing Hormone in Symptomless Autoimmune

Thyroiditis and in Borderline and Overt Hypothyroidism. *Acta Endocrinologica*, Vol. 75, No. 274, (1974).

Hall, R, C., Popkin, M, K., DeVaul, R., Hall, A, K., Gardner, E, R., Beresford, T, P. (1982). Psychiatric Manifestations of Hashimoto's Thyroiditis, *Psychosomatics*, Vol. 23, No. 4, (April, 1982), pp. (337-342).

Hegedus, L., Hansen, J, M., Rasmussen, U, F., Hansen, B, M., Mased, M, H. (1991). Influence of Thyroxine Treatment on Thyroid Size and Anti-Thyroid Peroxidase Antibodies in Hashimoto's Thyroiditis. *Clinical Endocrinology*, Vol. 35, No. 9, (September, 1991), pp. (235-238), doi: 10.1111/j.1365-2265.1991.tbo3528.x.

Hollowell, J, G., Staehling, N, W., Flanders, W, D., Hannon, W, H., Gunter, E, W., Spencer, C, A., Braverman, L, E. (2002). Serum TSH, T_4, and Thyroid Antibodies in the United States Population (1988 to 1994): National health and Nutrition Examination Survey (NHALES III). *The Journal of Endocrinology and Metabolism*, Vol. 87, (2002), pp. (489–499), doi: 10.1210/jc.87.2.489.

Hunt, P, J., Marshall, S, E., Weetman, A, P, Bunce, M, Bell, J, I., Wass, J, A., Welash, K, L. (2001). Histocompatability Leukocyte Antigens and Closely Linked Immunomodulatory Genes in Autoimmune Thyroid Disease. *Clinical Endocrinology*, Vol. 55, No. 4, (October, 2001), pp. (491-499), doi: 10.1046/j.1365-2265.2001.01356.x.

Hygek, E., Isaacson, P, G. (1988). Primary B-cell Lymphoma of Thyroid and its Relationship to Hashimoto's Thyroiditis. *Human Pathology*, Vol. 9, No. 11, (November, 1988), pp. (1315-1326), doi: 10.1016/s0046-8177(88)80287-9.

Kakourou, T., Kanaka-Gantenbein, C., Papadopoulou, A., Kaloumenou, E., Chrousos, G, P. (2005). Increased Prevelance of Chronic Autoimmune (Hashimoto's) Thyroiditis in Children and Adolescents Suffering from Vitiligo. *Journal of American Academy of Dermatology*, Vol. 53, No. 2, (August, 2005), pp. (220-223), doi: 10.1016/j.jaad.2005.03.032.

Kasagi, K., Kousaka, T., Higuchi, K., Ida, Y., Misaki, T., Miyamoto, S., Alam, M.S., Yamabe, H., Konishi, J. (1996). Clinical Significance of Measurements of Antithyroid Antibodies in the Diagnosis of Hashimoto's Thyroiditis: Comparison with Histological Findings. *Thyroid*, Vol. 6, No.5, (October, 1996), pp. (445-450), doi: 10.1089/thy.1966.6.445.

Kon, Y,C., Degroot, L,G. (2003). Painful Hashimoto's Thyroiditis as an indication for Thyroidectomy: Clinical Characteristics and Outcome in Seven Patients. *The Journal of Clinical Endocrinology and Metabolism*, Vol. 88, No.6, (June, 2003), pp. (2667-2672), doi: 10.1210/jc.2002-021498.

Kothbauer-Margreiter, I., Sturzenegger, M., Komor, J., Baumgartner, R., Hess, C, W. (1996). Encephalopathy Associated with Hashimoto's Thyroiditis: Diagnosis and Treatment. *Journal of Neurology*, Vol. 243, No. 8, (April, 1996), pp. (585-593), doi: 10.1007/BF00900946.

Kumar, N., Ray, C., Jain, s. (2002). Aspiration Cytology of Hashimoto's Thyroiditis in a Endemic Area. *Cytopathology*, Vol. 13, No. 1, (February, 2002), pp. (31-39), doi: 10.1046/j.1365-2303.2002.00366.x.

Limachi, F., Basso, S. (2002). Apoptosis: Life Though Planned Cellular Death Regulating Mechanisms, Control Systems and Relations with Thyroid Disease. *Thyroid*, Vol. 12, No. 1, (January, 2002), pp. (27-34), doi: 10.1089/105072502753451931.

Lima, M, A., Santos, B, M., Borges, M, F. (1998). Quantitative Analysis of C Cells in Hashimoto's Thyroiditis. *Thyroid*, Vol. 8, No. 6, (June, 1998), pp. (505-509), doi: 10.1089/thy.1998.8.505.

Li, Y., Bai, Y., Liu, Z., Ozaki, T., Taniguchi, E., Mori, I., Nagayama, K., Nakamura, H., Kakudo, K. (2009). Immunohistochemistry of IgG-4 can Help Sub classify Hashimoto's Autoimmune Thyroiditis. *Pathology International*, Vol. 59, No.9, (September, 2009), pp. (636-641), doi: 10.1111/j.1440-1827.2009.02419.x.

Marshall, G, A., Doyle, J, J. (2006). Long-term Treatment of Hashimoto's Encephalopathy. *Journal of Neuropsychiatric and Clinical Neurosciences*, Vol. 18, No. 1, (2006), pp. (14-20).

Martin,A., Davies, T, F. (1992). T Cells and Human Autoimmune Thyroid Disease: Emerging Data Show Lack of Need to Invoke Suppressor T Cell Problems. *Thyroid*, Vol. 2, No. 3, (1992), pp. (247-261), doi: 10.1089/thy.1992.2.247.

Male, D, K., Champion, B, R., Pryce, G., Matthews, H., Sheperd, P. (1985). Antigenic Determinants of Human Thyroglobulin Differentiated Using Antigen Fragments. *Journal of Immunology*, Vol. 54, No. 3, (March, 1985), pp. (419-427).

Mazokopakis, E, E., Papadakis, J, A., Papadomanolaki, M, G., Batistakis, A, G., Giannakopoulos, T, G., Protopapadakis, E, E., Ganotakis, E, S. (2007). Effects of 12 Months Treatment with I-Selenomethionine on Serum Anti-TPO Levels in Patients with Hashimoto's Thyroiditis. *Thyroid*, Vol. 17, No. 7, (August, 2007), pp. (609-612), doi: 10.1089/thy.2007.0040.

Mccohaney, W, M., Keating, F, R., Beahrs, O, H., Woolner, L, B. (1962). On the Increasing Occurrence of Hashimoto's Thyroiditis. *The Journal of Clinical Endocrinology and Metabolism*, Vol. 22, No. 542, (1962), doi: 10.1210/jcem-22-5-542.

Nagpal, T., Pande, s. (2004). Hashimoto's Encephalopathy: Response to Plasma Exchange. *Neurology India*, Vol. 52, (2004), pp. (245-247).

Nikiforova, M, N., Caudill, C, M., Biddinger, P., Nikiforov, Y, E. (2002). Prevalence of RET/PTC Rearrangements in Hashimoto's Thyroiditis and Papillary Thyroid Carcinomas. *International Journal of Surgical Pathology*, Vol. 10, No. 1, (January, 2002), pp. (15-22), doi: 10.1177/106689690201000104.

Padberg, S., Heller, K., Usadel, K, H, Schumm-Draaeger, P, M. (2001). One Year Prophylactic Treatment of Euthyroid Hashimoto's Thyroiditis Patients with Levothyroxine : Is there a Benefit. *Thyroid*, Vol. 11, No. 3, (March, 2001), pp. (249-255), doi: 10.1089/105072501750159651.

Peschen-Rosin, R., Schabet, M., Dichgans, J. (1999). Manifestation of Hashimoto's Encephalopathy Years Before Onset of Thyroid Disease. *European Neurology*, Vol. 41, No. 2, (1999), pp. (79-84), doi: 10.1159/000008007.

Pino Rivero, V., Guerra Camacho, M., Marcos García, M., Trinidad Ruiz, G., Pardo Romero, G., Gonzâlez Palomino, A., Blasco Huelva, A. (2004). The Incidence of Thyroid Carcinoma in Hashimoto's Thyroiditis: Our Experience and Literature

Review. *An Otorrinolaringol Ibero Am*, Vol. 31, No. 3, (2004), pp. (223-230). Review. Spanish

Pyne, D., Isenberg, D, A. (2002). Autoimmune Thyroid Disease in Systemic Lupus Erythematosus. *Annals of Rheumatology*, Vol. 61, (2002), pp. (70-102), doi: 10.1136/ard.61.1.70.

Rottem, M. (2003). Chronic Urticaria and Autoimmune Thyroid Disease: Is There a Link? *Autoimmune Reviews*, Vol. 2, No. 2, (March, 2003), pp. (69-72), doi: 10.1016/s1568-9972(02)00141-6.

Radetti, G., Gottardi, E., Bona, G., Corrias, A., Salardi, S., Loche, S. (2006). The Natural History of Euthyroid Hashimoto's Thyroiditis in Children. *Journal of Pediatrics*, Vol. 149, No. 6, (December, 2006), pp. (827-832), doi: 10.1016/j.peds.2006.08.045.

Shih, M, L., Lee, J, A., Hsieh, C, B., Liu, H, D., Kebebew, E., Clark, O, H., Duh, Q, Y. (2006). Thyroidectomy for Hashimoto's Thyroiditis: Complications and Associated Cancers. *Thyroid*, Vol. 18, No. 7, (July, 2006), pp. (729-734), doi: 10.1089/thy.2007.0384.

Staii, A., Mirocha, S., Todorova-Koteva, K., Glinberg, S., Jaume, J, C. (2010).Hashimoto's Thyroiditis is More Frequent than Expected when Diagnosed by Cytology which Uncovers a Pre-Clinical State. *Thyroid Research Journal*, Vol. 3, No.11, (2010).

Sostre, S., Reyes, M, M. (1991). Sonographic Grading and Diagnosis of Hashimoto's Thyroiditis. *Journal of Endocrinological Investigation*, Vol. 14, No. 2, (February, 1991), pp. (115-121).

Schiess, N., Pardo, C, A. (2008). Hashimoto's Encephalopathy. *Annals of New York Academy of Sciences*, Vol. 1142, , (October, 2008), pp. (254-265), doi: 10.1196/annals.1444.018.

Schmidt, M., Voell, M., Rahlff, I., Dietlein, M., Kobe, C., Faust, M., Schicha, H. (2008). Long-Term Follow-Up of Antithyroid Peroxidase Antibodies in Patients with Chronic Autoimmune Thyroiditis (Hashimoto's Thyroiditis) Treated with Levothyroxine. *Thyroid*, Vol. 18, No. 7, (2008), pp. (755-760), doi: 10.1089/thy.2008.0008.

Singh, B., Shaha, A, R., Trivedi, H., Carew, J, F., Poluri, A., Shah, J, P. (1999). Coexistent Hashimoto's Thyroiditis with Papillary Thyroid Carcinoma: Impact on Presentation, Management, and Outcome. *Surgery*, Vol. 126, No. 6, (December, 1999), pp. (1070-1077), doi: 10.1067/msy.2099.101431.

Tagami, T., Tamanaha, T., Shimazu, S., Honda, K., Nanba, K., Nomura, H., Yoriko, S, U., Usui, T., Shimatsu, A., Naruse, M. (2010). Lipid Profiles in Untreated Patients with Hashimoto's Thyroiditis and the Effects of Thyroxine Treatment on Subclinical Hypothyroidism with Hashimoto's Thyroiditis. *Endocrine Journal*, Vol. 57, No. 3, (December, 2009), pp. (253-258).

Takano, T., Miyauchi, A., Matsuzuka, F., Yoshida, H., Kumar, K., Amino, N. (2000). Diagnosis of Thyroid Malignant Lymphoma by Reverse Transcription- Polymerase Chain Reaction Detecting the Monoclonality of Immunoglobulin Heavy Chain Messenger Ribonucleic Acid. *Journal of Clinical Endocrinology and Metabolism*, Vol. 85, (2000), pp. (67-675), doi: 10.1210/jc.85.2.671.

Takasu, N., Komiya, I., Asawa, T., Nagasawa, Y., Yamada, T. (1990). Test for Recovery from Hypothyroidism during Thyroxine Therapy in Hashimoto's Thyroiditis. *Lancet*,

Vol. 336, No. 8723, (November, 1990), pp. (1084-1086), doi:10.1016/0140-6736(90)92567-2.

Takasu, N., Yamada, T., Takasu, M., Komiya, I., Nagasawa, Y., Asawa, T, Shinoda, T., Aizawa, T., Koizumi, Y. (1992). Disappearance of Thyrotropin-Blocking Antibodies and Spontaneous Recovery from Hypothyroidism in Autoimmune Thyroiditis. *The New England Journal of Medicine,* Vol. 326, (February, 1992), pp. (513-518), doi: 10.1056/NEJM199202203260803.

Takashi, A., Nobuyuki, A., De Groot, L.J. (2008). Hashimoto's Thyroiditis, In: *Thyroid Disease Manager,* Takashi, A., Nobuyuki, A, Endocrine Education, Inc., Retrieved from < Hashimoto's Thyroiditistp://www.thyroidmanager.org/Chapter8/chapter8.Hashimoto's Thyroiditisml#id2504737>.

Tunbridge, W, M., Evered, D, C., Hall, R., Appleton, D., Brewis, M., Clark, F., Evans, J, G., Young, E., Bird, T, Smith, P, A. (1977). The Spectrum of Thyroid Disease in a Community: The Wickham Survey. *Clinical Endocrinology,* Vol. 7, No. 6, (December, 1977), pp. (481-493).

Thomas, C, G., Rutledge, R, G. (1981). Surgical Intervention in Chronic (Hashimoto's) Thyroiditis. *Annals of Surgery,* Vol.193, No. 6, (June, 1981), pp. (769-776).

Unger, P., Ewart, M., Wang, B, Y., Gan, L., Koz, s., Burstein, D, E. (2003). Expression of P63 in Papillary Thyroid Carcinoma and in Hashimoto's Thyroiditis: A Pathological Link? *Human Pathology,* Vol. 34, NO. 8, (August, 2003), pp. (764-769), doi: 10.1016/s0046-8177(03)00239-9.

Vasconcellos, E., Pina-Girza, J. E., Fakhoury, T., Fenichel, G.M. (1999). Pediatric Manifestations of Hashimoto's Encephalopathy. *Pediatric Neurology,* Vol. 20, No.5, (May, 1999), pp. (394-398), doi: 10.1016/s0887-8994(99)00006-5.

Vickery, A, L., Hamlin, E (1961). Struma Lymphomatosa (Hashimoto's Thyroiditis): Observations on Repeated Biopsies in 16 Patients. *The New England Journal of Medicine,* Vol. 264 , (February, 1961), pp. (226-229).

Volpe, R., Clark, P, V., Row, V, V. (1973). Relationship of Age Specific Incidence Rates to Immunological Aspects of Hashimoto's Thyroiditis. *Canadian Medical Association Journal,* Vol. 109, No. 9, (November, 1973), pp. (898-901).

Wang, C., Crapo, L, M. (1997). The Epidemiology of Thyroid Disease and Implications for Screening. *Endocrinology and Metabolism Clinics of North America,* Vol. 26, No.1, (1997), pp. (189-218), ISSN 0889-852.

Wu, Z., Stephens, H, A., Sachs, J, A., Biro, P, A., Cutbush, S., Magzoub, M, M, Becker, C., Schwartz, G., Bottazzo, G, F. (1994). Molecular Analysis of HLA-DQ and DP Genes in Caucasoid Patients with Hashimoto's Thyroiditis. *Tissue Antigens,* Vol. 43, No. 2, (February, 1994), pp. (116-119).

Weetman, A, P., Walport, M, J. (1987). The Association of Autoimmune Thyroiditis with Systemic Lupus Erythematosus. *Oxford Journals Rheumatology,* Vol. 6, No. 5, (19897), pp (359-361), doi: 10.1093/rheumatology/26.5.359

Wilkinson, M., Sacker, L, S. (1957). The Lupus Erythematosus Cell and its significance. *British Medical Journal,* Vol. 2, No. 5046, (September, 1957), pp. (661-665).

Yoshida, H., Amino, N., Yagawa, K., Uemura, K., Satoh, M., Miyai, K., Kumahara, Y. (1978). Association of Serum Antithyroid Antibodies with Lymphocytic Infiltration of the

Thyroid Gland: Studies of Seventy Autopsied Cases. *The Journal of Clinical Endocrinology and Metabolism*, Vol. 46, No. 6, (June, 1978), pp. (859-862), doi: 10.1210/jcem-46-6-859.

Zois, C., Stavrou, I., Kaiogera, C., Svarna, E., Dimolitais, I., Seferiadis, K., Tsatsoulis, A. (2003). High Prevalence of Autoimmune Thyroiditis in Schoolchildren after Elimination of Iodine Deficiency in Northwestern Greece. *Thyroid*, Vol. 13, No. 5, (2003), pp. (485-489), doi: 10.1089/105072503322021151.

Different Faces of Chronic Autoimmune Thyroiditis in Childhood and Adolescence

Ljiljana Saranac and Hristina Stamenkovic
Pediatric Clinic, Faculty of Medicine Nis, University of Nis
Serbia

1. Introduction

The importance of the thyroid gland for the human body is largely due to its production of hormones necessary for appropriate energy levels and an active life. These products have pleiotropic effects, exerting an immense array of hormonal activities, playing a critical role in early brain development, somatic growth, bone maturation, and mRNA synthesis for more than a hundred proteins that constantly regulate the maintenance of each and every bodily function. They also have critical effects on energy metabolism and on the metabolism of nutrients and inorganic ions. To such an extent is every tissue impacted in one way or another by thyroid hormones that a given degree of thyroid dysfunction is highly likely to result in multiorgan failure, this often mimicking different diseases (Saranac et al., 2011).

2. Chronic autoimmune thyroiditis as multifaced disease

Chronic autoimmune thyroiditis (CAT) is multifaced disease. Its incidence has increased dramatically over the past few decades afflicting up to 2% of the general population. CAT as autoimmune disorder results from a complex interplay of genetic, environmental, and endogenous factors. Genetic factors are predominant and likely account for aproximately 80% of the liability to develop autoimmune thyroid disorders (AITD). However, at least 20% is due to environmental factors. The mechanisms whereby environmental factors may affect the onset and the course of AITD are, in many instances, obscure or, at least, incompletely understood, but gene-environment interaction seems a fundamental process for the occurrence of AITD (Weetman, 2003; Bartalena et al., 2007). In children, CAT is the most common cause of acquired hypothyroidism in nonendemic goitre areas (Fisher, 1990; Raillison et al., 1975; Tomer & Huber, 2009). Unlike overt goitrogenic form of CAT, atrophic one remains hidden or misdiagnosed for years. The clinical manifestations of acquired hypothyroidism in childhood differ from those in adults. The classic manifestations also occur in children, but are not so prominent (Table 1). Instead, the most important sign of acquired hypothyroidism in childhood is growth failure (Table 2). Weight tends to increase and in most instances weight for age is greater than height for age. The retardation of bone age in hypothyroidism usually equals or exceeds the retardation in linear growth (Fisher, 1999; Hall, 1989). Herein we present two cases of atrophic CAT with long course and delayed diagnosis.

Lack of energy	Hoarseness of the voice, slow speach	Hearing loss
Cold intolerance	Typical facial appearance	Uveal effusion
Acroparaesthesiae	Prolongation of the tendon reflexes	Muscle cramps
Dryness of the skin	Myxedoedematous, xantochromic skin	Muscle stiffness
Weight gain	Slowing of all intellectual funtions	Anorexia
Constipation	Diminished memory and somnolence	Ascites, pleural effusion
Bradycardia	Enlarged, indolent, dilated heart,	Pericardial effusion
Anaemia	Shortness of breath	Menstrual disorders
Infertility	Other endocrine dysfunction	Exocrine dysfunction

Table 1. Clinical signs of overt hypothyroidism

Growth retardation
Bone age retardation
Muscle hypertrophy pseudohypertrophy
Sexual disorders
Delayed puberty
Precocious puberty

Table 2. Clinical signs of acquired hypothyroidism unique to childhood (Fisher, 1990)

Segmental vitiligo, hypopigmented rings surrounding dark naevi ("halo naevi"), leucotrichia, premature greying of the hair, and alopecia areata are all, like typical vitiligo, associated with autoimmune disorders and are asigned as clinical markers of autoimmunity (Hall, 1989).

3. Examples from clinical praxis of overt, late diagnosed hypothyroidism in children

3.1 Case 1

A 14- year-and-7-month-old boy in pubertal age, but with no signs of pubertal development was referred to endocrinologic examination because of short stature. At admission his height was only 127 cm (- 4.3SD), his height age was 8 years with proportional delay in bone maturation. Muscular pseudohypertrophy and dry, xantochromic skin were present. His appearance was apathetic with an emotionally flat affect. Muscular pseudohypertrophy of solar muscles was present and this phenomenon has been referred to as the Kocher-Debre-Semelaigne syndrome. The hormonal status showed the hypothyroid state; low levels of TT4 and TT3 and extreme elevation of TSH level suggestive of feedback pituitary adenoma. The sella turcica was enlarged and the rare radiologic signs of neglected hypothyroidism were present: osteosclerosis of the skull base and "motocyclist's sunglasses sign" (Fig. 1). In addition epiphyseal dysgenesis and delayed bone maturation were observed (Fig. 2). Ultrasound scan showed atrophic thyrod gland. The severe impairment of linear growth led to dwarfism, characterized by limbs that are disproportionately short compared with the trunk. Besides the growth retardation, the child appeared younger than his age because of sexual infantilism (Fig. 3). The treatment with Na-l-thyroxine accelerated growth and resulted in normal final height and allowed for pubertal progression. This catch-up growth was adequate to compensate the preexistant growth retardation (Fig. 3).

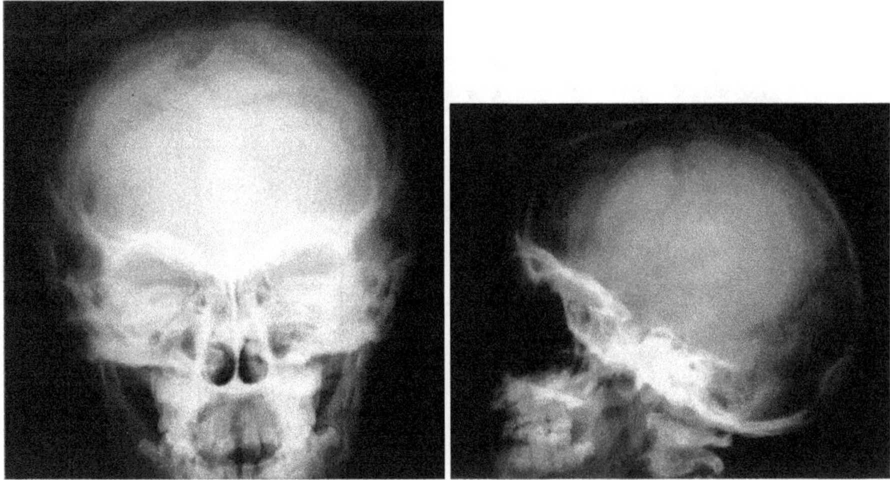

Fig. 1. Cranial radiologic image of the patient with neglected hypothyroidism.

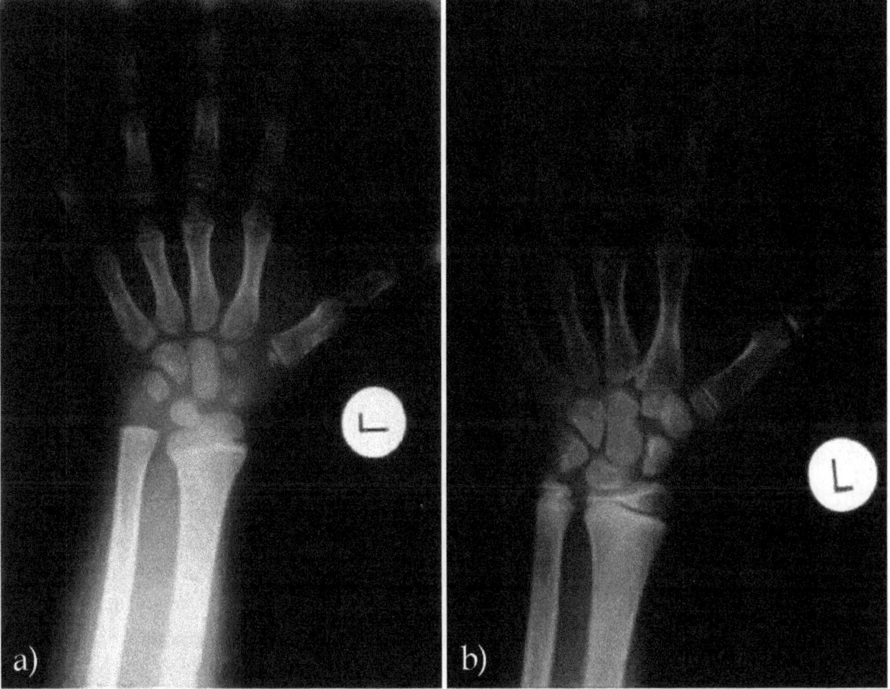

Fig. 2. Bone age retardation of hypothyroid patient (a) corresponds to 8 years versus chronological age of 14 years and 7 months. The treatment allowed for faster bone maturation (2 years for a year) (b).

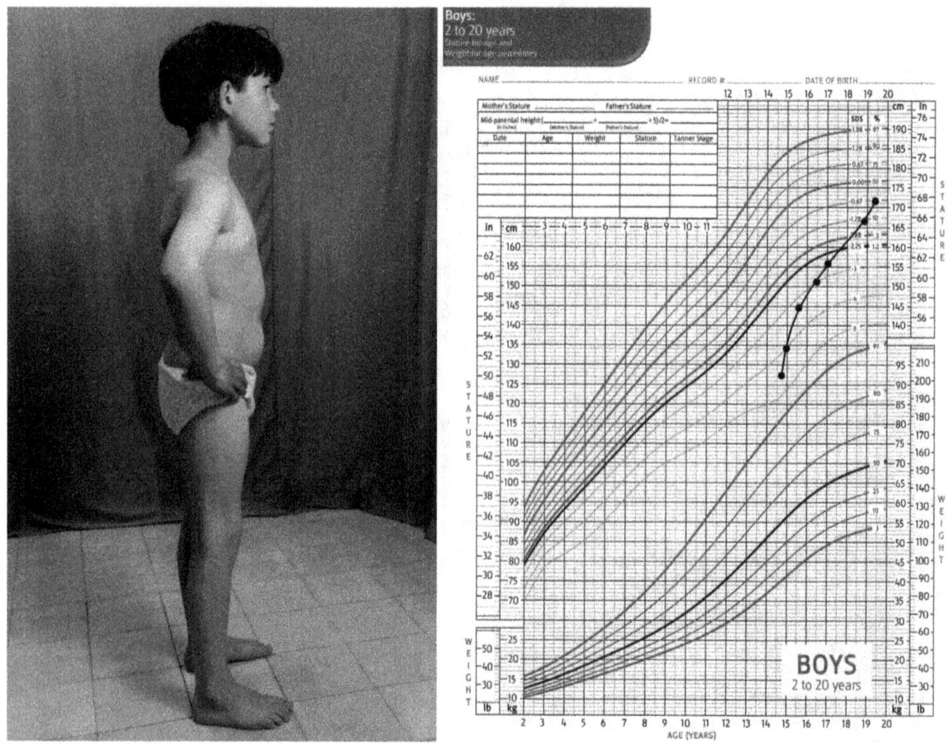

Fig. 3. Disproportionately short stature with pubertal delay and growth curve of the Case 1.

3.2 Case 2

In adolescent girl the diagnosis of atrophic CAT was overlooked and she was treated as exogenous form of obesity and liver disease. At admittion she was 13 years old, inert, apathetic, bradicardic and with dry skin. Weight gain during past 2 years was reported and she was put on unrewarding diets. Her height of 160 cm was within normal rang, P75 (+0.67), height age was 14 years, calculated ideal weight for heigt was 50 kg, so her body mass (BM) of 66kg showed +16 kg, BMI 26 kg (P95) corresponding to clinical obesity. The most prominent laboratory findings were elevated liver enzyms (oxalacetic and piruvic transaminase), lactat dehydrogenase and creatinin phosphokinase as well as triglycerids (Table 3). HBsAg Hepatitis C antigen was positive. A significant association between hepatitis C and AITD has been found (Fernandez-Soto et al., 1998; Testa et al., 2006). The treatment with hepatoprotectors and diet was obviously unsuccessful. After diagnosis of CAT with acquired hypothyroidism and introduction of thyroid hormone replacement therapy, simultaneously with maintenance of euthyroid state, liver enzyms normalized. Ultrasound image showed small gland with inhomogene structure and hypoechogenic zones (Fig. 4).

Glutamic oxalacetic transaminase	172 IU/l	TT4	23.04 nmol/l
Glutamic piruvic transaminase	269 IU/l	fT4	0 nmol/l
Creatinine phosphokinase	1291 mU/ml	TT3	0.21 nmol/l
Lactat dehydrogenase	677 mU/ml	fT3	0.52 pmol/l
Triglyceride	2.61 mmol/l	TSH	102 mU/l
Cholesterol	5.48 mmol/l	TPO Abs	>1000
		Tg Abs	>1000

Table 3. Laboratory data of the case 2.

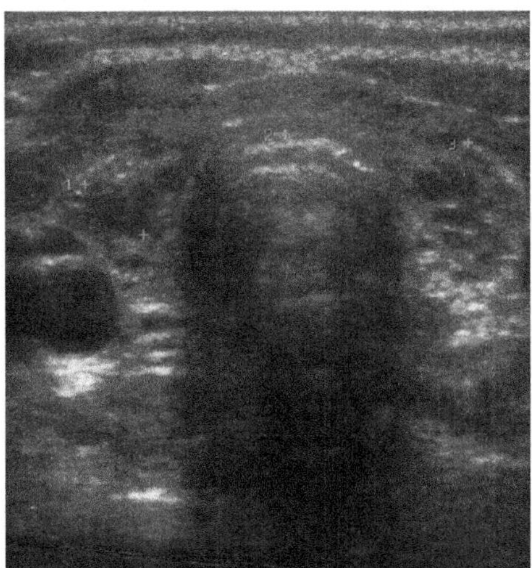

Fig. 4. Ultrasound trasphersal scan of the thyroid in atrophic CAT.

Both cases are illustration of thyroid hormone effects in almost all tissues in the body. Because the long-standing hypothyroidism the dose of Na-l-thyroxine was increased gradually to prevent cardiac failure. Most children respond well to the dose of 100 μg/m^2 body surface (Fisher, 1990; Fisher & Grueters, 2008). When clinical features, such as loss of body hair, raise the possibility of pituitary hypothyroidism, it is dangerous to treat the patient with thyroid hormone without checking the plasma cortisol and if necessary correcting adrenocortical deficiency (Hall, 1989).

Unlike insulin and cortisol levels, which fluctuate widely in response to food ingestion and stress, thyroid hormones are typically maintained at a constant level that keeps the metabolic machinery running in a proper metabolic rate. Thyroid hormones are crucial for survival both in rodents and humans (Zimmerman-Belsing et al., 2003). In many respects thyroid hormones may be viewed as tissue growth factors. Indeed, normal overal whole body growth does not occur in the absence of thyroid hormones despite adequate levels of growth hormone (GH). They influence the function of other endocrine systems. After 3 to 4 years of age thyroid hormone deficiency is not associated with mental retardation, but delayed somatic and linear bone growth. Bone maturation, measured as bone age, also is delayed, diaphyseal bone growth is reduced, and epiphyseal growth and mineralisation largely cease. The effects of thyroid hormones on somatic and skeletal growth are mediated by stimulation of growth hormone and growth factors synthesis and action. Thyroid hormone dependent effects known to be mediated by stimulation and acumulation of mRNAs coding for specific proteins include GH synthesis in pituitary cells, selected enzymes and proteins in liver, (including malic enzyme), beta-myosin heavy chain synthesis in cardiac tissue and Na/K-ATP-ase in a variety of tissues (Fisher, 1990; Fisher & Grueters, 2008). Growth hormone synthesis by pituitary cells is known to be thyroid hormone dependent. Other peptide growth factors besides insulin-like growth factors (IGF-s) may mediate the thyroid hormone effects on specific target tissues; epidermal growth factor, nerve growth factor and erythropoetin (Griffin, 1988; Fisher, 1990). Thyroid hormones also potentiate growth hormone stimulation of insulin- growth factor synthesis and action as well as GH and IGFs binding to the receptors and postreceptor events. Additionally TRH rise in primary hypothyroidism acts as suppressor of nocturnal growth hormone pulses. Chernausek and al. in 1989 documented the attenuation of spontaneous growth hormone secretion in hypothyroid state and proportional fall of IGF-I serum concentration.

Catch-up growth is defined as a linear growth rate greater than expected for age after a period of growth inhibition. Growth inhibiting conditions conserve the limited proliferative capacity of growth plate chondrocytes, thus showing the normal process of growth plate senescence. When the growth-inhibiting condition resolves, the growth plates are less senescent and therefore growth more rapidly than normal for age (Marino et al., 2008; Shao et al., 2006). If the hypothyroid state is prolonged prior to treatment, catch-up growth may be incomplete. Excessive dosage is marked by disproportionate advancement in skeletal age. (Fisher & Grueters, 2008).

3.3 Subclinical hypothyroidism

Some children with CAT expirience all thyroid dysfunction types during natural course of the disease: mild hyperthyroidism at diagnosis (hashitoxicosis), euthyroid state and gradual progression from subclinical to overt hypothyroidism. Another intriguing form of CAT could be subclinical hypothyroidism with mixed signs of hypo and hyperfunction ("autoimmune dysthyroidism"). Thus, clinical features do not always correspond to hormonal status. The reasons for diagnostic pitfalls, beacause of clinical ambiguity are chalanging for pediatricians and endocrinologists.

Even though subclinical hypothyroidism is defined as an asymptomatic disorder in whom euthyroid state is maintained due to TSH elevation, in our expirience this dysfunction type asigned as mild, subclinical or compensated, actually has clinical expression. Tunbridge recorded in adults clinical features that included cold intolerance, a dry skin, lack of energy, puffiness around the eyes, acroparaesthesiae and weight gain, and the signs elicited were those of periorbital swelling, scaling of the skin and a slow pulse rate (minor degrees of hypothyroidism) (Hall, 1989). In children even subclinical form of hypothyroidism has impact on growth, weight regulation, bone maturation and pubertal development.

While the mild clinical picture of hypothyroidism is expected in children, the appearance of opposite, hyperfunction signs in subclinicaly hypothyroid subjects, is intriguing. Possible explanation could be the rise of TRH with neurotransmiter properties that leads to release of TSH, PRL, FSH, and noradrenalin (NA). Tachycardia, nervouseness, emotional lability in subclinicaly hypothyroid subjects could be attribued to NA released in this way. The turnover of NA in brain of hypothyrod subjects is elevated (Jovanovic-Micic et al., 1991; Bauer et al., 2008).

The ambiguity in clinical picture could be explained by presence of heterogenic antibodies to TSH receptor in the same subject. Transient shift from blocking to stimulating antibodies may provoke hyperthyroid signs in hypothyroid subject (Song et al., 1996; Saranac et al., 2003, 2010).

4. Conclusion

CAT attracts clinician's attention for decades. Despite of a rapidly growing body of evidence on complexity of etiopathogenesis and clinical presentation of AITD, primary care physicians neglect or misdiagnose CAT. We believe that it is particularly important to draw attention to this problem in pediatric patients. An improved understanding of CAT clinical diversity could yield better diagnostic and treatment pathways.

5. References

Bartalena, L.; Tanda, ML.; Piantanida, E.; Lai, A.; Compri, E.; Lombardi, V. (2007). Environnment and thyroid autoimmunity, In: *The Thyroid and Autoimmunity: Merck European Thyroid Symposium Noordwijk*, Wiersinga, WM.; Drexhage, HA.; Weetman, AP, pp. 60-73, Thieme, ISBN 978-3-13-134661-2, Stuttgart

Bauer, M.; Goetz, T.; Glenn, T; Whybrow, C. (2008). The thyroid-brain interaction in thyroid disorders and mood disorders. *J Neuroendocrinol*, Vol.20, No.10, (October 2008), pp. 1101- 1114, ISSN 0953-8194, e-ISSN 1365-2826

Chernausek, SD. & Turner, R. (1989). Attenuation of spontaneous nocturnal growth hormone secretion in children with hypothyroidism and its correlation with plasma insulin-like growth factor I concentrations. *J Pediatr* Vol.114, No.6, (Jun, 1989), pp. 968-972, ISSN 0022-3476, e-ISSN 1097-6833

Fernandez-Soto, L.; Gonzales, A.; Escobar-Jimenez, F.; Vazquez, R.; Ocete, E.; Olea, N.; Salmeron, J. (1998). Increased risk of autoimmune thyroid disease in hepatitis C vs hepatitis B before, during, and after discontinuing interferon therapy. *Arch Intern Med*, Vol.158, No.13, (July 1998), pp. 1445-1448, ISSN 0003-9926, e-ISSN 1538-3679

Fisher, DA. (1990). The Thyroid, In: *Clinical Pediatric Endocrinology*, ed 2, Kaplan, SA, pp. 87-126, W. B. Saunders Company, ISBN 9780721652832, Philadelphia

Fisher, DA. & Grueters, A. (2008). Thyroid disorders in childhood and adolescence. In: *Pediatric Endocrinology*, ed 3, Kaplan., SA, pp. 237-253, Saunders Elsevier, ISBN 978-1-4160-4090-3, Philadelphia

Griffin, JE. & Ojeda, SR. (1988). The thyroid. In: *Textbook of Endocrine Physiology*, Griffin JE, pp. 222-244, Oxford University Press, ISBN 0-19-505442-3, New York

Hall, R. (1989). Thyroid, In: *Fundamentals of Clinical Endocrinology*, ed 4 Hall, R. & Besser, M, pp. 66-152, Churchill Livingstone, ISBN 9780443036491, London

Jovanovic-Micic, D.; Samardzic, R. & Beleslin D. (1991). Thyrotropin-releasing hormone: distribution, role and importance (article in Serbian). *Srp Arh Celok Lek*, Vol.119, No.9-10, (September-October 1991), pp. 263-270, ISSN 0370-8179

Marino, R.; Hedge, A.; Barnes, KM. et al. (2008). Catch-up growth after hypothyroidism is caused by delayed growth plate senescence. *Endocrinology*, Vol.149, No.4, (April 2008), pp. 1820-1828, ISSN 0013-7227, e-ISSN 1945-7170

Rallison, ML.; Dobyns, BM.; Keating, FR.; Rall, JE.; Tyler, FH. (1975). Occurence and natural history of chronic autoimmune thyroiditis in childhood. *J Pediatr*, Vol.86. No.5, (May 1975), pp. 675-682, ISSN 0022-3476, e-ISSN 1097-6833

Saranac, L.; Zivanovic, S. & Novak, M. High fT3 (free triiodothyronine), new syndrome or innocent bystander. *Endocrine Abstracts 2010: 22 P771 Abstr European Congress of Endocrinology*, Prague, April 24-28, 2010.

Saranac, L.; Miljkovic, M.; Stamenkovic, H.; Mileusnic-Milenovic, R.; Petrovic, G.; Kamenov, B. (2003). Late onset transient thyroid dysfunction in children born to mothers with autoimmune thyroid disease. *Facta Universitatis Series Medicine and Biology*, Vol.10, No.1, (March 2003), pp. 52-56, ISSN 0354 – 2017

Saranac, L.; Zivanovic, S.; Bjelakovic, B.; Stamenkovic, H.; Novak, M.; Kamenov, B. (2011). Why is the thyroid so prone to autoimmune disease. *Horm Res Paediatr*, Vol.75, No.3, (February 2011), pp. 157-165, ISSN 1663-2818, e-ISSN 1663-2826

Shao, YY.; Wang, L.; Ballock, RT. (2006). Thyroid hormone and the growth plate. *Rev Endocrin Metab Disord*, Vol.7, No.4, (December 2006), pp. 265-271, ISSN 1389-9155, e-ISSN 1573-2606

Song, YH.; Li, Y. & Maclaren, NK. (1996). The nature of autoantigens targeted in autoimmune endocrine diseases. *Immunol Today*, Vol.17, No.5, (May 1996), pp. 232-238, ISSN 0167-5699

Testa, A.; Castaldi, P.; Fanti, V.; Fiore, GF.; Grieco, V.; De Rosa, G. (2006). Prevalence ov HCV antibodies in autoimmune thyroid disease. *Eur Rev Med Pharmacol Sci*, Vol.10, No.4, (July-August 2006), pp. 183-186, ISSN 1128-3602

Tomer, Y. & Huber, A. (2009). The etiology of autoimmune thyroid disease: a story of genes and environment. *J Autoimmun*, Vol.32, No.3-4 (May-June 2009), pp. 231-239, ISNN 0896-8411

Weetman, AP. (2003). Autoimmune thyroid disease: propagation and progression. *Eur J Endocrinol*, Vol.14, No.1, (January 2003), pp. 1-9, ISSN 0804-4643, e-ISSN 1479-683X

Zimmerman-Belsing, T.; Brabant, G.; Holst, JJ.; Feldt-Rasmusen U. (2003). Circulating leptin and thyroid dysfunction. *Eur J Endocrinol*, Vol.149, No.4, (October 2003), pp.257-271, ISSN 0804-4643, e-ISSN 1479-683X

Part 3

Pregnancy and Childhood

Universal Screening for Thyroid Disorders in Pregnancy: Experience of the Czech Republic

Eliska Potlukova[1], Jan Jiskra[1], Zdenek Telicka[1], Drahomira Springer[2] and Zdenka Limanova[1]

[1]3rd Department of Medicine, General University Hospital and 1st Faculty of Medicine, Charles University in Prague, Czech Republic

[2]Institute of Clinical Biochemistry and Laboratory Diagnostics, General University Hospital, Prague, Czech Republic

1. Introduction

The role of the thyroid gland in pregnancy and the impact of thyroid disorders on the course of pregnancy and development of the offspring have drawn a considerable interest in the recent years, both in the medical and in the general society. About 10% of pregnant women are positive for autoantibodies against thyroperoxidase (TPOAb) (Glinoer 2007, Lazarus and Kokandi 2000, Springer 2009) and between 2 and 4% suffer subclinical or overt hypothyroidism (Casey 2005; Vaidya 2007, Springer 2009). Dysfunction of the maternal thyroid in pregnancy adversely affects the course of pregnancy and the psychomotor development of the offspring (Haddow 1999, Morreale de Escobar 2004). According to recent findings, even the mere positivity of TPOAb without concomitant thyroid dysfunction in pregnant women may have a negative impact on the psychomotor development of the child (Li 2010). Furthermore, up to one half of the TPOAb-positive (TPOAb+) pregnant women develop postpartum thyroiditis (PPT) which can lead to persistent hypothyroidism in about one third of women (Lazarus and Premawardhana 2008). According to recent findings of Stagnaro-Green, this proportion may be even much higher and persistent hypothyroidism may affect up to one-half of women with history of PPT (Stagnaro-Green 2011b). If unrecognised and untreated, late postpartum thyroid dysfunction, in most cases subclinical (SH) or overt hypothyroidism (OH) may have a long-term negative effect not only on the mother´s health, but also on the next pregnancies.

Since 2006, repeated attempts to implement a universal screening programme for thyroid disorders in the first trimester of pregnancy have been made in the Czech Republic. Moreover, the Czech Endocrine Society initiated a wide informational campaign concerning the importance of correct thyroid function in pregnancy in the media, including TV discussions, seminars and lectures for both the general population and the health professionals. Members of the Czech Endocrine Society together with colleagues from the Czech Society of Biochemistry have initiated several studies focused on various aspects of thyroid disorders among Czech pregnant women. In this review article, we present an overview of the data obtained in the recent years.

Impact of thyroid dysfunction on pregnancy and foetal health

The developing foetus is dependent upon the maternal thyroid hormone synthesis up to the 14th to 16th gestational weeks. Afterwards, its´ own thyroid gland starts to synthesise thyroid hormones, albeit in insufficient quantities. Thus, the first trimester of pregnancy is crucial in terms of adequate supply of maternal thyroid hormones to the embryo. Numerous retrospective and case-controlled studies confirmed detrimental effects of maternal overt hypothyroidism (OH) on the course of pregnancy and on foetal health.

Severe deficit of thyroid hormones leads to irreversible changes in foetal development. Impairment of neuronal differentiation leads to inadequate development of the central nervous system with resulting mental retardation. It may also lead to somatic defects including congenital cardiac defects and disrupted bone growth. These changes are most prominent in untreated congenital hypothyroidism (cretinism). Moderate thyroid hormone deficit may lead to less pronounced neurocognitive dysfunction. As Haddow et al. have shown in their well-cited study, children of untreated hypothyroid pregnant women had at age 7 to 9 years IQ below 85 points in 19% of cases in comparison with 5% of children of euthyroid or substituted mothers. The average IQ was 7 points lower in children of hypothyroid untreated mothers than in children of hypothyroid mothers substituted by levothyroxine (LT4) (Haddow 1999). Furthermore, iodine-deficient pregnant women are prone to hypothyroxinaemia. As Morreale de Escobar has shown, up to 70 % of children of iodine-deficient mothers may suffer from attention deficit hyperactive disorder (Morreale de Escobar 2004a,b).

Apart from neurocognitive foetal impairment, maternal untreated OH is associated with the risk of foetal loss in up to 60% (Abalovich 2002) and the risk of gestational hypertension in 22 % (Leung 1993), which was higher than in euthyroid women of women with subclinical hypothyroidism. According to Allan et al, women with OH have also an increased risk of foetal death (Allan 2000). Thus, it is of no doubt that untreated maternal OH may be detrimental for the maternal-foetal unit in the short-term and in the long-term sense.

Pros and cons of universal screening for thyroid disorders in pregnancy

Although maternal autoimmune thyroid disorders (AITD) fulfil many criteria used for identification of diseases subject to universal screening, this issue has been highly controversial. The main arguments for implementation of universal screening are the following: a) the impact of maternal hypothyroidism on the course of pregnancy and the health of offspring has been well described and the treatment is effective and simple; b) the prevalence of hypothyroidism in pregnancy is comparable with other universally screened diseases; c) the method of screening (laboratory measurement of thyroid parameters) is relatively simple and inexpensive – the financial costs depending on the choice of thyroid parameters screened; d) it is cost-effective (on condition that not only OH, but also SH decreases the offspring´s IQ (Dosiou 2008, Thung 2009); e) the risk-benefit ratio of the screening for each individual is acceptable. In the past, some authorities recommended universal screening but not the American Thyroid Association or the Association of American Obstetricians and Gynaecologists, who have consistently advocated a case-finding screening strategy focused on high-risk women (Abalovich 2007, Stagnaro-Green 2011) (Table 1).

Authority	Year	Recommendation
American Association of Clinical Endocrinologists	2002	Universal screening
Expert panel of American Thyroid Association, American Association of Clinical Endocrinologists and The Endocrine Society	2004	Case-finding screening
Second panel of American Thyroid Association, American Association of Clinical Endocrinologists and The Endocrine Society	2005	Universal screening
British Thyroid Association, Association of Clinical Biochemists, British Thyroid Foundation. UK guidelines for the Use of thyroid Function Tests	2006	Case-finding screening
American College of Obstetrics and Gynecology	2007	Case-finding screening
The Endocrine Society	2007	Case-finding screening
American Thyroid Association	2011	Case-finding screening

Table 1. Overview of recommendations for screening for thyropathy in pregnancy.

The main argument of the opponents to universal screening is the lack of randomised controlled trials demonstrating that treatment by LT4 of pregnant women with subclinical hypothyroidism increases the offspring´s IQ. Preliminary results of the first major study "The Control Antenatal Thyroid Screening Study" presented on ITC in Paris 2010 were rather disappointing (Lazarus 2010). The authors found only a non-significant difference in the prevalence of three-year-old children with IQ<85 of women unscreened vs. mothers screened and treated in case of SH in pregnancy (15% vs. 11.5%, p=0.09). However, the major drawback of this study is that pregnant women up to the 16th gestation week were included. Thus, we may suspect that in some women the treatment started too late, after the crucial changes in the embryonic/foetal brain have occurred. Another multicenter randomized placebo-controlled clinical trial is at present being conducted by the Maternal Fetal Medicine Unit of the National Institutes of Health in the USA. The primary outcome will be child IQ at 5 years of age. Results of this study should be available in 2015 and they may give a final answer to the question of universal screening for thyroid disorders in pregnancy.

The case-finding screening strategy

Due to the above-mentioned facts, the latest guidelines of the American Thyroid Association (ATA) recommend a case-finding screening targeted at women at high-risk for hypothyroidism in pregnancy (Stagnaro-Green 2011a). The new guidelines introduce age over 30 years and body-mass index over 40 kg/m2 among the risk factors. The other risk factors include: history of thyroid dysfunction or prior thyroid surgery, symptoms of thyroid dysfunction or the presence of goitre, TPOAb positivity, diabetes type 1 or other autoimmune diseases in history, history of miscarriage or preterm delivery, history of head of neck radiation, family history of thyroid dysfunction, use of amiodarone/lithium or recent administration of iodinated radiologic contrast, infertility and residence in an area of known moderate to severe iodine insufficiency. Thus, according to ATA, the first physician dealing with newly pregnant women should consider 12 different risk factors. If any of them were positive, he should order a blood test for thyroid-stimulating hormone (TSH). In our opinion, this form of screening is likely to be neglected due to practical reasons. It has been shown that the case-finding approach may miss up to one half of pregnant women in comparison with universal screening (Vaidya 2007, Horacek 2010, Jiskra 2011a); and it may be difficult to implement in the routine practice (Vaidya 2002). Moreover, in our view, assessment of only TSH is insufficient due to the above-mentioned risks carried by isolated hypothyroxinemia and TPOAb positivity.

2. Prevalence of thyroid disorders in pregnant Czech women

The Czech Endocrine Society together with the Czech Society of Biochemistry has repeatedly attempted to implement universal screening for AITD in the first trimester of pregnancy. In order to gain data on thyroid disorders in Czech pregnant women, two large studies including nearly 8 000 consecutive pregnant women (Springer 2009, Limanova 2011), have been conducted in the Czech Republic in the last years.

The first study by Springer et al. was performed between 2006 and 2008 and examined 5520 consecutive asymptomatic pregnant women in the 9th-11th gestational week. The aim of this study was to evaluate the prevalence of thyroid disorders in pregnant Czech women and to identify optimal reference intervals in evaluation of maternal thyroid function during the first trimester of pregnancy. The screening consisted of laboratory assessment of serum thyroid stimulating hormone (TSH), free thyroxine (FT4, only in those with pathological TSH/TPOAb) and autoantibodies against thyroperoxidase (TPOAb). All measurements were performed by chemiluminometric immunoanalysis on an ADVIA Centaur system (Siemens, Healthcare Diagnostics Inc, Tarrytown, NY, USA) in one centre (Institute of Clinical Biochemistry and Laboratory Diagnostics, General University Hospital in Prague). Women with positive screening result were advised to visit an endocrinologist within a few days. Based on the results obtained, Springer et al. set normal limits for TSH and TPOAb in pregnancy as following: TSH 0.06-3.67 mU/l; TPOAb <143 kU/l; the study did not attempt to set new reference ranges for FT4. In this cohort of pregnant women, 822 (14.9%) had at least one of the parameters outside of the normal range. Suppressed TSH was found in 141 (2.55%) women, while 299 (5.42%) had TSH over the reference interval; elevation of TPOAb was present in 549 (9.95%) women (Jiskra 2011a). The data are shown in detail in Table 2.

Thus, in this study, there was a higher prevalence of pregnant women with TSH elevation (4.48%) as compared to other iodine-sufficient countries, where the prevalence of pregnant women with TSH elevation reaches 2-3% (Casey 2005; Allan 2000; Vaidya 2007). Obviously, these numbers depend on the TSH upper limit of reference range used. In the Czech studies, the cut-off at 3.67 mU/l was used (Springer 2009). This value was determined as the 97.5th percentile of TSH values of 4337 women in the first trimester of pregnancy with no history of thyroid disease, anti-TPO level lower than 60 kU/l (=negative) and free bhCG lower than triple that of the median (56.6 mg/l). It is interesting to note that the 97.5th percentile in unselected women was higher (Table 3). At present, world authorities recommend to use the upper cut-off at 2.5 mUl (Stagnaro-Green 2011). Therefore, for the Czech population, this cut-off lies either too low; or there is a higher prevalence of hypothyroidism among Czech pregnant women; or our analytical method used for TSH measurements gives higher numbers than methods used by others. However, our analysis was performed using a well-established and widely used analyser (Advia Centaur, Siemens). Apparently, the cut-off at 2.5 mU/l would lead to large numbers of pregnant women positive in screening.

	Number of women screened
Total	5520
Positive in screening (at least one parameter)	822 (14.89%)
Hypothyroidism	299 (5.42 %)
Overt hypothyroidism	49 (0.89 %)
Subclinical hypothyroidism	250 (4.53 %)
TPOAb+ hypothyroidism	144 (2.61 %)
TPOAb- hypothyroidism	155 (2.81 %)
Transient gestational hyperthyroidism	99 (1.8 %)
Hyperthyroidism	141 (2.55 %)
Overt hyperthyroidism	19 (0.34 %)
Subclinical hyperthyroidism	122 (2.21 %)
TPOAb+ hyperthyroidism	23 (0.42 %)
TPOAb- hyperthyroidism	118 (2.14 %)
TPOAb positivity (>143 kIU/l)	549 (9.95 %)
Euthyroid TPOAb+	376 (6.81 %)
TPOAb+, normal TSH, decreased FT4	5 (0.09 %)
TPOAb+, normal TSH, elevated FT4	1 (0.02 %)

Hypothyroidism was defined as TSH >3.67 mIU/l (overt with decreased FT4 and subclinical with TSH >3.67 mIU/l and normal FT4). Hyperthyroidism was defined as decreased TSH <0.06 mIU/l (overt with TSH <0.06 mIU/l and FT4 >23.0 pmol/l and subclinical with TSH<0.06 mIU/l and normal FT4.

Table 2. Results of universal screening for thyroid disorders among Czech pregnant women in the 9th to 11th gestational weeks.

TSH mU/l	**N**	**Median**	**Minimum**	**Maximum**	**2.5th percentile**	**5th percentile**	**95th percentile**	**97.5th percentile**
Non-selected	5520	1.280	0	411.874	0.048	0.147	3.713	4.796
Selected group	4337	1.213	0	11.534	0.062	0.154	3.144	3.670

Selected group: pregnant women with no history of thyroid disease, anti-TPO level lower than 60 kU/l and free bhCG lower than triple that of the median (56.6 mg/l).

Table 3. Reference ranges for TSH in the 9th to 11th gestational weeks in Czech pregnant women.

After two years of preparations, a joint "Pilot Project" of the Czech Society of Endocrinology, the Society of Clinical Biochemistry and the General Insurance Company of the Czech Republic started in 2009 (Limanova 2011). The Pilot Project was supported by the General Insurance Company. The aim of the Pilot Project was to ascertain the optimal combination and economic feasibility of diagnostic tests, the timing of the blood test and the possibility of connecting the test with genetic-disorder screening in the first trimester of pregnancy. The purpose of the study was also to provide information about cooperation among gynaecologists, laboratories and endocrinologists. In the Pilot Project, TSH, FT4 and TPOAb were measured in 2937 consecutive pregnant women from 13 Czech regions with good laboratory background and cooperative endocrinologists. Contrary to the previous study, measurements were performed in regional laboratories and the reference ranges differed according to each laboratory. In this cohort, 569 (19.4%) woman were screened as positive. Abnormalities of TSH were found in 11% of women: elevation in 7.8% and suppression in 3.2%. Only 15 (0.5%) women with TSH suppression were diagnosed with true hyperthyroidism. Hypothyroxinemia was found in 3.7% and TPOAb positivity in 262 (8.9%) women. One hundred fifty-eight women (5.37%) had positive TPOAb with normal thyroid function. Thus, in this second study, we found an even higher prevalence of abnormally high TSH among pregnant women than in the study of Springer et al. However, due to the different analytical methods, these results cannot be directly compared. Cooperation with gynaecologists wasn´t always optimal despite the fact that they were provided with all necessary information well in advance. On the other hand, laboratories analysed the samples promptly, and many of them took part in providing publicity and further information to other cooperating health care professionals. In conclusion, the Pilot Project study showed that implementation of universal screening for thyroid disorders in pregnancy would be feasible in the Czech Republic, although the general knowledge on importance of correct thyroid function in pregnancy needs to be improved among practical gynaecologists.

The attempts to implement a universal screening programme for AITD in pregnancy in the Czech Republic have suffered a major blow due to the world financial crisis starting in 2009. In the future years, we will probably have to concentrate on implementation of the case-finding approach years among the official risk factors.

3. Ultrasound imaging and risk-assessment of positively screened pregnant women

Most of the studies on AITD in pregnancy deal only with laboratory parameters and it is not clear whether the thyroid ultrasound (TUS) image is of any consequence for the clinical outcomes of the pregnancy. Studies concerning TUS in pregnancy are scarce, mostly aimed at the assessment of thyroid volume. Therefore, in one of our studies, we focused on the relationship between TUS, laboratory parameters and the outcome of pregnancy. Between 2006 and 2009, we performed thyroid ultrasound in 186 pregnant women positively screened for thyroid disorders in the first trimester of pregnancy; i.e. they had abnormal TSH and/or positivity for TPOAb (Jiskra 2011a). The control group consisted of 67 age-comparable non-pregnant women with pathological TSH and/or TPOAb levels. Unexpectedly, we found that these positively screened pregnant women had rather small thyroid glands with the median volume of 8.5 ml. This is smaller than in age-comparable non-selected non-pregnant Czech women in the study of Dvorakova et al. (median 11.8 mL in group of women aged 31-35 years) (Dvorakova 2006). Furthermore, the thyroid volume in pregnant women did not differ from controls. This is in contrast to the findings of both Fister and Vila, who showed an increased thyroid volume in pregnancy in iodine-sufficient (Fister 2009) and iodine-deficient areas (Vila 2008). The finding of small thyroids in pregnant Czech women is probably linked to the saturation with iodine. Iodine supplementation of salt has been introduced in Czechoslovakia in 1950. Therefore, the present pregnant women are already the third generation who live in iodine-sufficient conditions.

In our study, we also found that only 49% of the TPOAb+ pregnant women had autoimmune pattern on TUS. This was significantly less than in non-pregnant TPOAb+ controls (74 %) (Fig.1). Apparently, alterations of immune system in pregnancy cause a different manifestation of autoimmunity in the thyroid tissue. Moreover, we found that the thyroid ultrasound pattern was associated with preterm delivery: TPOAb+ women without autoimmune pattern in TUS had significantly lower prevalence of preterm delivery than the TPOAb+ ones with autoimmune pattern (3.1 vs. 15.2 %). Therefore, autoimmune TUS image in TPOAb+ pregnant women seems to be associated with preterm delivery.

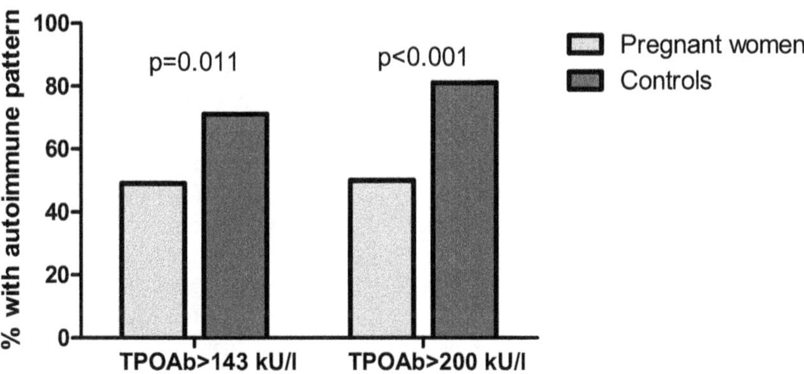

Fig. 1. Ultrasound autoimmune pattern in TPOAb-positive pregnant women and controls.

In the next study from 2011, we focused on the relationship between clinical history, laboratory findings and TUS pattern in positively screened pregnant women (Jiskra 2011b). In this study, 200 of the positively screened women from the cohort of Springer et al. were included (Springer 2009). We regarded women as high-risk if they had any of the following risk factors: family and/or personal history of thyroid disease (including presence of goitre and signs and symptoms suggestive for thyroid dysfunction), family and/or personal history for autoimmune disease, history of neck irradiation, previous miscarriages and preterm deliveries). After exclusion of transient gestational hyperthyroidism, only 74/159 (47 %) women were classified as high-risk for thyroid disease according to their history. There were no significant clinical and laboratory differences between the high- vs. low-risk women, except for higher proportion of FT4 < 75th percentile and a larger thyroid volume in the high-risk group. These finding were consistent with the results of Horacek et al. (Horacek 2010) who found that case-finding screening strategy would miss one half of the high-risk women.

4. Postpartum follow-up of positively screened women

Between 2009 and 2010, we invited all 822 positively screened women from the first cohort of 5520 pregnant women screened (the cohort of Springer et al.) for follow-up (Potlukova et al. 2011, manuscript in preparation). In order to gain as complete a picture of their clinical state and history as possible, we asked them to fill in a detailed internet-based questionnaire concerning their personal, family and gynaecological history. Furthermore, we invited them for a blood test including analysis of TSH, FT4 and TPOAb. The two main aims of the study were: a) to assess the prevalence of high risk-profile women in this group; b) to evaluate the postpartum thyroid function in this group with regard to the adequacy of treatment.

Of the 822 women invited, 237 (28.8%) joined the study. This group of positively screened women differed from the one analysed in our other two recent studies (Jiskra 2011a, b). The median age of participating women was 31 years at the time of screening in pregnancy. The median interval between delivery and follow-up reached 21 months. The analysis of questionnaires brought a major finding: the use of the new guidelines of American Thyroid Association (Stagnaro-Green 2011) for identification of high-risk women substantially increased the proportion of high-risk women among the positively screened. The "old" risk factors could identify only two thirds of the positively screened women: personal and family history of thyroid disease (only first-degree relatives), diabetes mellitus type 1, other autoimmune diseases in personal history, infertility and history of spontaneous abortion. However, if the "new" risk factor, age>30 years (in our analysis, 31 years and more), was added to the classical ones, 85% of the women could be classified as "high-risk" (Fig.2). This is a surprisingly high number, especially in the view of previous studies (Jiskra 2011b, Horacek 2010, Vaidya 2002). However, this effect of age could be partially due to selection bias, as the majority of women who answered the questionnaire had good education and therefore they tended to later pregnancies. We also tried to identify the most important risk factors in order to simplify the decision process which women should be screened. We found that four risk factor could identify 82% of the high-risk women: age 31 and more, personal and family history of thyroid disease and the presence of goitre (Fig.2).

In our follow-up study, we further found that one third of initially euthyroid TPOAb+ pregnant women had TSH outside of normal range at follow-up. In comparison to pregnancy, median TSH (as well as FT4) significantly increased at follow-up (Fig. 3). Thirty-eight (33.6%) of 113 initially euthyroid TPOAb+ women had TSH outside of normal range at follow-up (median 17 months after delivery): 13 (11.5%) had TSH<0,37 mU/l; 18 (15.9%) had TSH >4,0 and <10.0 mU/l (all had normal FT4). Seven (6.2%) had TSH>10.0 mU/l with three having a hypothyroxinemia. It is important to note that many of these women were inadequately treated: all of the women with TSH suppression at follow-up were simply overdosed by LT4; and half of those with TSH elevation at follow-up were treated by too low doses of LT4. Thus, TPOAb positivity even with normal thyroid function in pregnancy carries a high risk of hypothyroidism one and half years postpartum. This is in line with results of Stagnaro-Green, who found that 50% of women with PPT were hypothyroid one year after delivery (Stagnaro-Green 2011). Our results also show that monitoring and treatment of women with AITD in the peripartal period is commonly inadequate.

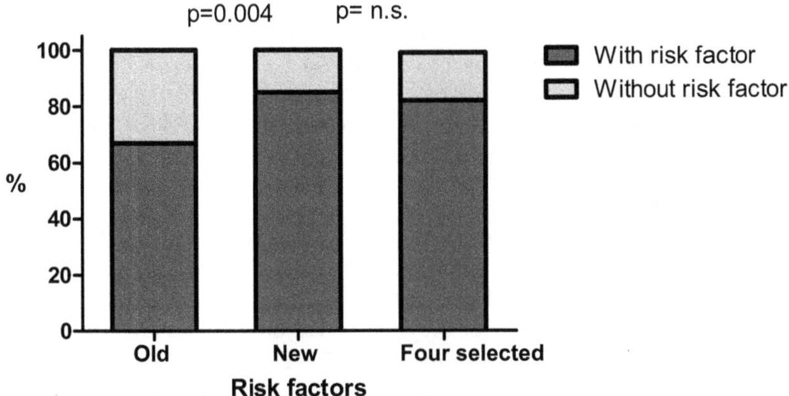

Fig. 2. **Proportion of positively screened pregnant women with at least one risk factor for hypothyroidism.** Old: risk factors according to Guidelines of ATA 2007; New: risk factor according to Guidelines of ATA 2011; Four selected: age, personal and family history of thyroid disease and the presence of goitre.

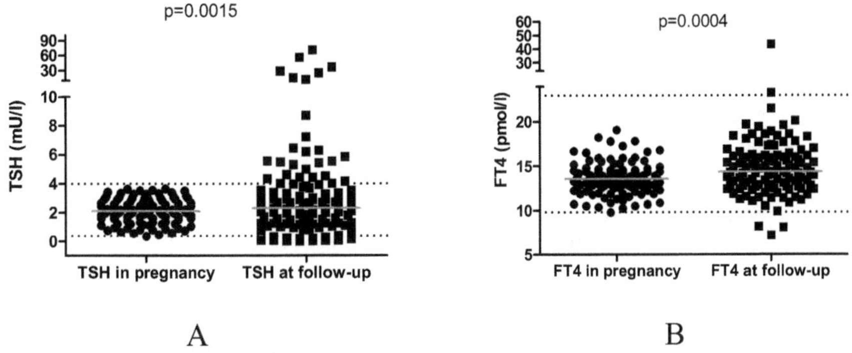

Fig. 3. **Postpartum development of the thyroid function in initially euthyroid TPOAb+ pregnant women.** A: Thyroid Stimulating Hormone (TSH); B: Free Thyroxine (FT4). Median time between delivery and follow-up was 17 months. Median values of TSH and FT4 are marked in grey. Reference intervals for non-pregnant women are marked by dotted lines.

5. Financial analysis

Two studies have dealt with the cost-effectiveness of universal screening for thyroid disorders in pregnancy and both found it cost-effective under condition that subclinical hypothyroidism decreases IQ of the offspring (Dosiou 2008, Thung 2009). In order to roughly assess the financial aspects of the universal screening in the Czech conditions, we performed a simple statistical analysis of the financial costs of the Pilot Project (Telicka

2010). The goal of this study was to find out the overall costs of the Pilot Project as compared to positively-screened tests and simulate the costs in the current situation when the screening is not paid by the insurances companies. Total costs of both TSH and TPOAb screening included in the Pilot Project were 1 373 218 CZK (15 280 €) for 2 651 tested women. The cost of one positive result in any tested parameter (TSH/TPOAb) amounted 2 243 CZK (91€) and the costs of one positive result for hypothyroidism was 1380 CZK (56€).

6. Conclusions

We have shown that the prevalence of thyroid disorders is relatively high among the Czech pregnant women in comparison with other developed iodine-sufficient countries. About one tenth of pregnant women are TPOAb+ and more than 4% have subclinical or overt hypothyroidism in the first trimester of pregnancy. We have also shown that one third of initially euthyroid TPOAb+ pregnant women have TSH outside of normal range one and half years after delivery. This was due to postpartum thyroiditis and in many cases inadequate treatment. Thus, TPOAb positivity may endanger not only the current, but also the next pregnancies.

Based on the ultrasound findings in the positively screened women, we can furthermore conclude that pregnant TPOAb positive women have less pronounced TUS changes than non-pregnant controls. Thus, sonography may only be a part of a more complex diagnostic procedure in the screening for thyroid disorders in pregnancy. However, it seems that pregnant women with autoimmune pattern in thyroid ultrasound have an increased risk of preterm delivery.

Moreover, in our studies we confirmed that targeted case-finding screening programme based on the "old" risk factors (Abalovich 2007) would miss one-half of pregnant women with thyroid disease. Also, high- and low-risk pregnant women have similar clinical and laboratory characteristics. However, these findings change if "new" risk factors including age over 30 years (Stagnaro-Green 2011) are used for identification of high-risk women. Age over 30 years increases the proportion of positively screened pregnant women with at least one risk factor to 85%; however, this may be an effect of selection bias.

Finally, the financial analysis showed that the costs of the screening for thyroid dysfunction in pregnancy are not high enough to rend the financial issue a main obstacle in an implementation of universal screening. Both TSH and TPOAb should be included in any screening programme.

The awareness on the thyroid problematics in pregnancy has improved in the general population thanks to the activities of the Czech Society of Endocrinology in the recent; however, some health care professionals dealing with pregnant women show lack of interest in this topic. In conclusion, our data provide a contribution to the published guidelines for management of thyroid disease in pregnancy and present a basis for a world-wide discussion.

7. Acknowledgements

These studies were supported by the grants of the Czech Health Ministry IGA NS 10662-3 and 10595-3.

8. References

Abalovich M, Gutierrez Z, Alcaraz G, Maccallini G, Garcia A, Levalle O. Overt and subclinical hypothyroidism complicating pregnancy. Thyroid 2002;12:63-68

Abalovich M, Nobuyuki A, Barbour L, Cobin RH, De Groof LJ, Glinoer D, Mandel SJ, Stagnaro-Geen A: Management of thyroid dysfunction during pregnancy and postpartum: an Endocrine Society clinical practice guideline. J Clin Endocrin Metab 2007; Aug;92(8 Suppl):S1-47

Allan WC, Haddow JE, Palomaki GE, Williams JR, Mitchell ML, Hermos RJ, Faix JD, Klein RZ. Maternal thyroid deficiency and pregnancy complications: implications for population screening. J Med Screen 2000; 7: 127-130

Casey BM, Dashe JS, Wells CE, McIntire DD, Byrd W, Leveno KJ et al. Subclinical hypothyroidism and pregnancy outcomes. Obstet Gynecol 2005; 105: 239-45

Dosiou C, Sanders GD, Araki SS, Crapo LM. Screening pregnant women for autoimmune thyroid disease: a cost-effectiveness analysis. Eur J Endocrinol 2008; 158: 841-851.

Dvoraková M, Bílek R, Cerovská J, Hill M, Novák Z, Vavrejnová V, Vlcek P, Vrbíková J, Zamrazil V. The volumes of the thyroid gland in adults aged 18-65 years in the Czech Republic--determination of the norms. Vnitr Lek 2006; 52: 57-63.

Fister P, Gaberscek S, Zaletel K, Krhin B, Gersak K, Hojker S (2009) Thyroid volume changes during pregnancy and after delivery in an iodine-sufficient Republic of Slovenia. Eur J Obstet Gynecol Reprod Biol 2009 145: 45-48.

Glinoer D. The regulation of thyroid function in pregnancy: pathways of endocrine adaptation from phsysiology to pathology. Endocr Rev 1997; 18: 404-33

Haddow JE, Palomaki GE, Allan WC, Williams JR, Knight GJ, Gangon J et al. Maternal thyroid deficiency during pregnancy and subsequent neuropsychological development of the child. N Engl J Med 1999; 341: 549-55

Horacek J, Spitalnikova S, Dlabalova B, Malirova E, Vizda J, Svilias I, Cepkova I, McGrath C, Maly J. Universal screening detects two-times more thyroid disorders in early pregnancy than targeted high-risk case finding. Eur J Endocrinol 2010;163: 645 – 650

Jiskra J, Bartakova J, Holinka S, Limanova Z, Springer D, Fait T, Antosova M, Telicka Z, Potlukova E. Low concordance between positive antibodies to thyroperoxidase and thyroid ultrasound autoimmune pattern in pregnant women. Endocr J 2011; *in press.*

Jiskra J, Bartakova J, Holinka S, Límanová Z , Springer D, Antosová M, Telicka Z and Potlukova E. Low prevalence of clinically high-risk women and pathological thyroid ultrasound among pregnant women positive in universal screening for thyroid disorders. Exp Clin Endocrinol Diabetes 2011; DOI http://dx.doi.org/10.1055/s-0031-1284369

Lazarus JH, Kokandi A. Thyroid disease in relation to pregnancy: a decade of change. Clin Endocrinol (Oxf) 2000; 53: 265-78

Lazarus J. Outcome of the CATS study. Oral presentation at the International Thyroid Congress (ITC), Paris, France, 2010, September 11-16. Symposium no. 18

Lazarus JH, Premawardhana LDKE. Postpartum Thyroiditis. In: Contemporary Endocrinology: Autoimmune Diseases in Endocrinology. AP Weetman (ed), Humana Press Inc. New Jersey, USA, 2008: 177-92

Leung AS, Millar LK, Koonings PP, Montoro M, Mestman JH. Perinatal outcome in hypothyroid pregnancies. Obstet Gynecol 1993; 81:349-353

Li Y, Shan Z, Teng W, Yu X, Li Y, Fan C, Teng X, Guo R, Wang H, Li J, Chen Y, Wang W, Chawinga M, Zhang L, Yang L, Zhao Y, Hua T. Abnormalities of maternal thyroid function during pregnancy affect neuropsychological development of their children at 25-30 motnhs. Clin Endocrinol (Oxf) 2010; 72: 825-829

Limanova Z, Springer D: Thyreopathy examination during pregnancy - results of pilot project. Cas Lek ces. 2011; 150: 389-393.

Morreale de Escobar G, Obregon MJ, del Rey FE. Maternal thyroid hormones early in pregnancy and foetal brain development. Best Pract Res Clin Endocrinol Metab 2004; 18: 225-48

Morreale de Escobar G, Obregon MJ, Escobar del Rey F. Role of thyroid hormone during early brain development: Eur J Endocrinol 2004; 151: U25–U37.

Springer D, Zima T, Limanova Z. Reference intervals in evaluation of maternal thyroid function during the first trimester of pregnancy. Eur J Endocrinol. 2009;160(5):791-7.

Stagnaro-Green A, Abalovich M, Alexander E, Azizi F, Mestman J, Negro R, Nixon A, Parce EN, Soldin OP, Sullivan S, Wiersinga W. Guidelines of the American Thyroid Association for the diagnosis and management of thyroid disease during pregnancy and postpartum. Thyroid 2011; 21: 1-45.

Stagnaro-Green A, Schwartz A, Gismondi R, Tinelli A, Mangieri T, Negro R. High rate of persistent hypothyroidism in a large-scale prospective study of postpartum thyroiditis in southern Italy. J Clin Endocrinol Metab 2011;96: 652-657

Telicka Z, Jiskra J, Springer D. Simple Method of Economical Analysis of Diagnosis Procedure (Used in Screening of Thyroid Gland Diseases in Pregnant Women) during the first trimester of pregnancy. European Journal for Biomedical Informatics. 2010; online: http://ejbi.cz/articles/201012/59/1.html

Thung SF, Funai EF, Grobman WA. The cost-effectiveness of universal screening in pregnancy for subclinical hypothyroidism. Am J Obstet Gynecol 2009; 267.e1-267.e7

Vaidya B, Bilous M, Hutchinson RS, Connolly, V, Jones S, Kelly WF et al. Screening for thyroid disease in pregnancy: an audit. Clin Med 2002; 2: 599-600

Vaidya B,Anthony S, Bilous M, Shields B, Drury J, Hutchison S et al. Detection of thyroid dysfunction in early pregnancy: Universal screening or targeted high-risk case finding? J Clin Endocrinol Metab 2007; 92: 203-7

Vila L, Legaz G, Barrionuevo C, Espinel ML, Casamitjana R, Muñoz J, Serra-Prat M, Puig-Domingo M. Iodine status and thyroid volume changes during pregnancy: results of a survey in Aran Valley (Catalan Pyrenees). J Endocrinol Invest 2008; 31: 851-855.

8

Treatment of Graves' Disease During Pregnancy

Teresa M. Bailey
Ferris State University College of Pharmacy
USA

1. Introduction

1.1 Etiology

Graves' disease is an autoimmune syndrome where thyroid stimulating antibodies bind to and activate the thyrotropin receptor on thyroid cells resulting in hyperthyroidism (Weetman, 2000; Jonklaas, 2011). Specifically, the production of thyroid-stimulating immunoglobulin (TSI) and thyroid-stimulating hormone-binding inhibitory immunoglobulin (TBII) act on the thyroid stimulating hormone receptor to cause thyroid stimulation or thyroid inhibition, respectively.

Graves' disease is the most common cause of hyperthyroidism in the United States with an estimated prevalence of 3 per 1,000 (Jonklaas, 2011, Abalovich, 2007). The occurrence of Graves' disease is similar in Caucasians and Asians, with a lower incidence in African Americans (Weetman, 2000; Jonklaas, 2011). Major risk factors for Graves' disease include female gender and genetic predisposition. Graves' disease is approximately eight times more common in women than men and often occurs in clusters in families (Weetman, 2000). An increased frequency of certain human leukocyte antigens (HLAs) has also been associated with Graves' disease. In Caucasians, HLA-D3 is present in approximately 50 percent of patients. The presence of both HLA-B8 and HLA-D3 indicates a fourfold increase in the risk of developing Graves' disease (Jonklaas, 2011).

1.2 Signs and symptoms

Common symptoms of hyperthyroidism may present as irritability, hyperactivity, altered mood, insomnia, fatigue, heat intolerance, increased sweating, palpitations, dyspnea, pruritis, weight loss with increased appetite, thirst and polyuria, increased stool frequency, oligomenorrhea or amenorrhea, and loss of libido. Hyperthyroidism signs may include fine tremor, hyperkinesis or hyperreflexia, warm, moist skin, palmar erythema, hair loss, muscle weakness and wasting, sinus hypertension, tachycardia, atrial fibrillation, and/or heart failure. When hyperthyroidism is left untreated, manifestations of Graves' disease may appear such as diffuse goiter, ophthalmopathy, retrobulbar pressure or pain, scleral injection, eyelid lag or retraction, exophthalmos, localized dermopathy, lymphoid hyperplasia, or thyroid acropachy. Conditions associated with Graves' disease may comprise of type 1 diabetes mellitus, Addison's disease, pernicious anemia, alopecia areata, vitiligo, myasthenia gravis, or celiac disease (Weetman, 2000).

1.3 Diagnosis

The American Association of Clinical Endocrinologists and the American Thyroid Association recommend reflect same (TSH) testing as an initial test for screening and evaluation of symptomatic disease (Bahn, 2011). Laboratory results in Graves' disease show an overall increase in both free triiodothyronine (FT_3) and free thyroxine (FT_4) with a disproportionate increase in triiodothyronine (T_3) to thyroxine (T_4). Values for serum T_3 and T_4 are elevated due to the saturation of thyroid binding globulin. However, levels for FT_3 and FT_4 are elevated to a greater extent than serum values. Reflect same (TSH) is suppressed to the undetectable range (Weetman, 2000; Jonklaas, 2011).

1.4 Treatment

Current treatments for Graves' disease include radioactive iodine, surgery, and antithyroid drugs such as propylthiouracil (PTU), methimazole, and carbimazole (a precursor molecule to methimazole not available in the US). Selection of the treatment modality varies greatly by geographic location with radioactive iodine being the treatment of choice in the United States and antithyroid drugs in most other countries (Weetman, 2000; Cooper, 2005; Jonklaas, 2011). In addition to geographic location, other aspects influence the selection of the most appropriate treatment such as: time to initial improvement, planning pregnancy, pregnancy or breastfeeding, size of the goiter, age of patient, likelihood of side effects, concurrent severe ophthalmopathy, interference with daily activities, and the likelihood of recurrence after treatment (Weetman, 2000).

1.4.1 Thioamides

Antithyroid drugs, thioamides, decrease thyroid hormone synthesis by inhibiting thyroid peroxidase catalyzed iodination of thyroglobulin and by inhibiting iodotyrosine coupling. Therefore, these drugs do not cure Graves' disease but only control hyperthyroidism. Propylthiouracil has an added mechanism of action by reducing the peripheral conversion of T_4 to T_3. The American Thyroid Association and the American Association of Clinical Endocrinologists recommend methimazole as the preferred antithyroid drug in any patient with Graves' disease except during the first trimester of pregnancy (Bahn, 2011).

The initial dosing of either thioamide is empirical. The American Thyroid Association recommends a starting dose of 10-40 mg of methimazole or 100-600 mg of PTU daily in nonpregnant women. The pharmacokinetics of the thiamides are distinct. Methimazole's onset of action is 12-18 hours with a duration of action of 36-72 hours. The peak plasma concentration of methimazole is reached within 1-2 hours of ingestion and the half-life is 4-6 hours after oral administration and has an oral bioavailability of 93% (Clark, 2006). Dosing depends on the severity of hyperthyroidism, 15 mg/day for mild up to 60 mg/day for severe hyperthyroidism. Based on the pharmacokinetics, the daily dose is divided into three doses, given every 8 hours. Methimazole is metabolized in the gastrointestinal system and first pass through the liver.

The peak plasma concentration of PTU is reached within 1-2 hours of ingestion and the elimination half-life is 1-2 hours. The oral bioavailability of PTU is 53-88% and the duration of action is 12-24 hours. Again, dosing depends on the severity of hyperthyroidism but usually is 100-300 mg/day divided into 3 doses, every 8 hours.

The pharmacokinetics of PTU and methimazole in pregnant women are similar to non-pregnant women (Clark, 2006). However, the metabolism and excretion of these drugs are increased in pregnant women with hyperthyroidism, due to an increased metabolic state of pregnancy. Therefore, during pregnancy women may require a higher daily dose of antithyroid drug, such as PTU 300-450 mg per day or methimazole 30-40 mg per day.

Propylthiouracil is highly protein bound (80-85%) whereas, methimazole has neglible protein binding. It was thought PTU was less likely to cross the placenta compared to methimazole (Clark, 2006). To address the theory that PTU has less fetal transfer than methimazole, Mortimer et al. evaluated the maternal to fetal transfer in nine isolated human placental lobules perfused with low and high doses of PTU and methimazole (Mortimer, 1997). Placentas were collected from euthyroid women with no history of antithyroid drug ingestion. All placentas were delivered at term by cesarean. Both PTU and methimazole readily crossed the placenta achieving steady state concentrations in approximately two hours. Both drugs demonstrated similar transfer kinetics, were nonsaturable, and were unaffected by the addition of bovine albumin to the perfusate. The authors concluded that PTU and methimazole had similar placental transfer kinetics. Therefore the rationale that PTU has less fetal transfer than methimazole was not supported in this well established model of drug transfer across the human placenta (Mortimer, 1997). So although, methimazole has neglible protein binding, methimazole has similar placental transfer compared to PTU.

Because propylthiouracil has a shorter half-life, higher protein binding, and less drug concentration in breast milk, some providers view PTU as a safer option in breastfeeding. However, the American Academy of Pediatricians considers both compatible with breastfeeding (AAP, 2001). Nonetheless, methimazole has been found sufficient amounts in breastfed infants to cause thyroid dysfunction. Low doses of methimazole (<20 mg/day) have not been shown to be a serious risk to nursing infants (Cooper, 2009; Marx, 2009). Doses of propylthiouracil of less than 300 mg a day is recommended (Marx, 2009; Abalovich, 2007). It is recommended to have the mother take the antithyroid drug after breastfeeding (Marx, 2009). Monitoring the infant's thyroid function while the nursing mother is taking either antithyroid drug is advised.

One of the serious, rare side effects of thioamides is agranulocytosis, presenting with a fever, sore throat and an absolute granulocyte count of less than 500 per cubic millimeter. Thioamide-induced agranulocytosis has an incidence of 0.1-0.4% among the thioamides, is not dose related, and usually occurs within the first 90 days of therapy. If suspected, a complete blood count should be drawn and the medication should be immediately discontinued. Unfortunately, there is a significant likelihood of cross reaction among the thioamides so switching to another thioamide should not be an option. Routine white blood count monitoring has not been helpful in prevention because the thioamide-induced agranulocytosis occurs rapidly. However, a baseline assessment of the patient's white blood cell count is recommended prior to initiation of the thioamide.

Other side effects include leucopenia, thrombocytopenia, hepatitis, and vasculitis. Vasculitis has been reported more often with PTU and results in glomerulonephritis and diffuse alveolar hemorrhage (Kang, 2006). Methimazole has been reported to have a 33% chance of cross reaction to PTU-induced vasculitis. More common side effects for both methimazole and PTU include fever, rash, arthritis, nausea, anorexia, and loss of taste or smell. (Weetman, 2000; Garcia-Mayor, 2010) The incidence of thioamide side effects is similar among pregnant and non-pregnant women. Side effects to methimazole are dose-related; PTU is less dose-related (Garcia-Mayor, 2010). Cross reactivity to thioamide-induced adverse events between the two agents may be as high as 50% (Garcia-Mayor, 2010).

2. Graves' disease in pregnancy

It is estimated that hyperthyroidism is present in approximately 0.1-0.2% of pregnancies (Miehle, 2003; Mestman, 2004; Galofre, 2009). Of those pregnancies, neonatal Graves' disease occurs in 1-5% of those babies (Fitzpatrick, 2010; Marx, 2008). Hyperthyroidism is the second most common endocrine disorder that occurs during pregnancy, following only diabetes mellitus (Mestman, 1998). Graves' disease is the most common cause of hyperthyroidism during pregnancy, accounting for 85-95% of the cases (Galofre, 2009; Ecker, 2000). Another cause of hyperthyroidism results from overstimulation of the thyroid gland via human chorionic gonadotropin (hCG). This syndrome, known as gestational transient thyrotoxicosis (GTT), occurs during the first half of gestation due to hyperemesis gravidarum and is less severe than hyperthyroidism due to Graves' disease (Glinoer, 2003).

2.1 Etiology

Thyroid function changes during pregnancy due to the elevated hCG, an increase in estrogen that increases circulating thyroid binding globulin levels which is the major transport protein for thyroid hormone, and a decrease in iodide due to increased renal clearance and losses due to the fetus and placenta (Marx, 2009). Before 12 weeks gestation, significant fetal brain development occurs through maternal thyroid hormones. After 12 weeks gestation, the fetal thyroid gland concentrates iodine and synthesizes thyroid hormone and continues fetal brain development (Morreale, 2000; Inoue, 2009; Abalovich, 2007).

2.2 Signs and symptoms

Pregnancy complicated by Graves' disease usually presents with symptoms appearing in the first trimester, improving in the second and third trimesters, and reappearing in the postpartum period (Mestman, 2004; Inoue, 2009). Significant fetal and maternal complications can occur if the condition is left untreated. Specifically, spontaneous abortion, preterm delivery, stillbirth, low birth weight, preeclampsia, heart failure, and thyroid storm are known complications (Mestman, 2004; Inoue, 2009; Marx, 2009). Low birth weight has been reported to occur nine times as often compared to pregnancies not complicated by hyperthyroidism (Millar, 1994). Neonatal hyperthyroidism, prematurity and intrauterine growth retardation may occur. A 5.6% incidence of fetal death or stillbirth and a 5% incidence of fetal and neonatal abnormalities have been reported (Hamburger, 1992). Unfortunately, fetal and neonatal risks associated with Graves' disease may be related to either the disease or the treatment of the disease. Since Graves' disease is mediated by antibodies that cross the placenta, the risk of immune-mediated hypothyroidism and hyperthyroidism may develop in the neonate (ACOG, 2002; Inoue, 2009). Women with Graves' disease have TSI and TBII that can stimulate or inhibit the fetal thyroid, causing fetal hyperthyroidism or hypothyroidism, respectively. There is no clinical correlation between the levels of antibodies and disease severity (Rashid, 2007). Occasionally, the antibodies may change during pregnancy from stimulation to inhibition of the TSH receptor (Laurberg, 2009).

2.3 Diagnosis

The American Association of Clinical Endocrinologists and the American Thyroid Association recommends measuring TSH but also FT_4 or free thyroxine index (FTI) in symptomatic pregnant women. The FT_4 rises in the first trimester due to the high circulating levels of human chorionic gonadotropin. Rarely hyperthyroidism during pregnancy is due to an abnormally high level of FT_3 instead of high FT_4. The TSH receptor antibody tests, TSI and TBII, may be helpful since these antibodies have been associated with infants born with hypothyroidism. If a pregnant woman has a low TSH but a normal FT_4, subclinical hyperthyroidism is diagnosed and requires no treatment since treatment in this group has not been shown to improve pregnancy outcomes (Abalovich, 2007).

2.4 Treatment

It has been shown that hyperthyroidism in a pregnant woman should be treated to lessen the fetal and neonatal risks. The highest complications were associated with the poorest control and the best control was associated with the least complications (Abalovich, 2007). Therefore, the goal of treatment is to achieve the high euthyroid or low hyperthyroid range (maternal FT_4 at or slightly higher than the upper limit of the normal nonpregnant reference range) and maintain this range throughout pregnancy in order to improve pregnancy outcomes (Chan, 2007). To accomplish this, antithyroid drugs are the preferred treatment during all stages of pregnancy. Radioactive iodine is contraindicated during pregnancy; inappropriate radioiodine administration given after 10-12 weeks destroys the fetal thyroid and results in neonatal hypothyroidism and cretinism (Gorman, 1999; Abalovich, 2007). Surgery is reserved for patients who require large doses of antithyroid drugs, or those who demonstrate poor medication adherence and continue to remain hyperthyroid (Cooper, 2005; Miehle &Paschke, 2003; Mestman, 2004; Mestman, 1998; Glinoer, 2003; Karabinas & Tolis, 1998; Masiukiewicz &Burrow, 1999; Atkins, Cohen & Phillips, 2000). If surgery is necessary, surgery is preferred during the second trimester to decrease the risk of spontaneous abortion (Galofre, 2009).

2.4.1 Thioamides

During pregnancy, women may require a higher daily dose of antithyroid drug. Propylthiouracil should be given 100-150 mg three times daily or methimazole 30-40 mg per day until the patient becomes euthyroid. Upon euthyroid, the dose may be reduced to the lowest amount to maintain the euthyroid state with serum T_4 at the upper end of normal and continued throughout pregnancy and labor. Improvement in FT_4 is usually seen in 4 weeks; whereas improvement in TSH occurs in 6-8 weeks (Galorfre, 2009). It is important not to overtreat because it may result in maternal or fetal hypothyroidsm (Casey, 2006). Therefore, monitoring is crucial; TSH and FT_4 every 2 weeks and then every 4-6 weeks when euthyroidism is achieved (Clark, 2006).

2.4.1.1 Teratogenicity

Historically, PTU has been the drug of choice when treating Graves' disease during pregnancy in the United States. Throughout the rest of the world, methimazole and carbimazole, are widely used to treat hyperthyroidism in pregnant women (Mandel, 2001; Dwarakanath, 1999). Methimazole has been linked to at least 25 reported cases of aplasia cutis, as well as at least 22 cases of esophageal or choanal atresia or a combination of both (Mestman, 2004; Mandel, 2001; Ferraris 2003; Hamburger, 1992; Van Dijke, 1987; Karlson, 2002; Seoud,2003; Kannan, 2008; Karg, 2004). Methimazole has been described as "methimazole embryopathy" in children exposed to methimazole during the first trimester of pregnancy, especially during the first 7 gestational weeks (Karlsson, 2002; Clementi, 1999). The embryopathy includes congenital anomalies such as choanal or esophageal atresia or aplasia cutis and developmental delay, hearing loss, and dysmorphic facial features (Chan, 2007).

An evaluation of 49,091 live births estimated the incidence of aplasia cutis in the general population to be 0.03% or 0.05% of congenital skin defects (Van Dijke, 1987). DiGianantonio and colleagues prospectively compared 241 women exposed to methimazole during pregnancy to 1,089 pregnant controls. No increased incidence of spontaneous or induced abortions or major congenital anomalies was reported in the methimazole cohort (DiGianantonio, 2001). Although a possible association between methimazole exposure during pregnancy and fetal congenital defects may exist, it has not been proven and may be secondary to hyperthyroidism (Briggs, 2011).

At least 7cases of congenital anomalies have been reported in newborns exposed to PTU. A causal relationship between PTU exposure and congenital anomalies has not been found (Briggs, 2011). The Israeli Teratology Information Service reported that the rate of major anomalies was comparable between PTU-exposed pregnancies and controls (Rosenfeld, 2009). At least 47 reports have been published describing PTU-related hepatic impairment in adults and children, approximately 0.1-0.5% in adults (Cooper, 1999; Cooper, 2009; Kontoleon, 2002; Patil-Sisodia, 2010). However, only one case has been reported of neonatal hepatitis secondary to transplacental propylthiouracil (Hayashida, 1990). Therapy with PTU should be discontinued since 25% of affected patients may progress to fulminant, fatal hepatic failure (Kontoleon, 2002; Patil-Sisodia, 2010). The incidence of PTU hepatic failure does not correlate to PTU dosage or duration or patient age (Patil-Sisodia, 2010).

The United States Food and Drug Administration classifies PTU and methimazole as Category D because of the potential for fetal hypothyroidism, rather than the potential teratogenicity. The American College of Obstetricians and Gynecologists (ACOG) recommends that either PTU or methimazole may be used to treat pregnant women with hyperthyroidism.

The "block and replace" regimen that adds levothyroxine with an antithyroid drug is not recommended in pregnant women (Marx, 2009). It was originally thought that the placental transfer of levothyroxine would prevent fetal hypothyroidism. Levothyroxine and methimazole administered concomitantly to pregnant women with Graves' disease has shown to reduce the incidence of postpartum hyperthyroidism (Hashizume, 1992). However, the necessary dose of the antithyroid drug is much higher when given with levothyroxine that fetal goiter and fetal hypothyroidism may still occur. Furthermore, the risk of fetal hypothyroidism is increased because the antithyroid medications but not levothyroxine cross the placenta (Rosenfeld, 2009).

2.4.1.2 Clinical trials

Clinical studies support that fetal thyroid function outcomes are similar between the two drugs (Mortimer, 1997; Marchant, 1977; Momotani, 1997). A retrospective chart review of 135 patients with a history or diagnosis of hyperthyroidism at a high risk obstetrics clinic over a 16 year time period (1974 to 1990) compared the use of PTU and methimazole to treat hyperthyroidism during pregnancy (Wing, 1994). Of the 135 patients, 99 (73.3%) received PTU and 36 (26.7%) received methimazole. Selection of the treatment agent was based solely on physician preference. Six of the patients received both PTU and methimazole and were therefore excluded from analysis.

Diagnosis of hyperthyroidism was based on history, physical exam, thyroid-stimulating hormone, free thyroxine index, and free triiodothyronine index. The time required to normalize free FT_4 levels and the incidence of congenital malformations or fetal hypothyroidism were evaluated. Maternal and fetal outcomes were obtained via retrospective chart review from clinic, labor, delivery, and postpartum records. Baseline characteristics for the two treatment groups were similar with respect to age, ethnicity, and parity.

Maternal results showed that gestational age had no effect on the time to free FT_4 normalization. The median time to normalization was 7 weeks for the methimazole-treated group and 8 weeks for the PTU-treated group ($p=0.34$). The Cox proportional hazard compared the time of normalization between the two groups after adjusting for the initial measurements with no statistical difference between the PTU-treated group and the methimazole-treated group ($p=0.52$). Of the 135 pregnancies, four infants (3%) were born with congenital anomalies to mothers treated with either PTU or methimazole. Of these four infants, three (3%) of the fetal anomalies occurred in the 99 women who were treated with PTU and one (2.7%) occurred in the 36 women treated with methimazole. Fetal anomalies reported were ventricular septal defect, patent ductus arteriosus, and severe pulmonic stenosis in the infants of the PTU-treated mothers, and congenital inguinal hernia in the infant of the methimazole-treated mother. No cases of aplasia cutis were reported in either group. Congenital hypothyroidism occurred in one infant of a PTU-treated mother. The authors concluded that the incidence of congenital anomalies were consistent with the national average of 2% to 5% in the general population. The authors concluded that both PTU and methimazole were equally safe and effective in the treatment of hyperthyroidism during pregnancy (Wing, 1994). Potential limitations to the study were mostly due to the retrospective design; unrandomized, unblinded, and non-placebo controlled. Selection bias in medication may have occurred as the choice of medication was based on physician preference. Also, small sample size resulted in inadequate power to evaluate the equivalence of the two medications.

Momotani et al. evaluated the effect of maternal ingestion of PTU and methimazole on fetal thyroid status using cord sera at delivery (Momotani, 1997). The authors identified 249 pregnant women with Graves' disease who received either PTU or methimazole during their pregnancy. Of these 249 women, 77 (30.9%) had received at least four weeks of therapy, 34 (44.2%) with PTU and 43 (55.8%) with methimazole. Controls consisted of 32 healthy women with no history of thyroid disease and who delivered at term.

Serum samples from mother and fetus were assayed for free FT_4 and TSH. No statistical difference was observed in mean fetal free FT_4 or fetal TSH between the PTU and methimazole treated groups. Low fetal free FT_4 was seen in 6% of the PTU group and 7% of the methimazole group. High fetal TSH rates were 21% in the PTU group and 14% in the methimazole group. The relationship between maternal dose and fetal thyroid status was not significant; low doses of PTU were associated with high TSH in 21% of infants and low doses of methimazole were associated with high TSH in 14% of infants. The authors concluded that the two agents were similar regarding the effects on fetal thyroid status, and the selection of PTU over methimazole to treat hyperthyroidism during pregnancy was not justified (Momotani, 1997). The trial appeared to be well designed and utilized a direct measure of fetal thyroid status at birth. Potential bias may have existed as medication selection was based solely on provider preference. The selection process was not explained regarding how pregnant women with Graves' disease and those who served as controls were identified.

Azizi et al. evaluated the methimazole's effect on intellectual development of children whose mothers received methimazole during pregnancy but not during lactation (Azizi, 2002). The authors identified 23 children, ages 3 to 11 years, of mothers who were treated with methimazole during pregnancy and 30 children, ages 3 to 11 years, of mothers who were not treated with methimazole during pregnancy. All mothers delivered at term and there were no congenital malformations in either group. Methimazole-exposed mothers received methimazole doses up to 20 mg per day. All neonates were euthyroid at the time of delivery.

No difference between the methimazole-treated group and the control in serum T_3, T_4, or TSH concentrations was observed. Physical characteristics such as weight and height were similar in both groups. A psychologist blinded to methimazole exposure used the Wechsler Preschool and Primary Scale of Intelligence (WPPSI) to detect a difference in verbal and performance IQ between the two groups. No difference in verbal or performance IQ between the two groups of children was shown. Total IQ for the methimazole-treated group was 117±11; IQ for the control group was 113±14. The authors concluded that no detrimental effects on the physical or intellectual development occurred in those children exposed to methimazole during pregnancy (Azizi, 2002). The main strength of this study was the single blinded psychologist evaluation of child intellect using the WPPSI exam. Unfortunately, the WPPSI is an intelligence test designed for children ages 2 years 6 months to 7 years 3 months and the study population included children 3-11 years of age. Other limitations to this study were a small sample size and low exposure dose of methimazole.

3. Conclusion

The selection of PTU over methimazole as the drug of choice to treat Graves' disease during pregnancy should not be based on misleading statements in the literature that PTU has less placental transfer than methimazole, that PTU leads to less fetal hypothyroidism, or that exposure to methimazole during pregnancy leads to a decreased intellectual function in children. The United States Food and Drug Administration classifies both PTU and methimazole as a Category D because of the potential for fetal hypothyroidism, rather than potential teratogenicity. The ACOG recommends that either PTU or methimazole may be used to treat pregnant women with hyperthyroidism. However, the Endocrine Society recommends PTU as a first line drug, especially during the first trimester (Abalovich, 2007). Clinical data shows that PTU and methimazole are equally efficacious in pregnant women with hyperthyroidism (Wing, 1994; Momotani, 1997). However, the possible association between methimazole and fetal anomalies such as aplasia cutis, esophageal atresia, and choanal atresia may present methimazole a less desirable first line treatment option than PTU. Although a causal relationship between methimazole and these fetal anomalies has not been established in clinical trials, the possibility of a relationship still exists. Therefore, in the absence of a compelling indication for the use of methimazole, PTU should still be considered as the first line agent in the treatment of Graves' disease during pregnancy. However, methimazole should be considered a viable second choice if the patient is intolerant to PTU, has an allergic reaction to PTU, or fails to become euthyroid on PTU.

4. References

AACE Thyroid Task Force. (2002). American Association of Clinical Endocrinologists medical guidelines for clinical practice for the evaluation and treatment of hyperthyroidism and hypothyroidism. *Endocr Pract* 2002 Nov-Dec;8(6):457-69.

Abalovich M, Amino N, Barbour LA, Cobin RH, De Groot LJ, Glinoer D, Mandel S, & Stagnaro-Green A. (2007). Management of thyroid dysfunction during pregnancy and postpartum: an endocrine society clinical practice guideline. *J Clin Endocrinol Metab* 2007;92(8):S1-S47.

American Academy of Pediatricians. (2001). Committee on Drugs. *American Academy of Pediatricians* 2001;108;776-89.

American College of Obstetricians and Gynecologists. (2002). Thyroid disease in pregnancy. ACOG Practice Bulletin No. 37. Clinical management guidelines for obstetrician-gynecologists. *Obstet Gynecol* 2002;100:387-96.

Atkins P, Cohen SB, & Phillips BJ. (2000). Drug therapy for hyperthyroidism in pregnancy. *Drug Safety* 2000;23:229-244.

Azizi F, Khamseh ME, Bahreynian M, & Hedayati. (2002). Thyroid function and intellectual development of children of mothers taking methimazole during pregnancy. *J Endocrinol Invest* 2002;25:586-589.

Bahn RS, Burch HB, Cooper DS, Garber JR, Greenlee MC, Klein I, Laurberg P, McDougall IR, Montori VM, Rivkees SA, Ross DS, Sosa JA, & Stan MN. (2011). Hyperthyroidism and Other Causes of Thyrotoxicosis: Management Guidelines of the American Thyroid Association and American Association of Clinical Endocrinologists.*Thyroid* 2011:21:593-646

Barbero P, Valdez R, Rodriguez H, Tiscornia C, Mansilla E, Allons A, Coll S, & Liascovich R. (2008). Choanal atresia associated with maternal hyperthyroidism treated with methimazole: a case-control study. *Am J Med Genet* 2008;146A:2390-2395.

Briggs GG, Freeman RK, Yaffe SJ, eds. (2011). *Drugs in pregnancy and lactation*, 9th ed. Philadelphia: Lippincott Williams and Wilkins, 2011.

Casey BM, & Leveno KJ. (2006). Thyroid disease in pregnancy. *Obstet Gynecol* 2006;108:1283-92.

Chan GW, & Mandel SJ. (2007). Therapy insight: management of Graves' disease during pregnancy. *Nature Clinical Practice Endocrin Metab* 2007;3(6):470-478.

Clark SM, Saade GR, Snodgrass WR, & Hankins GDV. (2006). Pharmacokinetics and pharmacotherapy of thionamides in pregnancy. *Ther Drug Monit* 2006;28(4):477-483.

Clementi M, Di Gianantonio E, Pelo E, Mammi I, Basile RT, & Tenconi R. (1999). Methimazole embryopathy: delineation of the phenotype. *Am J Med Genet* 1999;83:43-46.

Cooper DS. (2005). Antithyroid Drugs. *N Eng J Med* 2005;352:905-17.

Cooper DS. (1987). Antithyroid drugs: to breast-feed or not to breastfeed. *Am J Obstet Gynecol* 1987;157:234-5.

Cooper DS. (2009). Putting propylthiouracil in perspective. *J Clin Endocrinol Metab* 2009;94(6):1881-1882.

Di Gianantonio E, Schaefer C, Mastroiacovo P, Cournot M, Benedicenti F, Reuvers M, Occupati V, Robert E, Bellemin B, Addis A, Arnon J, & Clementi M. (2001). Adverse effects of prenatal methimazole exposure. *Teratology* 2001;64:262-266.

Dwarakanath CS, Ammini AC, Kriplani A, Shah P, & Paul VK. (1999). Graves' disease during pregnancy- results of antithyroid drug therapy. *Singapore Med J* 1999;40:70.

Ecker JL, & Musci TJ. (2000). Thyroid function and disease in pregnancy. *Curr Probl Obstet Gynecol Fertil* 2000;23:109-122.

Ferraris S, Valenzise M, Lerone M, Divizia MT, Rosaia L, & Blaid D. (2003). Malformations following methimazole exposure in utero: an open issue. *Birth Defects Res A Clin Mol Teratol* 2003;67:989-992.

Fitzpatrick DL, & Russel MA. (2010). Diagnosis and management of thyroid disease in pregnancy. *Obstet Gynecol Clin N Am* 2010;37:173-93.

Galorfre JC, & Davies TF. (2009). Autoimmune thyroid disease in pregnancy: a review. *J Women's Health* 2009;18(11):1847-56.

Garcia-Mayor RV, & Larranaga A. (2010). Treatment of Graves' hyperthyroidism with thionamides-derived drugs: review. *Med Chem* 2010;6(4):239-246.

Glinoer D. (2003). Management of hypo- and hyperthyroidism during pregnancy. *Growth Horm IGF Res* 2003;13:S45-S54.

Gorman CA. (1999). Radioiodine and pregnancy. *Thyroid* 1999;9:721-6.

Hamburger JI. (1992). Diagnosis and management of graves' disease in pregnancy. *Thyroid* 1992;3:219-224.

Hashizume K, Ichikawa K, Nishii Y, Kobayashi M, Sakurai A, Miyamoto T, Suzuki S, Takeda T. (1992). Effect of administration of thyroxine on the risk of postpartum recurrence of hyperthyroid Graves' disease. *J Clin Endocrinol Metab* 1992;75:6-10.

Hayashida CY. (1990). Neonatal hepatitis and lymphocyte sensitization by placental transfer of propylthiouracil. *J Endocrinol Invest* 1990;13:937-41.

Inoue M, Arata N, Koren G, & It S. (2009). Hyperthyroidism during pregnancy. *Can Fam Phys* 2009;55:701-703.

Jonklaas J & Talbert RL. (2011). Thyroid Disorders. In : DiPiro JT, Talbert RL, Yee GC, Matzke GR, Wells BG, Posey LM, eds. *Pharmacotherapy: A Pathophysiological Approach. 8th* ed. New York, NY: McGraw-Hill, 2011.

Kang AY, Baek YH, Sohn YJ, Lee SK, Son CH, Kim KH, & Yang DK. (2006). Diffuse alveolar hemorrhage associated with antineutrophil cytoplasmic antibody levels in a pregnant woman taking propylthiouracil. *Korean J Intern Med* 2006;21:240-243.

Kannan L, Mishra S, Agarwal R, Kartikeyan V, Gupta N, & Kabra M. (2008). Carbimazole embryopathy-bilateral choanal atresia and patent vitello-intestinal duct: a case report and review of the literature. *Birth Defects Research* 2008;82:649-651.

Karabinas CD, & Tolis GJ. Thyroid disorders and pregnancy. *J Obstet and Gynaecol* 1998;18:509-515.

Karg E, Bereg E, Gaspar L, Katona M, & Turi S. (2004). Aplasia cutis congenital after methimazole exposure in utero. *Pediatr Dermatol* 2004;21(4):491-494.

Karlson FA, Axelsson O, & Melhus H. (2002). Severe embryopathy and exposure to methimazole in early pregnancy. *J Clin Endocrinol Metab* 2002;87:947-948.

Kontoleon P, Ilias I, Koutras DA, Kontogiannis D, & Papapetrou PD. (2002). Successful treatment with carbimazole of a hyperthyroid pregnancy with hepatic impairment after propylthiouracil administration: a case report. *Clin Exp Obst Gyn* 2002;29:304-305.

Laurberg P, Bournaud C. Karmisholt J, & Orgiazzi J. (2009). Management of Graves' hyperthyroidism in pregnancy : focus on both maternal and foetal thyroid function, and caution against surgical thyroidectomy in pregnancy. *Euro J Endocrinol* 2009;160:1-8.

Lazarus JH. (2005). Thyroid disorders associated with pregnancy: etiology, diagnosis, and management. *Treat Endocrinol* 2005;4(1):31-41.

Mandel SJ, & Cooper DS. (2001). The use of antithyroid drugs in pregnancy and lactation. *J Clin Endocrinol Metab* 2001;86:2354-2359.

Marchant B, Brownlie BE, Hart DM, Horton PW, & Alexander WD. (1977). The placental transfer of propylthiouracil, methimazole and carbimazole. *J Clin Endocrinol Metab* 1977;45:1187-93.

Marx H, Amin P, & Lazarus JH. (1997). Hyperthyroidism and pregnancy. *BMJ* 2008;336:663-7.

Masiukiewicz US, & Burrow GN. (1999). Hyperthyroidism in pregnancy: diagnosis and treatment. *Thyroid* 1999;9:647-652.

Mestman JH. (2004). Hyperthyroidism in pregnancy. *Best Pract Res Clin Endocrinol Metab* 2004;18:267-288.

Mestman JH. (1998). Hyperthyroidism in pregnancy. *Endocrinol Metab Clin North Am* 1998;27:127-149.

Miehle K, & Paschke R. (2003). Therapy of hyperthyroidism. *Exp Clin Endocrinol Diabetes* 2003;111:305-318.

Millar LK, Wing DA, Leung AS, Koonings PP, Montoro MN, & Mestman JH. (1994). Low birth weight and pre-eclampsia in pregnancies complicated by hyperthyroidism. *Obstet Gynecol* 1994;84:946-9.

Momotani N, Yoshimura J, Ishikawa N, & Ito K. (1997). Effects of propylthiouracil and methimazole of fetal thyroid status in mothers with graves' hyperthyroidism. *J Clin Endocrinol Metab* 1997;82:3633-3636.

Morreale de Escobar G, Obregon MJ, & Escobar del Rey F. (2000). Is neuropsychological development related to maternal hypothyroidism or to maternal hypothyroxinemia? *J Clin Endocrinol Metab* 2000;85:3975-87

Mortimer RH, Cannell GR, Addison RS, Johnson LP, Roberts MS, & Bernus I. (1997). Methimazole and propylthoiuracil equally cross the perfused human term placental lobule. *J Clin Endocrinol Metab* 1997;82:3099-3102.

Patil-Sisodia K, & Mestman JH. (2007). Graves hyperthyroidism and pregnancy: a clinical update. *Endocr Pract* 2010;16(1):118-129.

Rashid M, & Rashid MH. Obstetric management of thyroid disease. *Obstet Gynecol* 2007;62(10):680-688.

Rosenfeld H, Ornoy A, Schechtman S, & Diav-Citrin O. (2009). Pregnancy outcome, thyroid dysfunction and fetal goiter after in utero exposure to propylthiouracil: a controlled cohort study. *Br J Clin Pharmacol* 2009;68(4):609-617.

Seoud M, Nassar A, Usta I, Mansour M, Salti I, & Younes K. (2003). Gastrointestinal malformations in two infants born to women with hyperthyroidism untreated in the first trimester. *J Perinat* 2003;20:59-62.

Van Dijke CP, Heydendael RJ, & De Kleine MJ. (1987). Methimazole, carbimazole, and congenital skin Defects. *Ann Intern Med* 1987;106:60-61.

Weetman AP. (2000). Graves' Disease. *N Eng J Med* 2000;343:1236-1248.

Wing DA, Millar LK, Koonings PP, Montoro MN, & Mestman JH. (1994). A comparison of propylthiouracil versus methimazole in the treatment of hyperthyroidism in pregnancy. *Am J Obstet Gynaecol* 1994;170:90-5.

9

Thyroid Function Following Treatment of Childhood Acute Lymphoblastic Leukemia

Elpis Vlachopapadopoulou[1], Vassilios Papadakis[2], Georgia Avgerinou[2] and Sophia Polychronopoulou[2]
[1]*Dept. of Growth and Development, Children's Hosp. "P.A. Kyriakou"*
[2]*Dept. of Pediatric Hematology-Oncology,. "Agia Sofia" Children's Hosp Athens, Greece*

1. Introduction

Acute lymphoblastic leukemia (ALL) is the most frequently encountered malignancy in childhood. Peak incidence is in early childhood. There is male predominance with 1.2:1 male to female ratio (Pui et al., 2006). Current therapeutic modalities have succeeded in assuring high cure rates. Treatment protocols involve mainly chemotherapy according to patient and leukemia risk classification. Irradiation therapy can be used as central nervous system (CNS) prophylaxis or as therapy for CNS involvement, although the use of CNS irradiation is reduced (Pui et al., 2009). Furthermore, allogeneic bone marrow transplantation can be used for very high risk patients or patients not responding to the treatment protocols (Pui et al., 2006).

Surveillance for long-term complications, following completion of chemotherapy is important, in order to prevent morbidity and to improve quality of life (Oeffinger et al., 2006). The vast majority of long-term sequelae are endocrine abnormalities involving the hypothalamic pituitary axis, the thyroid gland and the gonads. Growth hormone deficiency, precocious puberty, gonadal failure, hypothyroidism and thyroid cancer are the most likely long-term clinical presentations (Chemaitilly & Sklar, 2010).

The prevalence of hypothyroidism was found to be higher among childhood cancer survivors than in the general population, in a nation-wide registry of Finland. They reported the prevalence of hypothyroidism among cancer survivors, by reporting the clinically diagnosed hypothyroid patients who were receiving levothyroxine replacement therapy. Direct radiotherapy of the thyroid gland was related to a higher prevalence of hypothyroidism. Furthermore, they reported that females were more susceptible to hypothyroidism than males following childhood cancer (Madanat, 2008). Hypothyroidism, either primary or central, can be manifested in survivors of childhood malignancies (Madanat et al., 2007, Rose et al., 2006). The retrospective study by Madanat et al., reported that impaired thyroid function occurred in patients with a history of brain tumor, Hodgkin's disease, leukemia/non Hodgkin's lymphoma (NHL) and others. Age at diagnosis did not have an effect on the occurrence or time frame of development of thyroid hypofunction.

They found that radiotherapy combined with chemotherapy was associated with a higher risk for development of hypothyroidism, compared to chemotherapy alone (Madanat et al., 2007).

A recent report from the Japanese childhood cancer survivors program, reveals thyroid dysfunction in 18% of the patients, primary as well as central hypothyroidism. The vast majority of patients with primary hypothyroidism were irradiated to the neck area (Miyoshi et al., 2008).

Additional information derives from the registry of German patients, for the evaluation of side effects after radiation therapy in childhood and adolescence. The preliminary results of their report on the incidence of thyroid dysfunction come following a relatively short period of observation. The prevalence of thyroid dysfunction in patients treated for childhood ALL, is 11% which is much lower than the prevalence in patients treated for brain tumors. This is related to the lower dose of radiation given to the thyroid gland of ALL patients (Bőling et al., 2011).

Rose et al., reported on 62 patients with central hypothyroidism. Of those 10 patients (16%) had received chemotherapy only and none of these patients had hypothalamic tumors that would be clearly associated with endocrine dysfunction (Rose et al., 2006). Thus, they suggest that the occurrence of central hypothyroidism is more common than is thought, and they recommend a more vigilant and timely work-up in order to assure early identification and treatment of the hypothyroidism.

Thyroid dysfunction has been reported in survivors of childhood ALL in previous papers, but the incidence and the severity of thyroid dysfunction varies. ALL treatment protocols have evolved overtime, duration and intensity of the treatment, as well as medication combination and radiotherapy dose have changed. In a small group of Italian ALL patients, thyroid dysfunction was not appreciated during a 6 year follow-up period. However, a case of papillary thyroid cancer was identified (Neves Mascarenhas et al., 2006). In the paper published by Steffens et al, a retrospective analysis, primary hypothyroidism had occurred in patients treated for childhood ALL. The patients were divided in three groups, according to the therapeutic regime used: 1. chemotherapy only, 2. chemotherapy and cranial irradiation, and 3. combination of chemotherapy, cranial irradiation and bone marrow transplantation. Cases of hypothyroidism, as judged based on elevated serum TSH values were identified in all three groups but the higher incidence was appreciated in the latter group (Steffens M et al, 2008). Furthermore, there are reports of hypothyroidism in ALL patients, related to the use of craniospinal irradiation (Lando et al., 2001).

The papers presented, include pediatric patients diagnosed with ALL treated with different chemotherapeutic protocols with or without cranial irradiation and hemopoietic stem cell transplantation. The aim of the current retrospective study is to investigate a homogeneous group of children with ALL, treated with the same protocol (BFM). Patients with early death or relapse, as well as, patients who underwent hemopoietic stem cell transplantation in first remission were excluded from this analysis. Thyroid function was evaluated at diagnosis, at the end of chemotherapy, one to two years post chemotherapy completion and more than 3 years post treatment cessation. This study seeks to define the total prevalence of thyroid dysfunction in this homogeneously treated group of patients diagnosed with childhood acute lymphocytic leukemia.

2. Subjects and methods

The patient population included and analyzed retrospectively in this study, consists of the patient cohort with newly diagnosed acute lymphoblastic leukemia (ALL), treated according to the ALL-BFM protocols (ALL-BFM-90 and ALL-BFM-95 Protocols) from April 1994 to December 2010, in the Department of Pediatric Hematology-Oncology, at Agia Sofia Children's Hospital in Athens, Greece.

Acute lymphoblastic leukemia was diagnosed by bone marrow morphology and phenotype. Patients were assigned to the high risk (HR) treatment group if they had an absolute blast count on peripheral blood of more than 1.0 k/ul on day +8 of induction, following prednisolone treatment (prednisolone poor responders), no remission by bone marrow morphology on day +33 following induction or if they were found to have translocations t(4;11) or t(9;22) by karyotype or FISH at diagnosis bone marrow specimens. The rest of the patients were assigned to the median risk (MR) treatment group. Thus, standard risk (SR) patients were upgraded to the MR group (Schrapp et al., 2000, Moricke et al., 2008).

Figure 1 illustrates the outline of protocol ALL-BFM-90 and ALL-BFM 95 (Katsimpardi et al., 2006).

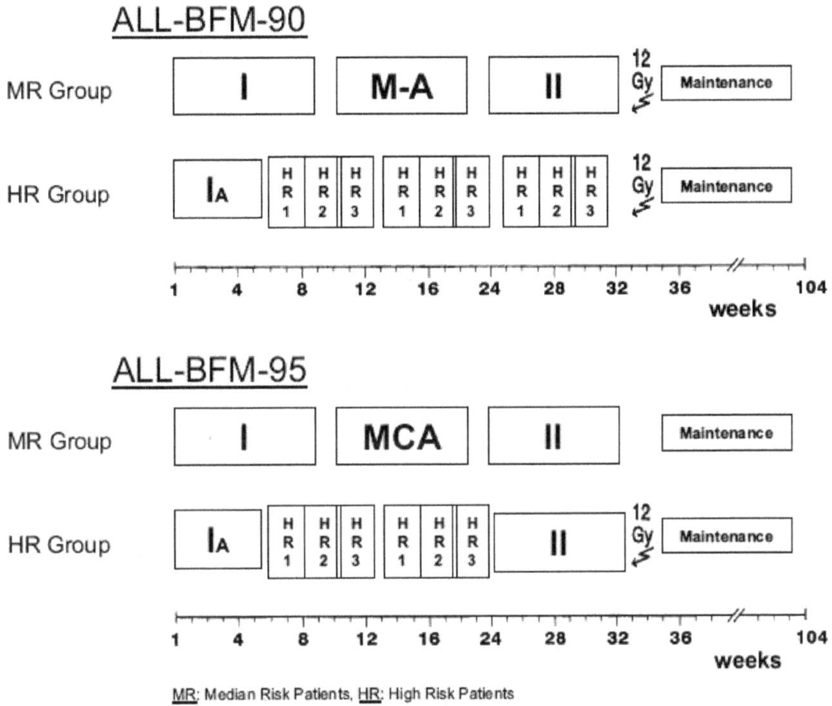

Fig. 1. ALL-BFM-95 and ALL-BFM-90 treatment protocol outline. From K Katsimpardi et al, Support Care Cancer (2006) 14: 277–284. DOI 10.1007/s00520-005-0884-6

Synopsis of the treatment schedule and strategy follows. Overall, treatment consisted of an induction, consolidation, reinduction and maintenance phase. The induction phase (Figure 1, Protocol I) was based initially on four drugs (prednisolone, vincristine, L-asparaginase and daunorubicin). Later (second phase of Protocol I, induction), two courses of 1 gr/m^2 of cyclophosphamide were administered at a 28-day interval, with 6-mercaptopurine p.o. and low dose aracytin i.v., for the interim time. This second part of the induction is omitted for all HR patients. The consolidation phase for MR patients (Figure 1, MA or MCA) was based on p.o. 6-mercaptopurine and 4 courses of high dose (5 gr/m^2) methotrexate i.v. The reinduction phase for the MR patients was similar to the induction phase (Figure 1, Protocol II), but with dexamethasone, vincristine, L-asparaginase and doxorubicin, initially. One dose of cyclophosphamide at 1 gr/m^2 with 14 days of 6-thioguanine and low dose i.v. aracytin followed (second phase of Protocol II).

Following only the initial phase of induction (Protocol IA), the high risk (HR) patient group received different, intensified treatment according to the protocol. Thus, patients treated according to the ALL-BFM-90 protocol received 9 blocks of treatment (in sequence: HR1, HR2, HR3 given in three series and no reinduction (ALL-BFM-90, Figure 1). Two of these HR blocks are based on high dose methotrexate (HR1, HR2) and one (HR3) is based on high dose aracytin. On the other hand, HR patients treated according to the ALL-BFM-95 protocol received 6 blocks of treatment (in sequence: HR1, HR2, HR3 given in two series). Then, reinduction with Protocol II followed, (ALL-BFM-95, Figure 1). Thus, Protocol II reinduction phase was common for MR and HR patients.

According to the protocols, all HR patients and all patients with T-precursor ALL received 12 Gy of cranial irradiation following the completion of the treatment that was described previously and prior to starting maintenance chemotherapy. MR patients were irradiated, as above, on the ALL-BFM-90 protocol but not on the ALL-BFM-95.

Allogeneic bone marrow transplantation (BMT) was recommended for a subset of HR patients, provided that a matched sibling donor was available.

Maintenance treatment consisted of 24 or 30 months in total for females and males respectively, of daily 6-mercaptopurine (50 mg/m^2) p.o./weekly methotrexate (20 mg/m^2) p.o. and monthly (28 day cycle) i.v. vincristine (1.5 mg/m^2), together with a five-day p.o. prednisolone (40 $mg/m^2/day$) pulse. Triple (methotrexate/ aracytin/ steroid, doses adjusted to age) intrathecal (IT) infusions every third pulse (84 days), were administered to patients not given CNS irradiation.

Overall, this ALL patient cohort has received more intensive treatment than the original ALL-BFM-90 and ALL-BFM 95 Protocol (Schrappe et al., 2000, Morriche et al., 2010). All SR group patients were treated according to the MR group (receiving additional 2 doses of anthracyclines) and maintenance treatment was increased in length (24 months for girls and 30 months for boys maintenance treatment in total) and was intensified with vincristine/ prednizolone monthly pulses and triple intrathecal infusions every third pulse. Detailed treatment schedule has been previously described. Details of the treatment schedule and patient outcome has been described before (Papadakis et al., 2003).

The purpose of this analysis is to evaluate the effect of ALL treatment on thyroidal function. Thus, in order to have a homogenously treated patient group, patients with early death or relapse and patients who underwent bone marrow transplantation in first remission according to the Protocol were excluded from the analysis.

Two hundred twenty- three patients, were treated for newly diagnosed ALL according to the BFM Protocol (ALL-BFM-90 and ALL-BFM-95 Protocols) from April 1994 to December 2010. From them 18 have not yet completed the prescribed chemotherapy and 5 suffered early death from toxicity and thus they were excluded from analysis. Additionally, 32 patients were excluded from the analysis, of which 17 underwent stem cell transplantation in first remission and 15 patients due to early relapse. Thus, 168 patients were eligible for analysis and the sex distribution was 93 males and 75 females.

The median age at diagnosis was 5.1 years (range, 1.0 to 16.7 years). Median duration of treatment and median age at completion of maintenance treatment was 3.2 years (range, 2.1 to 4.2 years) and 8.2 years (range, 4.0 to 19.6 years) respectively. A total of 26 patients received cranial irradiation.

Subjects who were diagnosed between April 1994 and April 1996 were treated according to the ALL-BFM-90 protocol (26 Patients) and those who were diagnosed beyond April 1996 according to the ALL-BFM-95 treatment protocol (142 Patients). Patients were sub-grouped into two groups according to risk, 149 patients were characterized as medium -risk and 19 as high -risk. From the patients included in the HR group, 5 were treated with BFM-90 and 14 with BFM-95 (patients who underwent transplantation were excluded).

A retrospective analysis of patient data extracted from their charts was performed. Time points at which the data were grouped together were: a. Diagnosis b. End of treatment, c. One year and d. More than three years after completion of prescribed treatment. For patients relapsing after cessation of treatment, the data up to the time of relapse were eligible for analysis.

Data of thyroid function that was evaluated were: serum levels of the thyroid stimulating hormone (TSH), triiodo-thyronine (T3) and thyroxine (T4), anti-thyroidal antibody levels and imaging of the thyroid gland by ultrasonography.

Serum levels of TSH, T3 and T4 were measured with current high resolution commercially available assays. For the purpose of this study, thyroid dysfunction was defined as either a T4 value below or a TSH value exceeding the defined normal range. By this definition, thyroid dysfunction includes cases of clinical, subclinical and central hypothyroidism.

3. Results

Out of the 168 eligible patients, 141 had at least one evaluation of thyroid function following completion of treatment. This cohort of patients evaluated consisted of 78 males and 63 female patients. Thirteen were treated according to the ALL-BFM 90 Protocol (all were assigned to MR treatment group) whilst 128 were treated according to the ALL-BFM 95 Protocol (115 MR, 13 HR treatment group). In regards to radiotherapy, 21 patients received cranial irradiation at a dose of 12 Gy, except for one earlier patient who received 16.8 Gy.

3.1 Data at diagnosis of leukemia

At the time of diagnosis, one 12.6 year old female patient, with known Down syndrome (trisomy 21), had been diagnosed with hypothyroidism and was already receiving T4 supplementation for years. This patient was excluded from further analysis.

		TOTAL	
		N	%
Patients		141	
Age at Diagnosis			
	Median	5.1	
	Range	1.0 - 16.7	
Sex			
	Male	78	55.3
	Female	63	44.7
Treatment			
	ALL-BFM 90	13	9.2
	ALL-BFM 95	128	90.7
Treatment Group			
	MR Group	128	90.7
	HR Group	13	9.2
	CT Only	117	83.0
	CT + RT	24	17.0

Table 1. Patient Characteristics of the Eligible Patients.
Abbreviations: MR, Median Risk; HR, High Risk; CT, Chemotherapy; RT, radiotherapy

Twenty -seven patients have thyroid function data at diagnosis. Of those patients, 19 out of 27 had values of thyroid hormones and TSH within normal range and with appropriate ratio. Another 6 patients (2 males and 4 females) had low T4 with corresponding low TSH value. Free T4 (FT4) was not measured. Those 6 patients are considered to have low thyroid function due to critical illness, that is acute lymphoblastic leukemia. The corresponding T4 (in μg/dl) and TSH (in μIU/ml) serum values were 5.2/3.0; 2.9/1.1; 3.0/2.5; 6.3/0.2 respectively. The nonthyroidal illness syndrome or euthyroid sick syndrome, describes a condition characterized by abnormal thyroid function tests encountered in patients with acute or chronic systemic illnesses. The laboratory parameters of this syndrome include low serum levels of T3 and high levels of reverse T3, with normal or low levels of T4 and normal or low TSH. Thyroid function usually returns to normal as, the acute illness resolves.

Additionally two patients (1 male and 1 female) had compensated hypothyroidism (elevated TSH values with T4 values within the normal range) which resolved spontaneously, as the patients did not receive substitution therapy, and repeat thyroid function tests were normal.

Of interest is the case of a 7.3 years old girl who at diagnosis was found to have hypothyroidism as evidenced by elevated TSH (10.5 μIU/ml) and thyroid sonogram with echogenicity changes characteristic of thyroiditis Hashimoto. However, antithyroglobulin and anti-Thyroid peroxidase antibodies were negative. One month later and while on treatment with high dose steroids and chemotherapy, the T4 and TSH serum values of 11.7 (in μg/dl) and 10,5 (in μIU/ml) found at diagnosis were reduced to 3.9 and 0.7, respectively. This change was attributed to steroid administration. At the last follow up 6.5 years from diagnosis and 3.8 years after the end of treatment, she remains euthyroid (T4 6.19 μg/dl, T3 124.8 ng/ml and TSH 1.98 μIU/ml) with minor changes on ultrasound.

Furthermore, one male patient, 13.6 years old, during the maintenance treatment phase of chemotherapy, was diagnosed with compensated hypothyroidism, during laboratory investigation for bilateral femoral neck necrosis. At initial evaluation he was found to have TSH values of 6.5 μIU/ml with normal values of T4 and T3. On a 4 month follow-up, TSH value had increased to 7.8 μIU/ml and he was started on substitution therapy with p.o. levothyroxine. He was found to have positive anti-thyroglobulin antibodies while thyroid gland ultrasonography depicted minor echogenicity changes. Thus, he was diagnosed with compensated hypothyroidism 2.3 years after commencement of leukemia treatment, due to thyroiditis Hashimoto, and he continues to be on replacement therapy. This patient is excluded from further analysis.

3.2 High risk patients who received cranial irradiation

Out of the 168 eligible patients, 25 have received cranial irradiation. Out of the 141 evaluable, analyzed patients, 24 had received cranial irradiation as prophylaxis. Even though CNS leukemia was not apparent at diagnosis, the patients either belonged to the high risk group or were diagnosed with T-cell ALL and were irradiated according to the protocol mandates. Radiotherapy dose was 12 Gy for 24 patients and 16.8 Gy in one of the ALL-BFM 90 patients. Thyroid function data was available in all 24 patients at some time-point following initiation of treatment and in some patients with serial values. Thyroid function measurements were available at a median time of 7.8 years (range, 2.0 to 12.9 years) after initiation of treatment and at a median time of 4.6 years (range, -0.9 to 10.0 years) after completion of treatment. All patients had thyroid function within normal limits and no borderline values (median TSH value of 2.85 μIU/ml, range 1.1 to 4.1 μIU/ml). One patient had borderline low T4 with normal TSH, raising suspicion for hidden central hypothyroidism, but further evaluation with TRH or night TSH surge was not performed.

At the same time, 5 of 5 patients with thyroid ultrasound evaluation, normal thyroid gland size and architecture was appreciated. The patient who had received 16.8 Gy of cranial irradiation, had normal function at one year following cessation of treatment and no further evaluation. All patients who were evaluated for thyroid function (in total, all 5 and 12 patients evaluated for thyroid function) at the end of treatment (5 patients) and one year later (12 patients), were also found to have values within normal limits.

3.3 Medium risk patients treated with chemotherapy only

3.3.1 Data at the completion of maintenance chemotherapy

Thyroid function evaluation was available in a total of 38 patients, 25 boys and 13 girls, with median age at evaluation of 8.5 years (range, 5.1 to 17.5 years) and at a median time of 3.4 years (range, 2.7 to 4.3 years) after initial diagnosis.

Twenty- six from the 38 patients, 68.5%, had thyroid function evaluation within the normal range. That is, serum values of T4 above or equal to 7.0 μg/dl and TSH values lower than 5.0 μIU/ml. Sonographic evaluation of the thyroid gland was performed in four of those patients and revealed thyroid glands of normal size and architecture.

Two patients (1 male, 1 female, 5.2%) have evidence of compensated hypothyroidism (T4 4.74 μg/dl, T3 138 ng/ml and TSH 6.75 μIU/ml the first and 7.05 μg/dl, 143.2 ng/ml and 5.23 μIU/ml the second, respectively).

Moreover, 10 patients (7 male, 3 female, 26.3%) with low values of T4 and inappropriately low values of TSH were appreciated, and they are considered to have hidden central hypothyroidism, that has not been further investigated. Of those, two patients with repeated values have the same serum T4 and TSH findings at 2.1 and 3.0 years after the end of treatment. To the contrary, three patients with low values of both T4 and TSH at 2 to 3 months after the end of treatment, reversed to normal values (T4 above 7 μg/dl and TSH below 5 μIU/ml) at follow-up measurements 4 to 12 months from the previous evaluation.

In total, thyroid dysfunction was appreciated in 12 patients (8 males, 4 females) accounting for 31.5% of the patients at the completion of chemotherapy. Of the above 12 patients with evidence of thyroid dysfunction, 6 had imaging by ultrasound, at the same time that hormonal measurements were drawn. All had normal sonographic findings, without evidence of nodules or altered echogenicity indicative of thyroiditis.

3.3.2 Data at one to two years following cessation of the treatment of leukemia

Thyroid function evaluation was available in a total of 38 patients, 24 boys and 14 girls, with median age at evaluation of 9.6 years (range, 4.6 to 20.9 years) and at a median time of 4.5 years (range, 3.0 to 5.1 years) after initial diagnosis and at a median time of 1.3 years (range, 0.9 to 2.1 years) after the end of treatment.

Thirty -one patients (81.6%) had normal values for thyroid function. In this group are included 3 patients with compensated hypothyroidism at the end of treatment, who reversed to normal values without any intervention.

Four patients, 3 males and one female, (10.5%) had evidence of hidden central hypothyroidism (low values of T4 and TSH). In this group are included 2 patients who were considered to have hidden central hypothyroidism at the end of treatment and their values remained similar at the current time point.

Additionally, 3 patients, 2 male and one female, (7.9%) had evidence of compensated hypothyroidism (T4 in μg/dl, and TSH in μIU/ml values of 9.2/5.2, 7.2/6.9, 10.1/7.1 respectively).

In total 18.4% of the patients have evidence of thyroid dysfunction when evaluated one-two years, following completion of chemotherapy.

In this patient cohort belong 5 patients described before with measurements at the end of treatment. Of those, 3 patients had evidence of compensated hypothyroidism at the end of treatment time -point, that reversed at the one to two year measurement and also, 2 patients with hidden, possibly central hypothyroidism who remained with the same findings (low values of TSH and T4).

3.3.3 Data at more than three years following cessation of the treatment of leukemia

Thyroid function evaluation was available in a total of 77 patients, 40 boys and 37 girls, with median age at evaluation of 14.0 years (range, 7.7 to 24.0 years) and at a median time of 9.1 years (range, 5.2 to 15.7 years) after initial diagnosis and at a median time of 5.7 years (range, 3.0 to 12.5 years) after the end of treatment. Figure 2a illustrates the results for all 77 patients.

Sixty- eight patients (88%) had normal values for thyroid function. Within this group of patients we have identified a group of 13 patients, asymptomatic, with low normal values of TSH and T4 in the low portion of normal values, together with normal values of total serumT3, that are being closely followed for evidence of central hypothyroidism **(Figure 2c).**

	TOTAL		End of Maintenance		1-2 years later		>3 years later	
	N	%	N	%	N	%	%	%
Patients	141		38	26,9	38	26,9	77	54,6
Age at Diagnosis								
Median	5,1		5,1		5,0		4,9	
Range	1,0 – 16,7		2,1 – 14,5		1,1 – 16,7		1,1 – 13,1	
Age at Evaluation								
Median(years)			8,5		9,6		14,0	
Range (years)			5.1 - 17.5		4.6 - 20.9		7.7 to 24	
Time Following Diagnosis								
Median(years)			3,4		4,5		9,1	
Range (years)			1,7 – 4,3		3.0 - 5.1		5.2 - 15.7	
Time Following End of Treatment								
Median(years)			0,2		1,3		5,7	
Range (years)			-0,2 – 0,9		0.9 - 2.1		3.0 - 12.5	
Sex								
Male	78	55,3	25	65,8	24	63,2	40	51,9
Female	63	44,7	13	34,2	14	36,8	37	48,1
Patients with Normal Findings			26	68,5	31	81,6	68	88,3
Patients with Abnormal Findings			12	31,5	7	8,4	9	11,7

Table 2. Patient Results. Medium risk patients treated with chemotherapy only

Interestingly, among these patients with normal thyroid function are two patients who reversed to normal values, as at two year follow-up were categorized as having compensated hypothyroidism, and have remained with normal values without any intervention up to 8.2 years later. The third female patient had increasing TSH values (from 5.2 to 6.8 μIU/ml) 3.9 years later and was referred to a local endocrinologist for further evaluation and treatment.

Two additional patients (a 24.4 year old female and a 13.7 year old boy) had previously been diagnosed with Hashimoto thyroiditis with borderline low T4 values and they were receiving p.o. treatment with levothyroxine at the time of last follow- up.

Additionally, a 15.8 year old girl had been receiving for a period of 6 months interferon-alpha 2b sc, as part of hepatitis C treatment and she was found to have TSH serum value of 18 μIU/ml. This is a possible side effect of the use of interferon-alpha. The medication was discontinued and the patient is being followed appropriately.

Furthermore, 6 patients (2 females and 4 males) were found to have low levels of serum T4 (less than 5.0 μIU/ml) together with normal to low normal values of TSH. These 6 patients are thought to have hidden central hypothyroidism. Three of them had normal thyroid sonograms. The patients need further evaluation with measurements of FT4, TBG to exclude TBG deficiency and depending on the results if FT4 is in the lower third of normal, perform a TRH test or measure TSH at night to assess whether there is normal night TSH surge, in order to exclude central hypothyroidism.

Among the group of patients with long- term follow- up 12% is found to have thyroid dysfunction of variable etiology.

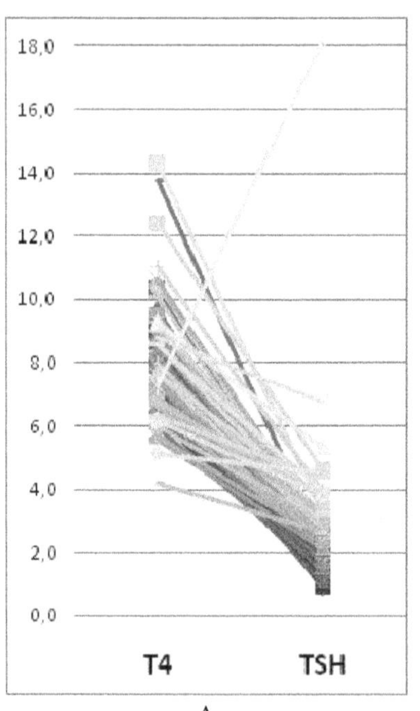

A

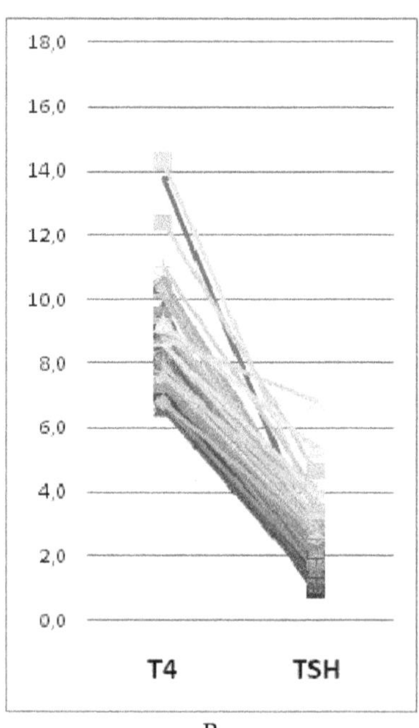

B

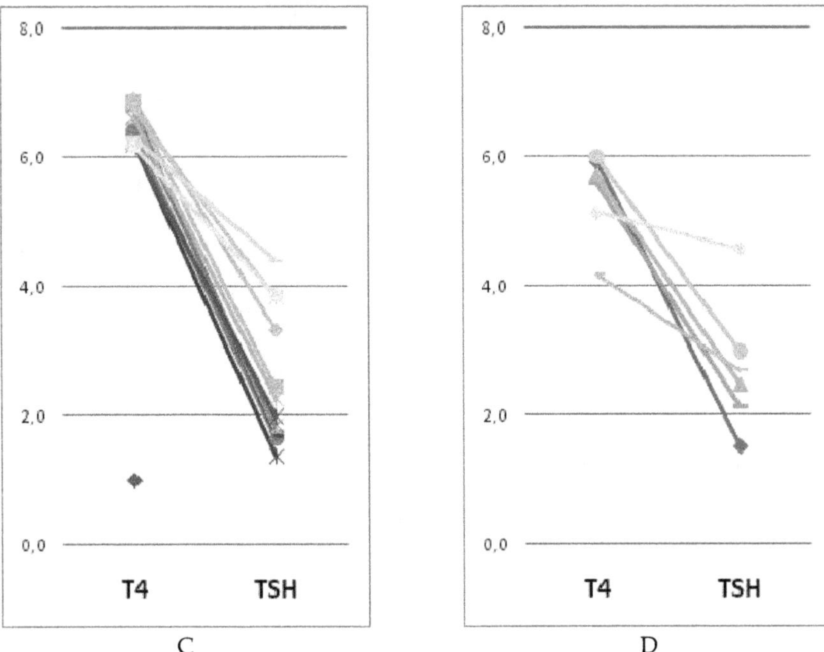

Fig. 2. Relation of the values of thyroid stimulating hormone (TSH, in μIU/ml) and thyroxine (T4 in μIU/ml) of patients more than three years after the end of treatment.
A: All 77 patients; B: 57 patients with normal values; C: 13 patients with low normal values; D: 6 patients with low values.

4. Discussion

Improvements in therapeutic protocols for childhood acute lymphocytic leukemia has led to very high survival rates above 85% with current treatment protocols (Conter et al., 2010, Moricke et al., 2010, Pui et al., 2009, Pui et al., 2010). High survival rates have been confirmed in the current cohort of Greek patients treated in a single department using BFM-90 and BFM-95 (Papadakis et al., 2003).

Hence, it is of great importance first, to identify the long term effects of therapeutic modalities, chemotherapy alone or in combination with prophylactic cranial irradiation and second, to find ways to either prevent them or detect them at the earliest possible in order to treat them appropriately and timely, assuring improved quality of life. Complications from the endocrine system account for the majority of long term- sequelae of cancer therapy in childhood (Chemaitilly & Sklar, 2010). As acute lymphoblastic leukemia is the commonest malignancy of childhood, it is essential to study all the possible complications of the survivors.

To our knowledge, most of the papers published to date, include patients treated for childhood ALL, in larger cohorts of childhood cancer survivors (Madanat et al., 2008). In addition, there are studies referring selectively to ALL patients, including patients treated with different protocols, as treatment guidelines were changing over time (Lando et al., 2001, Miyossi et al., 2008).

In this retrospective analysis, we aimed to recognize the prevalence of thyroid dysfunction in a cohort of Greek patients treated for childhood ALL, in a single center, according to the BFM-90 and BFM-95 treatment protocols. In the practice of this Center, as published previously (Papadakis et al., 2003), there are no patients assigned to the low risk group, meaning that a higher percentage of patients have received more intensive chemotherapy. Another factor that has to be appreciated, is that according to the current recommendations, the dose of cranial irradiation that the high risk group receives as prophylaxis of the central nervous system, is lower than the one administered in the previous decade. Furthermore, even smaller percentage of the patients treated for ALL are currently receiving cranial irradiation. An evaluation was performed at four time points as follows: at diagnosis, at the completion of chemotherapy, one to two years after completion of chemotherapy and at 3 years or later following completion of chemotherapy. Most of the previously reported data have no report on thyroid hormone values at diagnosis or at the end of therapy. The present data identifies the prevelance of thyroid dysfunction at all time points to occur at a relatively low percentage.

Of interest is the appreciation that a number of patients have thyroid dysfunction at diagnosis. A subgroup of the patients suffer from euthyroid sick syndrome related to the presence of a critical illness, that is acute lymphoblastic leukemia. Other patients have evidence of hypothyroidism or thyroiditis unrelated to the diagnosis of ALL. Therefore, we can suggest that evaluation of thyroid function which includes T4, FT4, T3, TSH as well as thyroid autoantibodies, should be added at the initial work-up, prior to chemotherapy initiation. Depending on the results, imaging of the thyroid gland by ultrasonography, has to be considered. This practice will permit us to identify thyroid dysfunction, preceeding therapeutic interventions, to assign specific etiology and differentiate among conditions that need to be treated, or euthyroid sick syndrome that usually needs no intervention and resolves spontaneously as the organism recovers.

As far as the high -risk group is concerned, which consisted of 24 patients who received intensified chemotherapy and cranial irradiation to12 Gy, thyroid function remains normal in the majority of subjects. As compared to previous reports, that radiation therapy increased the risk of hypothyroidsm development (Hancock, 1991) our findings can be attributed to the lower dose of radiotherapy that is administered as cranial and not craniospinal irradiation, thus exposing the thyroid gland to lower radiation dose. Data published previously, agrees that cranial radiation dose lower than 16 Gy is associated with lower risk of hypothyroidism development (Armstrong et al., 2010).

In the group of patients who were considered as medium- risk and received chemotherapy only we have appreciated the following findings. At the completion of chemotherapy, 68% of the evaluated patients have normal thyroid function. Of the patients who were considered to have some type of thyroid dysfunction, 5% have compensated hypothyroidism and 26% have possible hidden central hypothyroidism. It is of great interest that a third of them reversed to normal values 4 to 12 months later. These findings depict the importance of a more vigilant investigation to identify central hidden hypothyroidism using free T4 values, night TSH surge and in the patients that the results are equivocal, proceed to thyroid releasing hormone (TRH) stimulation test. Although, it is evident that in a percentage of patients there is spontaneous recovery, it is meaningful to identify patients with central hypothyroidism and treat them appropriately. Thus, both growth impairment and metabolic complications such as dyslipidemia and obesity can be prevented and the patients' well- being can be improved. Re-evaluation will be desirable in order to reassess the need for treatment continuation.

At one to two years following completion of chemotherapy, normal thyroid function was found in 81.6% of the patients. Among those patients with normal thyroid function appreciated, there are patients whose values were abnormal at the one year follow-up. The remaining 18.4% had mild thyroid dysfunction of variable etiology. Compensated hypothyroidism represents 7.9% of the whole group, whilst the remaining patients with thyroid dysfunction are assigned to the possible central hypothyroidism diagnosis.

The majority of the patients in the chemotherapy only treated group have normal thyroid hormone values at the 3 years and beyond follow-up examination. In the normal function group are included patients that were diagnosed to have compensated hypothyroidism at the one to two year time point evaluation. Spontaneous improvement and normalization of the findings is seen. Among the patients with normal values, we have characterized a subgroup of patients who had T4 in the lower third of normal values and low corresponding TSH. This patient subgroup accounts for 14% of the group with normal values.

Furthermore, 12% of the patients, a substantial and not to be underestimated group of patients, had thyroid dysfunction of different etiologies. Included in this group is a 2.5% that has compensated hypothyroidism and 7.5% have possible central hypothyroidism. The patients with abnormal findings have no clinically appreciable symptomatology of hypothyroidism, besides some patients who were obese. However, there is no detailed recording of height measurements, lipid profile evaluation and body fat measurements, that could reveal a subtle or hidden central hypothyroidism.

A limiting factor of this study is the fact that all the patents do not have measurements at all time points so that we could have a complete picture of evolution of thyroid function and possible dysfunction. This is an inherent characteristic of a retrospective study, with data collected from patient chart recordings and not a prospective patient evaluation. Moreover, there are additional laboratory investigations that could have been applied in order to clarify the exact nature of the dysfunction seen, which have not been performed timely. It is conceivable that this has led to some bias in our analysis. Moreover, a complete investigation at diagnosis which can depict patients with thyroid binding globulin deficiency, ectopic thyroid that was missed, cases of dysormonogenesis or thyroiditis Hashimoto will facilitate the clarification of thyroid dysfunction post therapy.

As our aim was to identify all cases of clinical, subclinical and central hypothyroidism, without exploring the mechanism behind diminished thyroid function, we relied on the adequacy of TSH and T4 testing. There are no records of the exact prevalence of acquired hypothyroidism, in the general Greek population. If we compare the percentage of hypothyroidism in survivors of childhood ALL to that reported in other populations, like the Finnish population reported by Madanat et al (Madanat et al., 2007), we observe a higher percentage of ALL survivors with thyroid dysfunction.

The findings of this study support the idea that chemotherapy alone has untoward effect on thyroid function. The mechanism of inducing such a thyroid dysfunction remains unclear. Whether this is a direct side- effect of the chemotherapy applied or whether the thyroid function is impaired due to the diagnosis of ALL and the chronic insult of years of treatment, remains to be discovered. The fact that the radiotherapy applied does not increase the risk of thyroid dysfunction can be attributed to the lower dose of irradiation and the limited field of radiation (cranial RT only). The prevalence of thyroid dysfunction in this study is higher, as patients with borderline values of low T4 and corresponding low TSH values were included in the thyroid dysfunction patient group, in an effort to increase the awareness for the patients with possible central hypothyroidism. The study will be continued and further investigations will be carried out in order to calculate the exact percentage of hypothyroidism and clarify the etiology.

Hence, the observations and data presented in this study support the idea that thyroid dysfunction is encountered with increased frequency in survivors of childhood ALL. Serial measurements of thyroid hormones, as well as, search for signs and symptoms of hypothyroidism is imperative during the diagnosis and the short and long- term follow- up of ALL survivors.

5. References

Armstrong G.T., Pan Z., Ness K.K., Srivastava D.and Robison L.L. 2010. Temporal trends in cause-specific late mortality among five-year survivors of childhood cancer *J. Clin.Oncol.* Vol 28, No 7, Mar 2010, pp 1224–1231

Bőling T., Geisenheiser A., Pape H., Martini C., Rϋbe C., Timmermann B., Fischedick K., Kortmann R.D., Gerb J., Koch R., Willich N. 2011. Hypothyroidism after head-and - neck radiotherapy in children and adolescents: Preliminary results of the "registry for the evaluation of side effects after radiotherapy in childhood and adolescence" (RISK) *Int. J. Radiation Oncology Biol. Phys.Dec 16 2010,*pp 1-5 Epub ahead of printing

Chemaitilly W., Sklar C.A. 2010. Endocrine complications in long-term survivors of childhood cancers. *Endocr Relat Cancer,* Vol 17, No 3, Jun 2010, pp 141-159.

Conter V., Bartram C.R., Valsecchi M.G., Schrauder A., Panzer-Grümayer R., Möricke A., Aricò M., Zimmermann M., Mann G., De Rossi G., Stanulla M., Locatelli F., Basso G., Niggli F., Barisone E., Henze G., Ludwig W.D., Haas O.A., Cazzaniga G., Koehler R., Silvestri D., Bradtke J., Parasole R., Beier R., van Dongen J.J., Biondi A., Schrappe M. 2010. Molecular response to treatment redefines all prognostic factors in children and adolescents with B-cell precursor acute lymphoblastic leukemia: results in 3184 patients of the AIEOP-BFM ALL 2000 study. *Blood.* Vol 115, No 16, Apr 2010, pp 3206-3214

Hancock S.L., Cox R.S., and McDougall I.R. Thyroid diseases after treatment of Hodgkin's disease. 1991. *N. Engl. J. Med.,* Vol 325, No 9, Aug 1991, pp 599–605

Katsimpardi K., Papadakis V., Pangalis A., Parcharidou A., Panagiotou J.P., Soutis M., Papandreou E., PolychronopoulouS., Haidas S. 2006. Infections in a pediatric patient cohort with acute lymphoblastic leukemia during the entire course of treatment.. *Support Care Cancer* Vol 14, No 3, Mar 2006, pp 277–284

Lando A., Holm K., Nysom K., Rasmussen A.K., Feldt-Rasmussen U., Petersen J.H. & Muller J. 2001. Thyroid function in survivors of childhood acute lymphoblastic leukaemia: the significance of prophylactic cranial irradiation. *Clinical Endocrinology* Vol 55, No 1, Jul 2001, pp 21–25

Madanat L.M., Lähteenmäki P.M., Alin J., Salmi T.T. 2007. The natural history of thyroid function abnormalities after treatment for childhood cancer. *Eur J Cancer*.Vol 43,No7, May 2007, pp 1161-1170.

Madanat L.M., Lähteenmäki P.M., Hurme S., Dyba T., Salmi T.T., Sankila R. 2008. Hypothyroidism among pediatric cancer patients: A nation-wide registry based study *Int J of Cancer* Vol 122, No 8, April 2008, pp 1868-1872

Miyoshi Y., Ohta H., Hashii Y., Tokimasa S., Namba N., Mushiake S., Hara J., Ozono K. 2008. Endocrinological analysis of 122 Japanese Childhood Cancer Survivors in a single Hospital *Endocrine Journal* ,Vol 55, No 6, Dec 2008, pp 1055-1063

Moricke A., Reiter A., Zimmermann M., Gadner H., Stanulla M., Dordelmann M., Loning L., Beier R., Ludwig W. D., Ratei R., Harbott J., Boos J., Mann G., Niggli F., Feldges A., Henze G., Welte K., Beck J. D., Klingebiel T., Niemeyer C., Zintl F., Bode U., Urban C., Wehinger H., Niethammer D., Riehm H., and Schrappe M. 2008. Risk-adjusted therapy of acute lymphoblastic leukemia can decrease treatment burden and improve survival: treatment results of 2169 unselected pediatric and adolescent patients enrolled in the trial ALL-BFM 95. *Blood* Vol 111, No 9, May 2008, pp 4477-4489

Möricke A., Zimmermann M., Reiter A., Henze G., Schrauder A., Gadner H., Ludwig W.D., Ritter J., Harbott J., Mann G., Klingebiel T., Zintl F., Niemeyer C., Kremens B., Niggli F., Niethammer D., Welte K., Stanulla M., Odenwald E., Riehm H., Schrappe M. 2010. Long- term results of five consecutive trials in childhood acute lymphoblastic leukemia performed by the ALL BFM group from 1981 to 2000 *Leukemia.* Vol 24, No 2, Feb 2010, pp 265-284

Neves Mascarenhas A., Papadia C., Alves Aquino C., Oba L., Ferreira M., Casulari L.A.. 2006. Treatment for acute lymphoblastic leukemia in children is associated with papillary carcinoma of thyroid, but not with thyroid dysfunction. *Minerva Pediatr.* Vol 58 No 5, Oct 2006, pp 469-476

Oeffinger, K.C., Mertens, A.C., Sklar, C.A., Kawashima, T., Hudson, M.M., Meadows, A.T., Friedman, D.L., Marina, N., Hobbie, W.,Kadan-Lottick, N.S., Schwartz, C.L., Leisenring, W. & Robison, L.L.. 2006. Chronic health conditions in adult survivors of childhood cancer. *New England Journal of Medicine*, Vol 355, No 15, Oct 2006, pp 1572–1582

Papadakis V., Panagiotou J. P., Polychronopoulou-Androulakaki S., Mikraki V., Parcharidou A., Tsitsikas C., Vrachnou E., Paterakis G, Maurou A., Sampani C., Soutis E.M., and Haidas S. 2003. Results of childhood acute lymphoblastic leukaemia treatment in Greek patients using a BFM-based protocol. *Haema* Vol 6, No2, Mar 2003 pp 208-216

Pui C.H. & Evans W.E. 2006. Treatment of acute lymphoblasticleukemia. *New England Journal of Medicine*, Vol 354, No 2, Jan 2006, pp 166–178

Pui C.H., Campana D., Pei D., Bowman W.P., Sandlund J.T., Kaste S.C., Ribeiro R.C., Rubnitz J.E., Raimondi S.C., Onciu M., Coustan-Smith E., Kun L.E., Jeha S., Cheng C., Howard S.C., Simmons V., Bayles A., Metzger M.L., Boyett J.M., Leung W., Handgretinger R., Downing J.R., Evans W.E., and Relling M.V. 2009. Treating childhood acute lymphoblastic leukemia without cranial irradiation. *New England Journal of Medicine* Vol 360, No 26, Jun 2009, pp 2730-2741

Pui C.H., Pei D., Sandlund J.T., Ribeiro R.C., Rubnitz J.E., Raimondi S.C., Onciu M., Campana D., Kun L.E., Jeha S., Cheng C., Howard S.C., Metzger M.L., Bhojwani D., Downing J.R., Evans W.E., Relling M.V. 2010. Long term results of St Jude Total Therapy Studies 11,.12,.13A, 13B and 14 for childhood acute lymphoblastic leukemia *Leukemia* Vol 24, No 2, Feb 2010, pp 371-382

Rose S.R., Lustig R.H., Pitukcheewanont P., Broome D.C., Burghen G.A., Li H., Hudson M.M., Kun L.E., Heideman R.L.. 1999. Diagnosis of hidden central hypothyroidism in survivors of childhood cancer. *J Clin Endocrinol Metab*. Vol 84, No 12, Dec 1999, pp 4472-4479

Schrappe M., Reiter A., Ludwig W.D., Harbott J., Zimmermann M., Hiddemann W., Niemeyer C., Henze G., Feldges A., Zintl F., Kornhuber B., Ritter J., Welte K., Gadner H., and Riehm H. 2000. Improved outcome in childhood acute lymphoblastic leukemia despite reduced use of anthracyclines and cranial radiotherapy: results of trial ALL-BFM 90. German-Austrian-Swiss ALL-BFM Study Group. *Blood*, Vol 95, No 11, Jun 2000, pp 3310-3322

Steffens M., Beauloye V., Brichard B., Robert A., Alexopoulou O., Vermylen Ch., Maiter D. 2008. Endocrine and metabolic disorders in young adult survivors of childhood acute lymphoblastic leukaemia (ALL) or non-Hodgkin lymphoma (NHL). *Clin Endocrinol (Oxf)*. Vol 69, No 5, Nov 2008, pp 819-827

10

Hypothyroidism and Thyroid Function Alterations During the Neonatal Period

Susana Ares[1], José Quero[1], Belén Sáenz-Rico de Santiago[2] and Gabriela Morreale de Escobar[3]
[1]*Neonatology Unit. Hospital LA PAZ. Madrid*
[2]*Department of Didactics and school Organization of the Faculty of Education of the Complutense University of Madrid.*
[3]*Instituto de Investigaciones Biomédicas. Universidad Autónoma de Madrid*
Spanish Preterm Thyroid Group
Spain

1. Introduction

The thyroid hormones, T_4 and 3,5,3′-triiodothyronine (T_3), are necessary for adequate growth and development (Greenberg AH et al., 1974; Zimmermann, 2011), throughout fetal and extrauterine life. These hormones regulate many metabolic processes: somatic growth, cardiac, pulmonary and bone maturation, central nervous system maturation, and neuronal differentiation, regulate oxygen consumption, and protein, lipid and carbohydrate metabolism. There is evidence that thyroid hormones are necessary for surfactant synthesis and lung maturation (Biswas S et al., 2002). Brain and lung maturation have received special attention, because of the potentially irreversible or life-threatening consequences associated with early thyroid hormone deficiency (Kester MA et al., 2004; De Vries et al., 1986). The importance of thyroid hormones to perinatal neural development is well established but their relation to the developmental sequelae of preterm birth is being recently studied. During the first half of gestation the thyroid hormone available to the fetus is predominantly of maternal origin. T_4 from the mother is the most important source of T_3 for the fetal brain and protects it from a possible hormone deficiency until birth. Once fetal thyroid secretion starts, fetal supplies are of mixed fetal and maternal origin. Although fetal thyroidal secretion is believed to constitute an increasing proportion of the hormone available to the developing fetus, maternal transfer of T_4 may still contribute significantly to fetal needs (20-50% of normal values) up to term, mitigating the consequences of inadequate fetal thyroid function. The transfer of iodine is also difficult to quantify, but the iodine content of the fetal thyroid increases progressively from less than 2 µg at 17 weeks of gestation up to 300 µg at term (Figure 1). Thyroid function in premature infants is immature at birth. Preterm infants often have low thyroxine (T4 and FreeT4) levels postnatally, a condition referred to as transient hypotiroxinemia of prematurity. Transient hypotiroxinemia can be found in approximately 35% of all premature newborns and in 50% babies born with less than 30 weeks. This occurs during an important period for brain development and low T4 levels could be a negative factor contributing to the neurodevelopment problems of very preterm infants. The number of extremely low birth weight babies (ELBW) is high. Interventions have increased the population at risk. The precocious diagnosis and treatment of the alterations of thyroid function during the neonatal period, could have beneficial effects in the prevention of developmental abnormalities. Iodine is a trace element which is essential for the synthesis of thyroid hormones. The iodine intake of newborns is entirely dependent on the iodine content of breast milk and the formula preparations used to feed them. An inadequate iodine supply (deficiency and excess) might be especially dangerous in the case of premature babies. The minimum recommended dietary allowance (RDA) is different depending on age groups. The iodine intake required is at least 15 μg/kg/day in full-term infants and 30 μg/kg/day in preterms. Newborn infants are in a situation of iodine deficiency, precisely at a stage of psychomotor and neural development which is extremely sensitive to alterations of thyroid function (Ares et al., 1994, 1995, 2004, 2005, 2007; Zimmermann MB, 2004, 2009)

2. Thyroid function in the fetus and newborn

T_4, free T_4 (FT_4) and T_3 of preterm and term neonates increased with PMA, whereas thyroglobulin (Tg) decreased and thyroid-stimulating hormone (TSH) did not change. Serum FT_4, T_3, Tg and TSH of neonates were affected negatively, independently of age, by different neonatal factors, including a low iodine intake. It is often presumed that the low thyroxine levels in premature infants are a continuation of levels experienced in utero, a

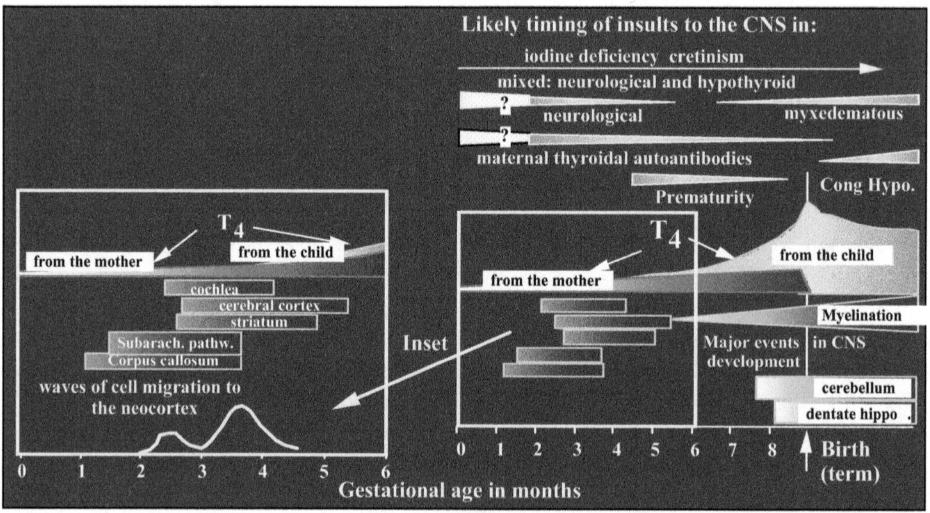

Fig. 1. Shows the overlapping changes in input thyroid hormones in utero and postnatally immediately with the start of important phases of development human brain during pregnancy. At the top T4 represents the amount needed by the fetus that is entirely from maternal origin until the middle of the pregnancy, and maternal origin and fetal thereafter. They represent only the needs of T4, and from it derives the brain T3 during these phases of development.

condition referred to as transient hypotiroxinemia of prematurity, but data derived from blood obtained by cordocentesis have shown that TSH and T4 levels sampled from fetuses are higher than those found in premature infants of the same gestational age (Figure 2). Neonatal lterations in thyroid function and hypothyroxinemia of prematurity are thought to be caused by several reasons. These include the incomplete maturation of the hypothalamic-pituitary-thyroid axis and relative immaturity of the type I iodothyronine deoidinase enzyme systems, the untimely interruption of maternal transfer of thyroid hormones to the fetus across the human placenta, maternal antibodies, postnatal drugs (dopamine, heparine, corticoids...) and neonatal disease. Quite prominent among these causes are iodine deficiency during gestation and the neonatal period, and peri- and post-natal exposure to an iodine excess, usually caused by iodine-containing antiseptics and radiologic contrast media. The percentage contribution of iodine deficiency to thyroid dysfunction may be greater in the more immature infants who have a very low iodine supply: Serum FT4, T3, Tg and TSH of preterm neonates were affected negatively, independently from age, by a low iodine intake. Iodine deficiency contributes to about 30% of the hypothyroxinaemia in enterally and parenterally fed preterm infants of 27–30 weeks gestation (Morreale G 1990, Morreale G 2002, Delange 2001, 2004, Fisher 1969, 1970, 1981)

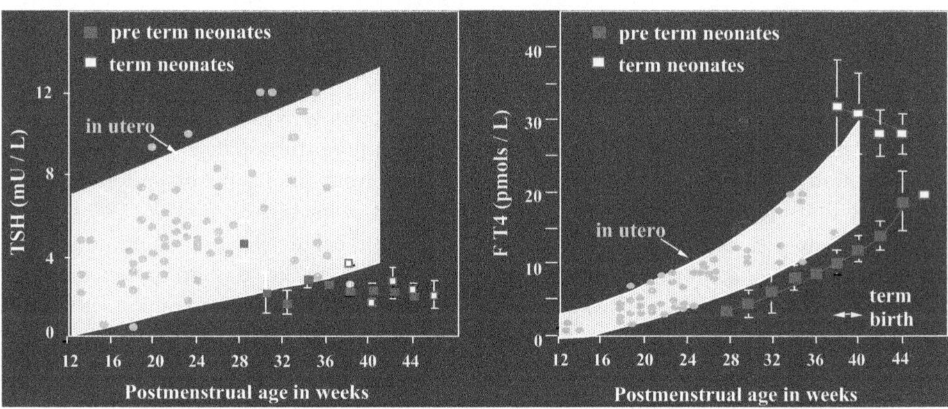

Fig. 2. Concentrations of FT4 of preterm and term neonates are superimposed on data published for fetuses in utero (by Thorpe-Beeston et al.1991) The shaded area corresponds to the 95 % confidence intervals for the fetal FT4 and TSH data (G Morreale de Escobar, S Ares 1998).

3. Iodine requirements during the first month of life

Iodine is a trace element which is essential for the synthesis of thyroid hormones. If maternal iodine deficiency in pregnancy is severe, fetal brain damage will occur. This damage is irreversible after birth. Mild/moderate iodine deficiency during pregnancy and early postnatal life is associated with neuro/psycho-intellectual deficits in infants and children. The severity is not only related to the degree of iodine deficiency, but also to the developmental phase during which it is suffered, the most severe being the consequence of iodine deficiency during the first two trimesters of pregnancy. An inadequate iodine supply might be especially dangerous in the case of premature infants, who are prematurely deprived of the maternal supply of hormones and iodine, before their own gland has been able to accumulate as much iodine as in term newborns. The iodine intake of newborns is entirely dependent on the iodine content of breast milk and the formula preparations used to feed them. The minimum recommended dietary allowance (RDA) for different age groups has recently been revised. Taking into consideration new information regarding iodine metabolism in premature and term newborn infants, to meet such requirements the iodine content of formulas for premature newborns should contain 20 μg/dl, and that of first and follow-up preparations 10 μg/ dl. We refer here to these new recommendations as those of the ICCIDD (International Council for the Control of Iodine Deficiency Disorders). The availability of iodine during the peri- and post-natal period of development should both ensure the minimal requirements and should not exceed the minimum amounts blocking their thyroid function. The requirement of iodine in neonates was evaluated from metabolic studies. To reach adequate intake the iodine content of formulas for premature newborns ought to contain 20 μg / dl, that of all other preparations 10 μg / dl. The recommended intake of iodine in neonates reflects the observed mean iodine intake of young infants exclusively fed human milk in iodine replete areas. However, it is well established that the iodine content of breast milk is critically influenced by the dietary intake of the pregnant and lactating mother (Delange F et al.,1985b; Delange F et al., 1993; Semba RD, 2001; Dorea JG, 2002). The iodine requirement in neonates was evaluated from metabolic studies by determining the values which resulted in a situation of positive iodine balance, which is required in order to insure a progressively increasing intrathyroidal iodine pool in the growing young infant (Delange F et al., 1993). In our unit we studied thyroid gland volume by ultrasound and we found that the volume varied from 0.3-1.3 ml in preterm infants during the first month of life and 0.9 ml in term infants at birth (Ares S et al., 1995). These studies indicate that the iodine intake required in order to achieve a positive iodine balance is at least 15 μg/kg/day in full-term infants and 30 μg/kg/day in preterms. This corresponds approximately to 90 μg/day and is consequently twice as high as the 1989 recommendations of 40-50 μg/ day (National Research Council, 1999; Delange F, 2004).

4. Iodine deficiency

Iodine is a trace element that is essential for the synthesis of thyroid hormones. An inadequate iodine supply (deficiency and excess) might be especially dangerous in the case of premature babies. The minimum recommended dietary allowance is different depending on age groups. Premature infants are in a situation of iodine deficiency, precisely at a stage of psychomotor and neural development that is extremely sensitive to alterations of thyroid function. The iodine intake does affect the circulating levels of FT4, T3, Tg and TSH in preterm infants, independently of their age. Circulating levels are lower in preterm than in term neonates of comparable age and iodine intake (or balance), at least up to 44 weeks PMA and an intake of 80 μg / day. T_4, free T_4 (FT_4) and T_3 of preterm and term neonates increased with age, whereas thyroglobulin (Tg) decreased and thyroid-stimulating hormone (TSH) did not change. Serum FT_4, T_3, Tg and TSH of preterm neonates were affected negatively, independently of age, by a low iodine intake . The percentage contribution of iodine deficiency to hypothyroxinaemia may be greater in the more immature infants who have a very low iodine supply: Serum FT4, T3, Tg and TSH of preterm neonates were affected negatively, independently from age, by a low iodine intake. Iodine deficiency contributes to about 30% of the hypothyroxinaemia in enterally and parenterally fed preterm infants of 27–30 weeks gestation (Figure 1 and Figure 2) (Ares S et al., 1994; Ares S et al., 1995; Ares S et al., 1997; Morreale de Escobar G et al., 1998; Ares S et al., 2004).

5. Iodine excess

In normal individuals, the acute and chronic excess of iodinerarely leads to profound clinical thyroid dysfunction, because of the rapid activation of several autoregulatory mechanisms. However, in some individuals, such as newborns, the escape from the inhibitory effect of large doses of iodine is not achieved and clinical (symptomatic hypothyroidism) or subclinical hypothyroidism (asymptomatic hypothyroidism or altered serum thyroid parameters) The most frequently identified sources of excess iodine leading to problems in neonates result from the use of iodine-containing disinfectants (10,000 microg of iodine/mL) and from radiograph contrast media (250-370 mg of iodine/mL) given for radiological examination. The total concentration of iodine in plasma comprises the iodine in circulating T4 and T3, plus the circulating iodide and any iodine contained in contrast media, or other contaminating compounds. The minimum amount of iodine that can cause a Wolff–Chaikoff effect in premature and term neonates has not been clearly defined, as it may depend on a variety of factors, including the chemical form in which the iodine overload is supplied (Wolff J, Chaikoff IL, 1969; Ares et al., 2008) . There is a marked individual variability in the sensitivity to iodine-overload. Urinary iodine concentrations above 16 microg/dL, 20 microg g/dL, and 25 microg g/dL may impair thyroid function in neonates. Some iodinated contrast agents, such as ipodate and iopanoic acid, are well-known inhibitors of all known iodothyronine deiodinases.

6. The role of thyroid hormones on human central nervous system during fetal and postnatal life

The close involvement between human brain development and thyroid hormones is widely accepted (Morreale de Escobar G et al., 2000, 2004). The effects of T_3 on the central nervous system are mediated by the regulation of the expression of genes that synthesize proteins implicated in cerebral neurogenesis, neuronal migration and differentiation, axonal outgrowth, dendritic ontogeny, and synaptogenesis. They are also necessary for cerebellar neurogenesis (predominantly during early postnatal life), gliogenesis (predominantly during late fetal life to 6 months postnatally), and myelogenesis (during the second trimester of gestation to 2 years of postnatal life). Low T_4 levels during neonatal life, especially if persistent, could be a negative factor contributing to the neurodevelopmental problems of very preterm infants. Indeed, retrospective studies have shown a relationship between hypothyroxinemia and developmental delay and an increased risk of disabling cerebral palsy (De Vries et al., 1986; den Ouden AL et al., 1996; Lucas A et al., 1988, Lucas A et al., 1996; Meijer WJ et al., 1992; Lucas A et al., 1996; Reuss ML et al., 1996).

7. Alterations of the thyroid function during the neonatal period risk factors

There are many more associations of postnatal factors with transient alterations of thyroid function than had previously been considered in newborn infants. A oblique preventative approach may be necessary through reduction in the incidence or severity of individual illness(es). Similarly, alternatives to those drugs that interfere with the hypothalamic-pituitary-thyroid axis should be evaluated (e.g. other inotropics instead of dopamine) (Table 1 and 2)

1. Abrupt withdrawal of maternal iodine, T4 and TRH from placenta.
2. The adaptive response of the thyroid axis at the interruption of the placental circulation is insufficient.
3. Incomplete development of the hypothalamic-pituitary-thyroid axis:
- Insufficient secretion of TRH
- Immature thyroid response to TSH
- Lower retention of iodine in the thyroid. Inefficient Thyroglobulin Iodination until week 34.
- Lower circulating levels of TSH, T4, FT4, T3 and FT3
4. Low synthesis and serum concentration of T4 binding globulin (TBG)
5. Underdevelopment of 5 'DI -deiodinase, especially in the liver
6. Decreased peripheral conversion of T4 to T3 in tissues
7. Increased frequency of serious morbidity, and therapeutic management of drugs. Multiple influences over the hypothalamic-pituitary-thyroid axis.
8. Frequent postnatal malnutrition
9. Undeterminated iodine intake and excretion.
10. Iodine deficiency or excess.

Table 1. Causal factors of transient alterations of thyroid function in the preterm newborn.

7.1 Hypothyroidism in the newborn

Neonatal hypothyroidism is defined as decreased thyroid hormone production in a newborn. In very rare cases, no thyroid hormone is produced. In primary hypothyroidism, TSH levels are high and T_4 and T_3 levels are low. If the baby was born with the condition, it is called congenital hypothyroidism. If it develops soon after birth, it is called hypothyroidism acquired in the newborn period. Hypothyroidism in the newborn may be caused by: a missing or poorly developed thyroid gland, a pituitary gland that does not stimulate the thyroid gland or thyroid hormones that are poorly formed or do not work. The most common cause of hypothyroidism in the newborn is complete absence or underdevelopment of the thyroid gland. Endemic cretinism is caused by iodine deficiency, and is occasionally exacerbated by naturally occurring goitrogens. Dysgenesis of the thyroid gland, including agenesis (ie, complete absence of thyroid gland) and ectopy (lingual or sublingual thyroid gland) may be a cause. The incidence of congenital hypothyroidism, as detected through newborn screening, is approximately 1 out of every 3,000 births, but the incidence is different depending on the country, sex, race, ethnicity, gestational age,....

Girls are affected twice as often as boys. Less commonly, the thyroid gland is present but does not produce normal amounts of thyroid hormones. Although initial preliminary studies were performed using thyroid-stimulating hormone (TSH) levels in cord blood, mass screening was made feasible by the development of radioimmunoassay for TSH and thyroxine (T4) from blood spots on filter paper, obtained for neonatal screening tests. Some infants identified as having primary congenital hypothyroidism may have transient disease and not permanent congenital hypothyroidism. Family history should be carefully reviewed for information about similarly affected infants or family members with unexplained mental retardation. Neonatal screening for congenital hypothyroidism in premature infants is not as well established as in term newborns regarding age and number of samples. Congenital hypothyroidism is more common in infants with birthweights less than 2,000 g or more than 4,500 g. and in multiple births. Inborn errors of thyroid hormone metabolism include dyshormonogenesis. Most cases are familial and inherited as autosomal recessive conditions. These may also include the following: thyroid-stimulating hormone (TSH) unresponsiveness (ie, TSH receptor abnormalities), impaired ability to uptake iodide, peroxidase, or organification, defect (ie, inability to convert iodide to iodine), Pendred syndrome, a familial organification defect associated with congenital deafness,

DRUG	METABOLISM	Thyroid function
Dopamine > 1 mcg / kg / min	Decrease: secretion of TSH	Decrease synthesis of thyroid hormones in the thyroid
Fenobarbital	Increased metabolism of T4	Decreased T4 and FT4 Increased secretion of TSH in patients treated with T4
Glucocorticoides (dosis altas)	Increased secretion of TSH in patients treated with T4 Altered conversion of T4 to T3 decreased TBG, T3 and TSH	Decreased T_4, T_3 and TSH
Furosemide	Decreases binding of T4 to TBG decreased T4, and increased FT4	Decreases T4 and increased circulating FT4
Heparine	Increases active lipoprotein lipase in plasma and concentration of free fatty acids which displaces T4 from TBG and increases free T4	Decreases binding of T4 to TBG decreased T4, and increased FT4
Octeotride		Decreased secretion of thyroid hormones in the thyroid
Oral Iron sulfate	Inhibition of intestinal L-T4 absorption (when supplemented)	decreased: T4, FT4 and increased TSH FT4 increased requirements in hypothyroidism

Table 2. Effects of some drugs used during the neonatal period on thyroid function.

Thyroglobulin defect (ie, inability to form or degrade thyroglobulin), Deiodinase defect. Thyroid hormone resistance (ie, thyroid hormone receptor abnormalities) may also be a cause. TSH or thyrotropin-releasing hormone (TRH) deficiencies are also noted. Hypothyroidism can also occur in TSH or TRH deficiencies, either as an isolated problem or in conjunction with other pituitary deficiencies (eg, hypopituitarism). If present with these deficiencies, hypothyroidism is usually milder and is not associated with the significant neurologic morbidity observed in primary hypothyroidism. Initially, the newborn may have no symptoms. Later, the newborn may become sluggish (lethargic) and have a poor appetite, low muscle tone, constipation, a hoarse cry, and a bulging of the abdominal contents at the bellybutton (an umbilical hernia). The morbidity from congenital hypothyroidism can be reduced to a minimum by early diagnosis and treatment. Untreated infants will have delayed development, intellectual disability, and short stature. Because early treatment can prevent intellectual disability, all newborns should receive a screening blood test in the hospital early after birth to evaluate thyroid function. Many newborns with hypothyroidism require thyroid hormone given by mouth for their entire life. Treatment is directed by a doctor who specializes in treating children with problems of the endocrine system (a pediatric endocrinologist).*(LaFranchi S 2001, LeFranchi S et all. 1977,* La Franchi S 2011, Rovet JF 1999, Rovet JF 1999, Rovet JF et al. 2000)

7.2 Transient neonatal hypothyroidism

Transient hypothyroidism occurs when thyrotropin (TSH) levels are elevated but thyroxine (T_4) and triiodothyronine (T_3) levels are low but the thyroid gland is present, and there is another factor that causes this alteration· TSH usually increases when T_4 and T_3 levels drop. TSH prompts the thyroid gland to make more hormones. In subclinical hypothyroidism, TSH is elevated but below the limit representing overt hypothyroidism. Somteimes, the levels of the active hormones will be within the laboratory reference ranges.In maternal autoimmune disease, transplacental passage of antibodies cause transient or permanent hypothyroidism. Temporary hypothyroidism can be due to the Wolff-Chaikoff effect. A very high intake of iodine can produce a blockage in the synthesis of thyroid hormones. Although iodide is a substrate for thyroid hormones, high levels reduce iodide organification in the thyroid gland, decreasing hormone production. The antiarrhythmic agent amiodarone can cause hyper- or hypothyroidism due to its high iodine content. Iodine in contrast agents or skin disinfectants can cause hypothyroidism or hyperthyrotropinemia in premature neonates (Lopez –Sastre et all. 1999, Delange 1988, Webwer G 1998).

7.3 Hiperthyrotropinemia

Physiologically, at birth occurs a sudden rise of TSH in normal newborns and premature infants, and the concentrations usually go down to within 1-2 weeks. Transient hyperthyrotropinemia is characterized the persistence of elevated TSH, but normal levels of T4. The duration of the disorder varies from a few days to several months. The etiology is unknown in most cases (idiopathic). Occasionally, it appears as result of an excess of iodine or deficiency and is more frequent in preterm infants. Generally the disorder does not require treatment, but it must be monitored in order to exclude primary hypothyroidism. Hypothyrotropinemia occurs when thyrotropin (TSH) levels are elevated but thyroxine (T_4) and triiodothyronine (T_3) levels are normal. TSH prompts the thyroid gland to make more hormone. TSH is elevated but below the limit representing overt hypothyroidism. The levels of the active hormones will be within the laboratory reference ranges. Some infants will require thyroxine substitution therapy depending on the age, concomitant illness, TSh levels … and should be evaluated individually.

7.4 Hypothyroxinemia of prematurity

Transient hypothyroxinaemia of prematurity (THOP) is the most common thyroid dysfunction in preterm infants and is defined by temporary low levels of T4, T3 and normal or low TSH. Low T4 levels in preterm infants are associated with persistent neurodevelopmental deficits in cognitive and motor function. Thyroid hormone substitution trials to date are underpowered and show inconsistent results; the question remains that if low T4 levels simply an epiphenomenon or not. The aetiology of transient hypothyroxinaemia is multifactorial and the components amenable to correction form the basis of the therapeutic strategy: rectification of iodine deficiency in parenteral nutrition; a reduction of non-thyroidal illnesses and attenuation of their severity; and substitution of drugs that interfere with the hypothalamic-pituitary-thyroid axis. Thyroxine substitution therapy should only be done in the context of clinical trials and only in those infants who are severely hypothyroxinaemic. Some studies that investigated THOP and disabling cerebral palsy (CP) found an increased risk of CP in the 15% of infants < 33 weeks gestation who had the lowest thyroxine levels. A relative risk of 4 for CP translates into an etiologic fraction of 75%, and a population attributable risk of 31%. This means that 75% of all disabling CP in children with THOP, and nearly a third of disabling CP in all infants below 33 weeks gestation age are associated with low thyroid hormone levels. Approximately 20,000 births each year in the United States are of < 28 weeks gestation and 70% of them (~14,000) now survive. Approximately 12% of survivors (nearly 1,700 children) will have disabling cerebral palsy. In addition, several studies measured IQ or its equivalent, and found a reduction of 7-8 points (or more than half a standard deviation for the population) in children of mothers with subclinical hypothyroidism during pregnancy independently of THOP suggesting the problem may be more widespread. Thus, in theory, treatment of THOP alone could lead to the prevention of as many as 500-600 cases of CP in this gestational group. Paneth reviewed relationships among THOP, adverse neurological outcomes, and other perinatal variables, and described six different ways in which these sets of variables could be related to each other, only some of which implied a causal role for THOP in neurological adversity (Paneth et all. 1998). However, unlike many other risk factors uncovered in population-based clinical research, this association is supported by a solid body of laboratory and clinical evidence, including the well-known adverse effects on the brain of thyroid and iodine deficiency. From population surveys, perinatal, developmental, human, animal and cell culture data, there is clearly a CNS *"window of vulnerability"* for brain damage in ELBW neonates. What is not yet known, and what cannot be established by any means other than a properly powered interventional trial, is whether the strong association of THOP with impaired neurodevelopment is in fact causal. Since previous work could not prove the need to treat due to sample size and concern that excessive treatment is itself a risk, outright intervention is not advocated at this time. On the other hand, if a physician were to choose to treat, we would recommend following a hospital-based structured protocol to *supplement* endogenous production without suppressing TSH release to enable future reflection on results rather than risk random intervention based on physician-to-physician bias (Van Wassenaer 1997, 1998, La Gamma 2006, 2009, Meijer WJ et al., 1992)

7.5 Low T3 syndrome

In terms of fetal thyroid function, fetal T3 levels are low throughout gestation, and increase during the third trimester, reaching only 50% of adult levels, due to increased conversion of T4 in T3 inverse (rT3). The state of low concentrations of T3, often observed in newborns, would be a reflection of fetal status. As in other ages, levels of T3 may fall in the presence of concomitant diseases and undernutrition. In some newborn infants hypoxemia, acidosis, hypocalcemia and infection, postnatal malnutrition have been found to be associated to low T3 levels by inhibiting the peripheral conversion of T4 to T3, leading to prolong (1-2 months at a time) the low values observed in adaptation to extrauterine life. Low serum total T3 is the most common abnormality in infants with neonatal illness, observed in about 70% of hospitalized patients. Serum total T3 levels can range from undetectable to normal in critically ill patients, with the mean total T3 level being approximately 40% of normal. It is believed that low serum T3 is a result of decreased production of T4, rather than increased degradation or increased disposal of T3. Unlike T4, which is produced solely in the thyroid, about 80% of circulating T3 is produced by extrathyroidal conversion of T4 to T3 by 50-monoiodinases present in organs such as the liver and kidney. Thus, there are two mechanisms by which T3 production may be reduced: decreased activity of the 5-monoiodinases that convert T4 to T3, and decreased delivery of T4 substrate for conversion to T3. Peeters et al. [16] provided evidence in support of the first mechanism with studies showing reduced tissue expression and activity of type 1 and 2 monodeiodinases (5-monoiodinases that convert T4 to T3) in liver and skeletal muscle biopsies obtained from ICU patients within minutes after death. Their results also showed increased tissue expression and activity of 50-monoiodinase activity (causing increased conversion of T4 to rT3) in the critically ill patients. There is also evidence to suggest that decreased thyroxine transport over the cell membrane may play a role in lowered T3 production in ill newborns.

7.6 Hyperthyroidism in the newborn

Rarely, a newborn may have hyperthyroidism, or neonatal Graves' disease. This condition usually occurs if the mother has Graves' disease during pregnancy or has been treated for it before pregnancy. In Graves' disease, the mother's body produces antibodies that stimulate the thyroid gland to produce increased amounts of thyroid hormone. These antibodies cross the placenta and similarly affect the fetus. An affected newborn has a high metabolic rate, with rapid heart rate and breathing, irritability, and excessive appetite with poor weight gain. The newborn, like the mother, may have bulging eyes (exophthalmos). If the newborn has an enlarged thyroid gland (goiter), the gland may press against the windpipe and interfere with breathing at birth. A very rapid heart rate can lead to heart failure. Graves' disease is potentially fatal if not recognized and treated by a pediatric endocrinologist. Doctors suspect hyperthyroidism based on the typical symptoms and confirm the diagnosis by detecting elevated levels of thyroid hormone and thyroid-stimulating antibodies from the mother in the newborn's blood. The results of a screening test of thyroid function done in all newborns may reveal hyperthyroidism. Newborns with hyperthyroidism are treated with drugs, such as propylthiouracil, that slow the production of thyroid hormone by the thyroid gland. This treatment is needed only for a few months because the antibodies that cross the placenta from the mother eventually disappear from the infant's bloodstream.

7.7 Thyroid function in term and preterm infants in relation to neonatal illness and medication

Many abnormalities along the pituitary–thyroid axis have been observed in critical illness associated with sepsis, myocardial infarction, cardiopulmonary bypass, and surgery. Such abnormalities include an attenuated response of thyroid stimulating hormone (TSH) to thyrotropin releasing hormone(TRH), decreased pulsatile TSH release, and decreased serum thyroid hormone levels. In mild illness, decreased serum total and free triiodothyronine (T3) are the predominant abnormalities. However, as the duration and severity of illness increase beyond 3-5 days, decreased serum total and free thyroxine (T4) levels are also observed. Decreased circulating levels of thyroidbinding globulin (TBG), decreased serum binding of T4, and decreased 5-monoiodinase activity, (the enzyme that converts T4 to T3) are also important contributing factors for the low thyroid hormone state of critical illness. It is not known how immaturity and disease influence postnatal thyroid function in infants <30 wk of gestational age. Is important to investigate the influences of disease and gestational age on the time course of thyroid hormones. Transient hypothyroxinemia is common in extremely premature infants, but has not been extensively investigated in ill term and preterm infants. Free thyroxine (FT4) levels in term and late preterm infants with respiratory distress would be inversely related to severity of illness. Further research is warranted to determine whether T4 supplementation would be beneficial in term and late preterm infants with respiratory distress. (Paul DA et al. 1998; Paul DA et al 2010, Judy L et al. 2009, Simpson 2005, Williams 2005)

7.8 Thyroid dysfunction related to congenital cardiac defects

Congenital heart disease is the most common form of congenital defect at birth. There are evidences that exists a very narrow relation between the thyroid gland and the heart during fetal development. Thyroid hormones are necessary for the functioning of the heart in the fetal and postnatal life. Cardiopulmonary bypass induces marked and persistent depression of circulating thyroid hormones in infants, possibly contributing to postoperative morbidity (cardiac low output, ventricular left dysfunction, vascular increased resistance and respiratory difficulty…) The aims to prevent thyroid dysfunction in affected newborns are to improve heart hemodynamics, vascular resistance and metabolism during the neonatal period and the prevention of long-term disabilities in the neurodevelopment of these newborns. Based on previous studies available, it appears that L-T4 replacement should be considered in patients with hypothyroidism in presence of cardiac defects in the attempt to reverse these negative prognostic factors and improve the cardiovascular function (del Cerro 2000, Mainwaring RD et al. 2001, Mainwaring RD et all. 2002, Klemperer JD 2002, Portman MA et al. 2004, Holzer R et al. 2004, Lynch BA et al. 2004, Fazio S et al. 2004, Dimmick S et al. 2004)

8. Conclusion

Neonates and especially preterm infants are a very important population at risk of suffering the consequences of thyroid dysfunction. Alterations of thyroid function in premature infants, leading to low circulating levels of T_4 or T_3, have been associated with impairment of neural maturation, as measured by nerve conduction velocity and by lower scores in the Bayley mental and motor scales (De Vries et al., 1996; den Ouden AL et al., 1996; Lucas A et al., 1988; Meijer WJ et al., 1992; Lucas A et al., 1996; Reuss ML et al., 1996). Iodine deficiency and excess may well be frequent causes of inadequate thyroid hormone levels and should be avoided. Such a close follow-up becomes mandatory if an iodine overload cannot be prevented. Premature infants in many countries are now in a situation of iodine deficiency, precisely at a stage of development that is very sensitive to alterations of thyroid function. The recommended intake of iodine for preterm infants based on balance studies is 30 μg /kg/day. Enteral and parenteral nutritional fluids are the principal sources of iodine intake in these infants. The volume of food ingested by the infant is small, iodine content in formula preparations is insufficient, parenteral nutrition does not supply enough iodine. Pregnant and lactating women and neonates are the main targets of the effects of iodine deficiency because of the impact of maternal, fetal and neonatal hypothyroxinemia on brain development of the progeny (Morreale de Escobar G et al., 2004; Lavado-Autric R et al., 2003; Morreale de Escobar G et al., 1998; Morreale de Escobar G et al., 2000). The neurological damage is clearly preventable if pregnant mothers are tested for thyroid function during the first trimester and by giving pregnant women, or even before pregnancy, sufficient iodine to avoid hypothyroxinemia. If the mother has adequate iodine nutrition, breast milk is the best source of iodine for the newborn. However, based on data from the literature and on metabolic considerations, it is proposed that the recommended dietary intake of iodine is 250-300 μg/day for pregnant women, 225-350 μg/day for lactating women, and 90 μg/day for neonates and young infants (Zimmermann M et al., 2004). This problem is not exclusive to Spanish premature babies as the iodine content of many formulas in other countries is also inadequate. Therefore, supplements should be added if iodine intake is found to be inadequate. Breast milk appears to be the best source of iodine for the premature infant (Ares S et al., 1994; Ares S et al., 1995; Ares S et al., 1997; Ibrahim M et al., 2003, Zimmermann 2010). Prevention of iodine deficiency and follow-up is recognized as a priority. The number of extremely low birth weight infants is high. Correction of their iodine deficiency and thyroid dysfunction and their consequences appears, at present, to be an intervention with promising possibilities (Ares S et al., 1995; van Wassenaer AG et al., 1997; Vanhole C et al., 1997; La Gamma EF et l., 2006). However, too little is yet known of the different factors involved in the metabolism of iodine and thyroid hormones during late fetal life and their adjustment to the conditions faced by newborn infants to be able to standardize possible treatment protocols. Future research would be facilitated if newborn infants and preterm babies were followed during their stay in intensive care units with respect to their iodine nutrition and thyroid function (T_4, FT_4, T_3, TSH, thyroid binding globulin TBG, Tg) as carefully as they are followed for other organ functions (Morreale de Escobar G et al., 1998; Rapaport R, 2002; Ares S et al., 2007) (Figure 3)

The high prevalence of thyroid function alterations that demanded treatment and delayed TSH elevation in premature infants and in term newborns reinforce the need for a specific protocol, based on retesting procedures, for neonatal screening. In conclusion, in view of more reliable recent information on thyroid function and physiology of newborn infants, the iodine content of many formulas for feeding infants appears to be inadequate. Most ill newborns and premature babies do not ingest the amount of iodine recommended from 1992 by the ICCIDD, the WHO, and the European Community (Delange F, 2001; Delange F, 2004; WHO, UNICEF, ICCIDD, 2001). Producers of such formulas should be urged to comply with the new recommendations and to control that their products do so irrespective of the country where they are being used. This review focuses on neonatal transient hypothyroxinaemia, a condition characterized by temporary postnatal reductions in concentrations of Total T4 or Free T4, with normal or low concentrations of thyroid stimulating hormone (TSH). There is neither an agreed quantitative definition, nor an agreed mode of measurement for the condition. Transient hypothyroxinaemia is not routinely monitored yet it is thought to affect about 50% of preterm infants; it was thought to be without long-term sequelae but observational studies indicate that neurodevelopment may be compromised. The aetiology of transient hypothyroxinaemia is complex. There are significant contributions from the withdrawal of maternal–placental thyroxine transfer, hypothalamic–pituitary–thyroid immaturity, developmental constraints on the synthesis and peripheral metabolism of iodothyronines and iodine deficiency. It is not possible to distinguish clinically, or from laboratory measurements, whether transient hypothyroxinaemia is an independent condition or simply a consequence of non-thyroidal illness and/or drug usage. An answer to this question is important because studies of thyroid hormone replacement have been instigated, with mixed results.

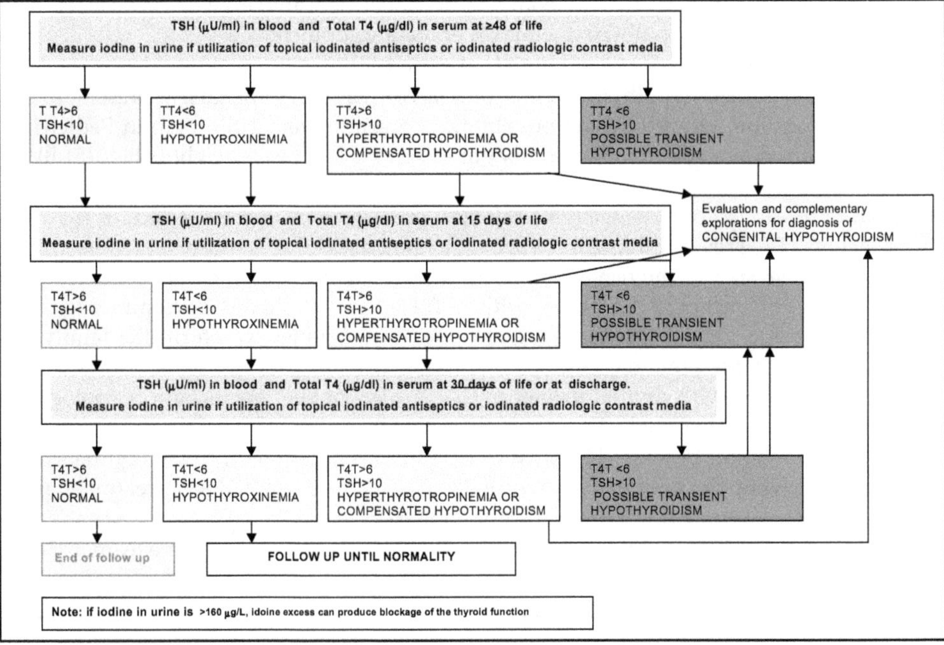

Fig. 3. Proposed protocol for monitoring neonatal thyroid function in special circumstances.

Until the aetiology of transient hypothyroxinaemia is better understood it would seem prudent not to routinely supplement preterm infants with thyroid hormones. Iodine deficiency, non-thyroidal illness and drug usage are the most modifiable risk factors for transient hypothyroxinaemia and are the clear choices for attempts at reducing its incidence. The high prevalence of thyroid function alterations that demanded treatment (1:242) and delayed TSH elevation in premature infants reinforce the need for a specific protocol, based on retesting procedures, for neonatal screening. The purpose of the present protocol is to systematically include the determination of T4 in blood spotted on DBS paper, in order to detect hypothyroxinemia, elevation of TSH, and other alterations in thyroid function and to establish the necessity to incorporate a routine into the Neonatal Thyroid Screening Program that would obtain a special screening specimen in infants at high risk of suffering alterations of their thyroid function (Table 3).

• An adequate iodine intake should be ensured in newborn infants. • Enteral and parenteral nutrition fluids are the principal sources of iodine intake in these infants. • If the mother has adequate iodine nutrition breast milk is the best source of iodine for the newborn. The volume of food ingested by the infant is low. The iodine content in formula preparations must be taken into account.Parenteral nutrition does not supply the preterm newborn with enough iodine to meet the recommendations.Supplements should be added if iodine intake is found to be inadequate. Most of the preterm babies are at high risk of iodine deficiency. Neonates and expecially preterm infants are a very important population at risk of suffering the consequences of both iodine deficiency and excess, because of the impact of neonatal hypothyroxinemia on brain development. • Iodine deficiency and excess ought to be avoided. • Correction of their hypothyroxinemia, and its consequences appears, at present, to be an intervention with promising possibilities.Prevention and Follow-up in Pediatrics is recognized as a priority. The number of extremely low birth weight babies (ELBW) is increasing. • Future research would be facilitated if: very premature infants are tested for thyroid function (T4, Free T4, T3, TSH, TBG, Tg) immediately after birth and repeatedly during their stay in intensive care units, and as carefully as they are followed for other organ functions. All babies with a TSH>10mU/l should be commenced on thyroxine at a dose of 10-15 micrograms/kg/day. Arrange to inform the family of the results on the same day and make arrangements to start thyroxine if necessary. • Early treatment with thyroxine (before 10 - 21 days of age) is crucial if neurological disability is to be avoided. • Treatment should be started as soon as diagnosis is confirmed (preferably the same day) following discussion with the endocrine team. Do not delay treatment if a member of the endocrine team cannot be contacted. • If the laboratory TSH is between 4 and 10, please discuss with endocrine team.

Table 3. Summary and key points.

List of Abbreviations:

- ICCIDD: International Council for Control of Iodine Deficiency Disorders
- thyroxine (T4)
- 3,5,3'-triiodothyronine (T3)
- thyroglobulin (Tg)
- thyroid stimulating hormone (TSH)
- thyroid binding globulin (TBG)
- gestational age in weeks (GA)
- body weight (BW)
- Transient hypothyroxinaemia of prematurity (THOP)
- cerebral palsy (CP)
- ELGAN—extremely low gestational age neonate

9. References

Ares S, Escobar-Morreale HF, Quero J, et al: Neonatal hypothyroxinemia: effects of iodine intake and premature birth. J Clin Endocrinol Metab 82:1704-1712, 1997

Ares S, Garcia P, Quero J, et al: Iodine intake and urinary excretion in premature infants born after less than 30 weeks of gestation. J Clin Pediatr Endocrinol 17(3):509, 2004

Ares S, Pastor I, Quero J, et al: Thyroid gland volume as measured by ultrasonography in preterm infants. Acta Pediátr 84:58-62, 1995

Ares S, Pastor I, Quero J, et al: Thyroidal complications, including overt hypothyroidism, related to the use of non-radiopaque silastic catheters for parentheral feeding of prematures, requiring injection of small amounts of an iodinated contrast medium. Acta Paediatr 84:579-578, 1995

Ares S, Quero J, Durán S, et al: Iodine content of infant formulas and iodine intake of premature babies. Arch Dis Child 71:184-191, 1994

Ares S, Quero J, Morreale de Escobar G, and the Spanish Preterm Thyroid Group: Iodine during the neonatal period: too little, too much? J Pediatr Endocrinol Metab 20:163-166, 2007 (suppl 1)

Ares S, Quero J, Morreale de Escobar G: Neonatal iodine deficiency: clinical aspects. J Pediatr Endocrinol Metab 18:1257-1264, 2005

Ares S, Saénz de Pipaón M, Ruiz-Díaz AI, et al: Hypothyroidism and high plasma and urine iodine levels related to the use of gastrografin. Curr Pediatr Rev 4:194-197, 2008

Biswas S, Buffery J, Enoch H, et al: A longitudinal assessment of thyroid hormone concentrations in preterm infants younger than 30 weeks' gestation during the first 2 weeks of life and their relationship to outcome. Pediatrics 109(2):222-227, 2002

De Vries LS, Heckmatt JZ, Burrin JM, et al: Low serum thyroxine concentrations and neural maturation in preterm infants. Arch Dis Child 61:862-866, 1986

del Cerro Marín MJ, Fernández A, García-Guereta L, et al: Alteraciones de la función tiroidea en niños con cardiopatía congénita tras la realización de cateterismo con contrastes yodados. Rev Esp Cardiol 53: 517-524, 2000

Delange F, Bourdoux P, Chanoine JP, et al: Physiology of iodine nutrition during pregnancy, lactation, and early postnatal life, in Berger H (ed): Nestle Nutrition Workshop Series, vol 16. New York, NY, Vevey/ Raven Press, 1988, 205-214

Delange F, Canoine JP, Abrassart C, et al: Topical iodine, breastfeeding and neonatal hypothyroidism (letter). Arch Dis Child 63:106, 1988

Delange F, Dalhem A, Bourdoux P, et al. Increased risk of primary hypothyroidism in preterm infants. J Pediatr 105:462-469, 1984

Delange F: Iodine deficiency as a cause of brain damage. Postgrad Med J 77:217-220, 2001

Delange F: Optimal iodine nutrition during pregnancy. Lactation and the neonatal period. Int J Endocrinol Metab 2:1-12, 2004

Delange F: Requirements of iodine in humans, in Delange F, Dunn JT, Glinoer D (eds): Iodine Deficiency in Europe. A Continuing Concern. New York, NY, Plenum Press, 1993, pp 5-16

Dembinski J, Arpe V, Kroll M, et al: Thyroid function in very low birthweight infants after intravenous administration of the iodinated contrast medium iopromide. Arch Dis Child Fetal Neonatal Ed 82:215-217, 2000 den Ouden AL, Kok JH, Verkerk PH, et al: The relation between neonatal thyroxine levels and neurodevelopmental outcome at age 5 and 9 years in a national cohort of very preterm and/or very low birth weight infants. Pediatr Res 39:142-145, 1996

Dimmick S, Badawi N, Randell T. Thyroid hormone supplementation for the prevention of morbidity and mortality in infants undergoing cardiac surgery. Cochrane Database Syst Rev. 2004;(3):CD004220

Dorea JG: Iodine nutrition and breast-feeding. J Trace Elem Med Biol 16:207-220, 2002

Fazio S, Palmieri EA, Lombardi G, Biondi B. Effects of thyroid hormone on the cardiovascular system. Recent Prog Horm Res. 2004;59:31-50.

Fisher DA, Hobel CJ, Garza RBS, Pierce CA. Thyroid function in the preterm fetus. Pediatrics 1970; 46: 208-216.

Fisher DA, Odell WD, Hobel CJ, Garza R. Thyroid function in the fetus. Pediatrics 1969; 44: 526-535.

Fisher DA. Ontogenesis of hypothalamic- pituitary-thyroid function in the human fetus. En: Delange F, Fisherm DA, Malvaux P (eds.). Pediatric Thyroidology. Karger, Basel 1985; 19-32.

Greenberg AH, Najjar S, Blizzard RM. Effects of thyroid hormones on growth, differentiation and development. In: Greep RO, Astwood DH, eds. Handbook of Physiology, Section 7, Vol. III. Washington, DC: American Physiological Society, 1974; 377-390.

Holzer R, Bockenkamp B, Booker P, Newland P, Ciotti G, Pozzi M. The impact of cardiopulmonary bypass on selenium status, thyroid function, and oxidative defense in children. Pediatr Cardiol. 2004; 25(5):522-8.

Ibrahim M, Morreale de Escobar G, Visser TJ, et al: Iodine deficiency associated with parenteral nutrition in extreme preterm infants. Arch Dis Child 88:F56-F57, 2003

Judy L. Shih and Michael S.D. Agus Thyroid function in the critically ill newborn and child Current Opinion in Pediatrics 2009, 21:536–540

Kester MHA, de Mena RM, Obregon MJ, et al: Iodothyronine levels in the human developing brain: major regulatory roles of iodothyronine deiodinases in different areas. J Clin Endocrinol Metab 89:3117-3128, 2004

Klemperer JD. Thyroid hormone and cardiac surgery. Thyroid. 2002 Jun;12(6):517-21.

La Gamma EF, van Wassenaer A, Golombek SG, et al: Neonatal thyroxine supplementation for transient hypothyroxinemia of prematurity: beneficial or detrimental? Treatments Endocrinol 5(6):335-347, 2006

La Gamma EF, van Wassenaer AG, Ares S, Golombek SG, Kok JH, Quero J, Hong T, Rahbar MH, de Escobar GM, Fisher DA, Paneth N. Phase 1 trial of 4 thyroid hormone regimens for transient hypothyroxinemia in neonates of <28 weeks' gestation. Pediatrics. 2009 Aug;124(2):e258-68. Epub 2009 Jul 5.

LaFranchi S. Congenital hypothyroidism: etiologies, diagnosis, and management. *Thyroid.* Jul 1999;9(7):735-40.

LaFranchi SH, Buist NR, Murphey WH, Larsen PR, Foley TP Jr. Transient neonatal hypothyroidism detected by newborn screening program. *Pediatrics.* Oct 1977;60(4):539-41.

Lavado-Autric R, Auso E, Garcia-Velasco JV, et al: Early maternal hypothyroxinemia alters histogenesis and cerebral cortex cytoarchitecture of the progeny. J Clin Invest 111(7):1073-1082, 2003

LeFranchi S. Hypothyroidism. In: Kliegman RM, Stanton BF, St. Geme III JW, Schor NF, Behrman RE, eds. *Nelson Textbook of Pediatrics*. 19th ed. Philadelphia, Pa: Saunders Elsevier; 2011;chap 559.

Lopez-Sastre JB, Rivas-Crespo MF: The newborn should be protected from dangerous transient induced thypotiroidism. Acta Paediatr 84: 1211, 1995

Lucas A, Morley R, Fewtrell MS: Low triiodothyronine concentration in preterm infant and subsequent intelligence quotient (IQ) at 8 year follow up. BMJ 312:1132-1133, 1996

Lucas A, Rennie J, Baker BA, et al: Low plasma triiodothyronine concentrations and outcome in preterm infant. Arch Dis Child 63:1201- 1206, 1988

Lynch BA, Brown DM, Herrington C, Braunlin E. Thyroid dysfunction after pediatric cardiac surgery. J Thorac Cardiovasc Surg. 2004 May;127(5):1509-11.

Mainwaring RD, Healy RM, Meier FA, Nelson JC, Norwood WI..Reduction in levels of triiodothyronine following the first stage of the Norwood reconstruction for hypoplastic left heart syndrome.Cardiol Young. 2001 May;11(3):295-300

Mainwaring RD, Nelson JC. Supplementation of thyroid hormone in children undergoing cardiac surgery. Cardiol Young. 2002 May;12(3):211-7

Meijer WJ, Verloove-Vanhorick SP, Brand R, et al: Transient hypothyroxinemia associated with developmental delay in very preterm infants. Arch Dis Child 67:944-947, 1992

Morreale de Escobar G, Ares S: The hypothyroxinemia of prematurity. J Clin Endocrinol Metab 83:713-715, 1998

Morreale de Escobar G, Escobar del Rey F: Thyroid physiology in utero and neonatally, in Rubery E, Smales E (eds): Iodine Prophylaxis Following Nuclear Accidents. Oxford: Pergamon Press, 1990, pp 3-32

Morreale de Escobar G, Kester M, Martinez de Mena R, et al: Iodothyronine metabolism in human fetal brain. J Endocrinol Invest 25:29, 2002 (suppl)

Morreale de Escobar G, Obregon MJ, Escobar del Rey F: Is neuropsychological development related to maternal hypothyroidism or to maternal hypothyroxinemia? J Clin Endocrinol Metab 85:3975-3987, 2000

Morreale de Escobar G, Obregón MJ, Escobar del Rey F: Role of thyroid hormone during early brain development. Eur J Endocrinol 151:U25-U37, 2004

National Research Council, Food and Nutrition Board. Recommended Dietary Allowances. Washington, DC: National Academy Press, 1989; 213-217 and 285.

Paneth, N: Does transient hypothyroxinemia cause abnormal neurodevelopment in premature infants? Clin Perinatol 1998; 25:627-637

Paul DA, Mackley A, Yencha EM Thyroid function in term and late preterm infants with respiratory distress in relation to severity of illness. Thyroid. 2010 Feb;20(2):189-94

Portman MA, Fearneyhough C, Karl TR, Tong E, Seidel K, Mott A, Cohen G, Tacy T, Lewin M, Permut L, Schlater M, Azakie A. The Triiodothyronine for Infants and Children Undergoing Cardiopulmonary Bypass (TRICC) study: design and rationale. Am Heart J. 2004 Sep;148(3):393-8.

Rapaport R. Thyroid function in very low birth weight newborn: rescreen or reevaluate. J Pediatrc 2002;140:287-289

Reuss ML, Paneth N, Pinto-Martin JA, et al: The relation of transient hypothyroxinemia in preterm infants to neurologic development at two years of age. New Engl Med 334:821-826, 1996

Rovet JF, Ehrlich R. Psychoeducational outcome in children with early-treated congenital hypothyroidism. *Pediatrics*. Mar 2000;105(3 Pt 1):515-22.

Rovet JF. Congenital hypothyroidism: long-term outcome. *Thyroid*. Jul 1999;9(7):741-8.

Rovet JF. Long-term neuropsychological sequelae of early-treated congenital hypothyroidism: effects in adolescence. *Acta Paediatr Sppl*. Dec 1999;88(432):88-95.

Semba RD, Delange F: Iodine in human milk: perspectives for infant health. Nutr Rev 59:269-278, 2001

Simpson J, Williams FLR, Delahunty C, van Toor H, Wu SY, Ogston SA, Visser TJ, and Hume R: Serum thyroid hormones in preterm infants and relationships to indices of severity of intercurrent illness, J Clin Endocrinol Metab 2005; 90:1271-1279

Thorpe-Beeston JG, Nicolaides KH, Felton CV, et al: Maturation of the secretion of thyroid hormone and thyroid-stimulating hormone in the fetus. New Engl J Med 324:532-536, 1991

Van Wassenaer AG, Kok JH, de Vijlder JJ, et al: Effects of thyroxine supplementation on neurologic development in infants born at less than 30 weeks' gestation. N Engl J Med 336:21-26, 1997

van Wassenaer AG, Kok JH, de Vijlder JJ, et al: Effects of thyroxine supplementation on neurologic development in infants born at less than 30 weeks' gestation. N Engl J Med 336:21-26, 1997

van Wassenaer AG, Kok JH, Dekker FW, deVijlder JJ: Thyroid function in very preterm infants: influence of gestation age and disease. Pediatr Res 1997;42:604-609.

Vanhole C, Aerssens P, Naulaers G, et al: L-thyroxine treatment of preterm newborns: clinical and endocrine effects. Pediatr Res 42:87-1997

Weber G, Vigone MC, Rapa A, et al: Neonatal transient hypothyroidism: aetiological study. Arch Dis Child Fetal Neonatal 79:70-72, 1998

WHO, UNICEF, ICCIDD: Assessment of the iodine deficiency disorders and monitoring their elimination. Geneva: WHO Publication, WHO/NHD/01.1. 2001, pp 107

Williams FLR, Ogston SA, van Toor H, Visser TJ, and Hume R, with collaboration from the Scottish Preterm Thyroid Group: Serum thyroid hormones in preterm infants: associations with postnatal illnesses and drug usage, J Clin Endocrinol Metab 2005; 90:5954-5963

Wolff J: Iodine goiter and the pharmacological effect of excess iodide. Am J Med 47:101-124, 1969

Zimmermann M, Delange F: Iodine supplementation of pregnant women in Europe: a review and recommendation. Eur J Clin Nutr 58:979-984, 2004

Zimmermann MB The role of iodine in human growth and development. Semin Cell Dev Biol. 2011 Jul 23

Zimmermann MB, Crill CM. Iodine in enteral and parenteral nutrition. Best Pract Res Clin Endocrinol Metab. 2010 Feb;24(1):143-58. Review.

Zimmermann MB. Iodine deficiency. Endocr Rev. 2009 Jun;30(4):376-408. Epub 2009 May 21. Review.

11

Neonatal-Prepubertal Hypothyroidism on Postnatal Testis Development

S.M.L. Chamindrani Mendis-Handagama
Department of Biomedical and Diagnostic Sciences,
The University of Tennessee College of Veterinary Medicine, Knoxville, Tennessee,
USA

1. Introduction

Thyroid hormones stimulate oxidative metabolism in many tissues in the body, however, testis is not one of them. Therefore, in this sense, testis is not considered as a target organ for thyroid hormones. However, recent findings clearly show that thyroid hormones have important functions on the testis development during neonatal-prepubertal life. Testis is an exocrine organ because it produces sperm and it is also an endocrine organ, because it produces hormones. In this chapter, general organization of the adult mammalian testis is first described to understand the organization of the adult testis. Thereafter, the general organization of the mammalian testis at birth is described, followed by how the neonatal-prepubertal hypothyroidism affects the testis development during this period, Esbablishment of the Sertoli and Leydig cell numbers in the adult testis during the neonatal-prepubertal life, is critical to the general maintenance and reproductive functions of the adult mammalian male; thyroid hormones play a crucial role in these processes. The effects of hypothyroidism on neonatal-prepubertal testis are discussed in this chapter using the observations generated with rodent models, focusing on testicular testosterone secretory capacity and sperm production, which are an essential function to the male mammal.

The hormone testosterone is essential for the mammalian male for maintenance and proper functioning of many organ systems of the body such as muscle, bone and skin, in addition to its requirement for the reproductive function. Leydig cells in the testis are the primary source of testosterone in the male mammal. There are two populations of Leydig cells in mammals studied to date; fetal and adult Leydig cell populations. Fetal Leydig cells are differentiated during the fetal life and are still present at birth. However, the adult population of Leydig cells differentiate postnatally from the mesenchymal stem cells in the testis to establish the adult population Leydig cells of the sexually mature testes; they are the main source of testosterone during adult life. Therefore, establishing the adult population of Leydig cells in the postnatal testis, which occurs during the neonatal-prepbertal life, is an essential process in the mammalian testis for the well being of the adult mammalian male. Research with several rodent species has shown that Leydig stem cell differentiation in the postnatal testis is arrested with hypothyroidism, but can be stimulated by supplementation with thyroid hormones. Transient neonatal hypothyroidism causes larger testis at adulthood, although the process of Leydig cell differentiation is arrested during the period of hypothyroidism. Differentiated Leydig cells in these animals after the hypothyroid period is withdrawn, are smaller in size but two-fold in number compared to the euthyroid animals. Therefore, the fertility and circulating testosterone levels in these transiently neonatal animals at adulthood are similar to euthyroid animals. Under hypothyroid conditions during the neonatal -prepubertal period, fetal Leydig cells continue to function normally with no change in their testicular testosterone secretory capacity, although the postnatal differentiation of adult population of Leydig cells are absent. However, prolonging the hypothyroid condition beyond the neonatal-prepubertal period fails to maintain the fetal population of Leydig cells; they undergo cell atrophy and loose their testosterone secretory capacity, in addition to the arrest in differentiation of adult population of Leydig cells. During the hypothyroid period, in the neonatal-prepubertal animals, Sertoli cells in the seminiferous tubules fail to mature, but continue to proliferate. When the hypothyroid status is withdrawn, these Sertoli cells mature and are now greater in number per testis compared to a euthyroid testis, because they were subjected to prolonged proliferative period because of hypothyroidism. Because of this reason, testes of transiently hypothyroid animals become larger in volume and weight at adulthood and produce greater numbers of sperm compared to the control animals.

These studies have revealed the importance of thyroid hormone for postnatal testis development in the mammalian testis.

2. Thyroid hormones

J.F. Gudernatsch (1912) provided the first evidence for thyroid hormones and their task in cellular differentiation. It is established now that thyroxine (T_4) and triiodothyronine (T_3) are produced by the thyroid gland and triiodothyronine is at least five times more potent than thyroxin. The most characteristic effect of thyroid hormones is their ability to stimulate oxidative metabolism in tissues in the body. However, in this sense, testis is not considered as a target organ for these hormones. Thyroid hormone secretion is regulated by the thyroid hormone releasing hormone and the thyroid stimulating hormone from the hypothalamus and the anterior pituitary, respectively.

3. General organization of the adult mammalian testis

Testes produce sperm for reproductive function and androgens (male hormones) which are necessary for general maintenance of many organ systems in the male and the reproductive function which includes libido. Testis has two compartments. The tubular compartment or the seminiferous tubules and the testis interstitium which lies out side of the tubular compartment (Figure 1). As stated earlier testis has exocrine and endocrine functions. Seminiferous tubules are comprised of Sertoli cells and germ cells (Figure 1). The testis interstitium has Leydig cells, which are the primary source of androgens (male hormones) of the adult mammalian male, the blood vessels, lymphatics, and many other cell types (Figure 1), such as fibroblasts, macrophages and plasma cells. Testes are encapsulated by three distinct layers; the innermost tunica vasculosa, the outer most tunica vaginalis and the tunica albuginea is in the middle. All of these are structures are suspended in the scrotum in many mammalian species (Davis et al., 1970).

3.1 Seminiferous tubules

The seminiferous tubules are of two kinds, the convoluted seminiferous tubules, which have Sertoli and germ cells, and the straight seminiferous tubules, which are continuous with the rete testis (Banks,1986). Rete testis is connected with the efferent ducts and continuous with the epididymis, which is continuous with the ductus deference/vas deference that is connected to the male urethra which leads to the external orifice of the penis. In this review, only the structural organization of the convoluted seminiferous tubules and the Leydig cells are described, because of the relevancy to the title of this chapter,

Convoluted seminiferous tubules. comprise approximately 90-92% of the volume of the adult testicular parenchyma in mammalian species studied to date (Mendis-Handagama et 1987, 1988, 1990). Beyond this point, convoluted seminiferous tubules will be referred to as seminiferous tubules throughout this chapter. Each seminiferous tubule is separated from the testis interstitum by a well defined basement membrane (Figure 1). Sertoli cells (Figure 1), first described by Sertoli in 1865, reside on the basement membrane of each seminiferous tubule and extend from the basement membrane to the lumen of the seminiferous tubules. Different stages of male germ cells are found in the seminiferous tubules (Figure 1); spermatogonia, primary spermatocytes, secondary spermatocytes, round apermatids and elongated spermatids. Sertoli cells together with the germ cells form the seminiferous epithelium, which is a stratified epithelium. In addition to the Setoli cells, spermatogonia (stem cells for male germ cells) are also reside on the basement membrane of the seminiferous tubules. All the other germ cells are attached to the Sertoli cells with their differentiation and maturation and move towards the lumen. Sertoli cells, spermatogonia and primary spermatocytes are diploid cells and secondary spermatids, round spermatids and elongated spermatids are haploid cells.

Sertoli cells provide seminiferous tubular integrity. Moreover, The adjacent Sertoli cells in each seminiferous tubule form Sertoli-Sertoli junctions (tight junctions, Brokelman, 1963; Flickinger and Fawcett, 1967; Nicander, 1967; Rosas, 1970) close to the basement membrane, which divides each seminiferous tubule into two compartments; the basal compartment and the adluminal compartment (Banks, 1986). More importantly, Sertoli-Sertoli cell junctions form the blood-testis barrier to protect the developing germ cells (Dym, 1973; Setchell and Waites, 1975). The basement membrane and the associated myoid cells of the seminiferous tubules contributes to the blood-testis barrier to a lesser extent (Dym and Fawcett, 1970; Fawcett et al., 1970). Sertoli cells function as 'nurse' cells for the developing germ cells; they provide nutrition and hormones (androgens) required for spermatogenesis, which is the process of producing sperm from spermatogonia. Different species demonstrate different cellular associations during the cycle of the seminiferous epithelium; six stages in the human (Clermont, 1963), twelve stages in the monkey (Clermont, 1969), and 14 stages in the rat (Leblond and Clermont, 1952)

Sertoli cells produce tubular fluid (Setchell and Waites, 1975). They transport and maintain a high concentration of androgens in the seminiferous tubules and secrete androgen binding protein (ABP; French and Ritzen, 1973) and the hormone inhibin (de Kretser et al., 2002), which are important in maintaining spermatogenesis. Also, it serves as a phagocytic cell to recycle residual bodies that arise as a byproduct of spermatogenesis (Lacy. 1967). It is also reported that Sertoli cells have a significant role in the process of spermiation, i.e. release of sperm into the seminiferous tubular lumen (Sapsford and Rae, 1968; Fawcett and Phillips, 1969). It is also important to document that the testicular size and sperm producing capacity of a testis is positively correlated with the number of Sertoli cells in the testis (Berndtson et al., 1987; Moura et al., 2011).

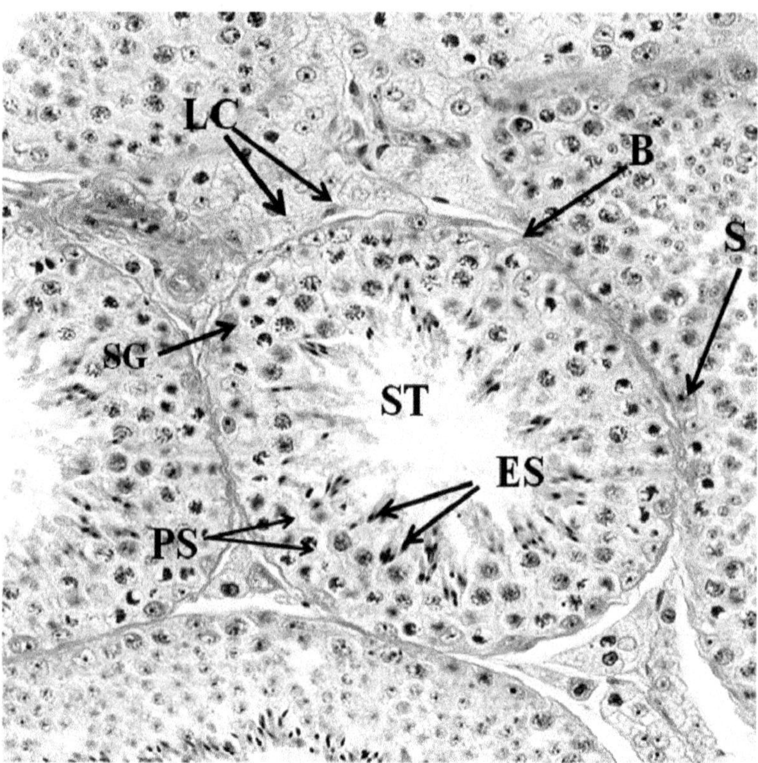

Fig. 1. A representative light micrograph of an adult dog testsis to show general organization of the testis parenchyma. LC=Leydig cells in the testis interstitium, ST=seminiferous tubules, B-basement membrane, S=nucleua of a Sertoli cell, SG=spermatogonia, PS=primary spermatocytes, ES=elongated spermatids.

3.2 Testis interstitium

The testis interstitium can be considered as the skeletal frame work of the testis and is approximately 8-10% of the adult testicular parenchyma (Mendis-Handagama et 1987, 1988, 1990). Leydig cells reside in the testis interstitium (Figure 1). Among species, variations are seen in Leydig cell number, size, morphological characteristics and their relationship to blood vessels and other surrounding structures; these are unique to each species (Fawcett et al., 1973) and will not be discussed in this review. Luteinizing hormone (LH) produced by the gonadotrophs of the anterior pituitary gland, is considered as the primary regulator of Leydig cell structure and function in the adult testis.

It is universally accepted that Leydig cells, which were first discovered in 1850 by Franz Leydig as large polygedral cells, are the source of androgens. Bouin and Ansel (1903) are credited with the concept that the primary androgen secreted by the testis is testosterone. In 1929, Gallagher and Koch also showed that the primary androgenic hormone secreted by the adult tests is testosterone. Later, Christensen and Mason (1965) and Hall et al., (1969), demonstrated that the principal site of testosterone synthesis in the testis is Leydig cells. Although the testosterone production by the Leydig cells is greatly influenced by the environment of the testis interstitium, this review will be primarily focused on Leydig cells.

The volume percentage (2-6%), the absolute volume (depends on the testis size), number (2-4500x10^6) and the size (1500-3000μm) of Leydig cells in the adult testis varies among species (Kaler and Neaves, 1978; Mori and Christensen, 1980; Mori et al., 1980; Johnson and Neaves, 1981; Mori et al., 1982; Mendis-Handagama et al., 1987, 1988 and 1990). The steroidogenic enzyme 3β- hyroxy steroid dehydrogenase (3βHSD) was exclusively localized histochemically in Leydig cells of mice (Baillie, 1964) , the rat (Levy et al , 1959) and in many other mammalian species (Wattenburg, 1958) . At present 3βHSD is used as a marker for Leydig cells (Ariyaratne and Mendis-Handagama, 2000; Ariyaratne et al., 2000a-d; Figure 2). Moreover, 11β-hydroxy steroid dehydrogenase 1 (11β-HSD1) is a marker for postnatally differentiated adult type Leydig cells, which is present as early as postnatal day 21 in the newly formed adult Leydig cells in the rat testis (Mendis-Handagamaet al., 1998; Figure 3) and will be discussed later in this review.

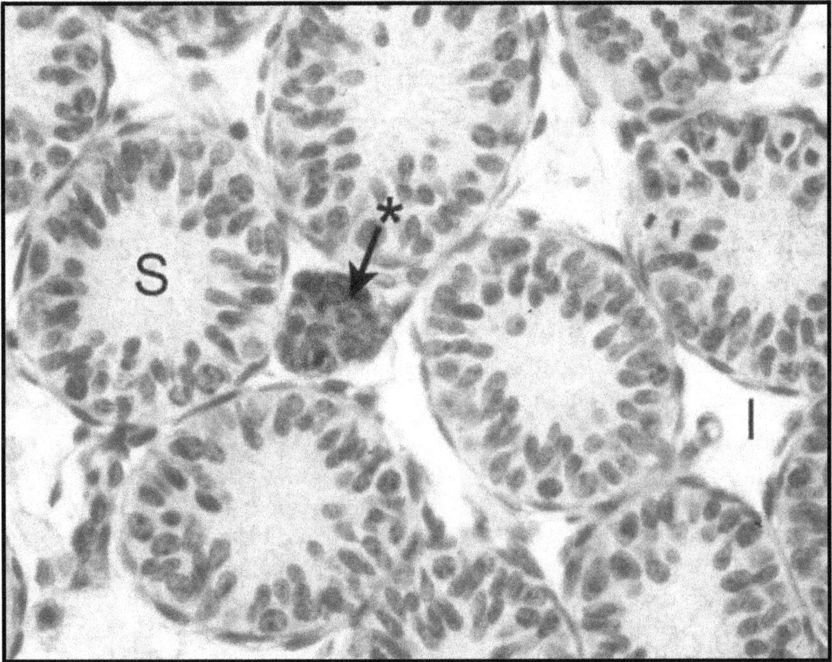

Fig. 2. A representative light micrograph of a 7 day old rat testis. S=seminiferous cord, I=testis interstitium, The arrow with an asterisk (*) depicts a cluster of fetal Leydig cells immunulabeled for 3β-HSD.

4. General organization of the mammalian testis at birth

4.1 Seminiferous cords

At birth, tubular compartment of the testis does not contain a lumen and therefore, referred to as the seminiferous cords (Figure 4). These cords contain only two types of cells; the Sertoli cells, which are located on the basement membrane of the cord and the gonocytes (Figure 4). Sertoli cell nucleus is much smaller than the nuclei of gonocytes which are easily distinguishable from the Sertoli cells due to their large and circular appearance in section (Figure 4).

During the postnatal growth of the testis, the immature Sertoli cells undergo cell proliferation, although at a steadily declining rate, until the adult Sertoli cell population is established. Studies on rats have shown that the migration of gonocytes to the basement membrane and become spermatogonia from that point onwards and the differentiation of spermatogonia to primary permatocytes in the neonatalprepubertal testis are associated with the restriction of Sertoli cell proliferation, but before the blood-testis barrier is formed (Vitale et al., 1973). Sertoli cell proliferation gives a stable population of Sertoli cells in the adult testis (Bishop and Walton, 1960; Attal and Courot, 1963; Sapsford, 1963). With the initiation of spermatogenesis occuring soon after birth in rodents and at various later times in ruminants and primates, the immature Sertoli cells in the seminiferous cords undergo maturation and gain adult type Sertoli cells observed in the adult testis (Sapsford, 1963; Flickinger,and Fawcett, 1967; Vitale et al., 1973; Nagano and Suzuki, 1976; Ramos and Dym, 1979). Sertoli cell maturation in the developing testis is also accompanied by formation of the blood-testis barrier (Vitale et al., 1973; Nagano and Suzuki, 1976; Ramos and Dym, 1979).

4.2 Testis interstitium

In this section of the review, the author focuses on the Leydig cells in the neonatal-prepubertal testis interstitum. The fetal population of Leydig cells differentiate during the fetal life and is still present at birth (Figure 5) in all species studied to date (Lording and de Kretser, 1972; Mendis-Handagama et al., 1987; Kerr and Knell, 1988; Chemes, 1996;

Ariyaratne and Mendis-Handagama, 2000; O'Shaughnessy et al., 2002, 2003) and continue to be present in the postnatal testis in rodents studied to date (Kerr and Knell, 1988; Ariyaratne and Mendis-Handagama, 2000; O'Shaughnessy et al., 2002, 2003). However, in humans, it is reported that fetal Leydig cells undergo cell atrophy postnatally (Chemes, 1996).

Leydig cells in the adult testis, which are identified as the mature adult Leydig cells are differentiated postnatally during the neonatal pre-pubertal period (Roosen-Runge and Anderson, 1959; Mancini et al., 1963; Niemi and Kormano, 1964; Baillie, 1964; Lording and de Kretser, 1972; Mendis-Handagama et. al., 1987; Ariyaratne et al., 2000d) from the peritubular mesenchymal cells (Figure 6), which are the stem cells of adult Leydig cells. The peritubular mesenchymal stem cells differentiate through a series of cell stages in the Leydig cell lineage (progenitor cells, newly formed adult Leydig cells, immature adult Leydig cells) and become the mature adult Leydig cells (Figure 6). In this differentiation process, a spindle-shaped peritubular mesenchymal cell, which does not have the steroidogenic potential, gradually achieve appropriate enzymes and receptors for steroid hormone biosynthesis and steroidogenic potential and finally become a large polyhedral mature adult Leydig cells (Figure 6); a non-steroidogenic mesenchymal stem cell gaining the steroidogenic status, e.g. gaining 3β -HSD enzyme activity can be visualized by performing immunocytochemistry (Figure 7).

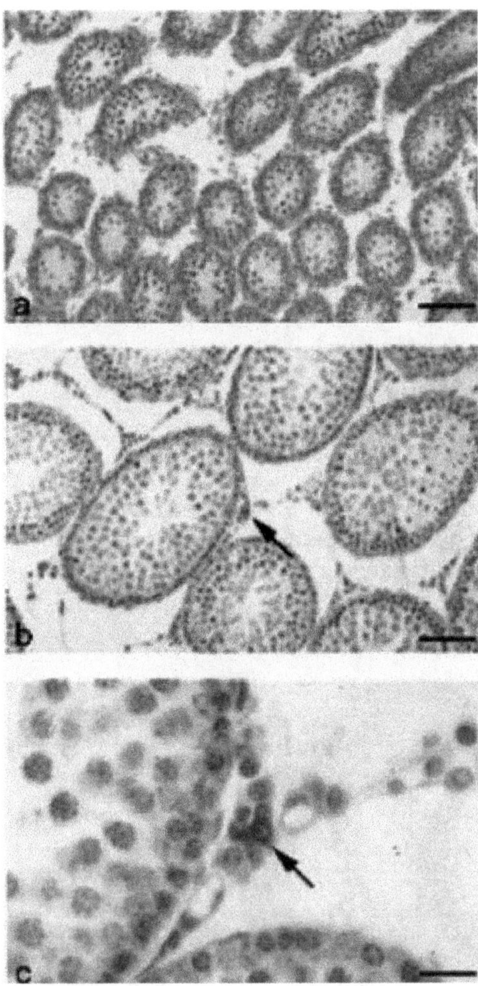

Fig. 3. Representative light micrographs to show the presence and absence of Leydig cells immunolabeled for 11β-HSD1 (marker for adult Leyidig cells) immunocytochemistry in testis interstitium of 21-day-old rats. (**a**) Low power micrographs of a hypothyroid rat where 11β-HSD1 positive cells are absent (bar=5.38μm) and (**b**) a control rat where 11β-HSD1 positive cells (newly formed adult Leydig cells are present (bar= 5.38μm).
(**c**) A higher-power view of the region located by the arrow in **b**. of a 21-day-old control rat I, Seminiferous tubule diameter is much reduced in the PTU/hypothyroid rat testis shown in (a). Bar= 5.12 μm. (Used with permission from the publisher, Mendis-Handagama et al., 1998, Biol. Reprod.59: 351-357.

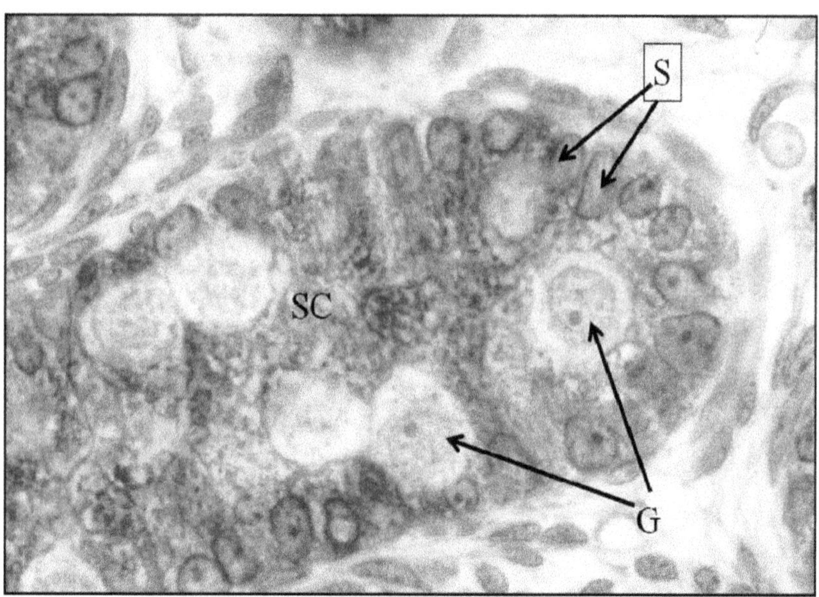

Fig. 4. Representative high power light micrograph of a I day old rat testis immunolabeled for anti-Mullerian hormone (brown stain) .SC=seminiferous cords, G=Gonoctes/Germ cells,, S=nuclei of Sertoli cells, (Used with permisiion from the publisher, Mendis-Handagama et al., 2008, Histology and Histopathology, 23:151-156, Figure modified).

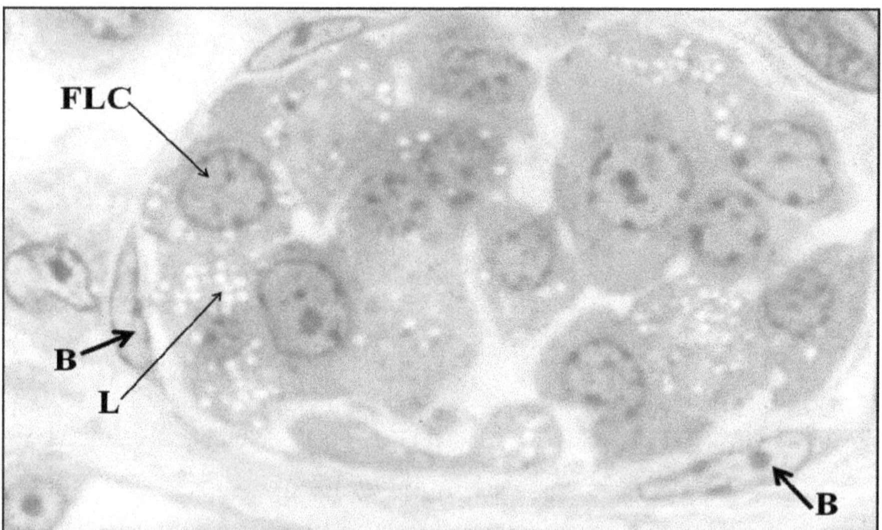

Fig. 5. Representative light micrograph to demonstrate fetal Leydig cells (FLC) in a 1 day old rat testis. L=cytoplasmic lipid droplets in fetal Leydig cells. B=basement membrane components surrounding a fetal Leydig cell cluster, a characteristic feature associated with fetal Leydig cells.

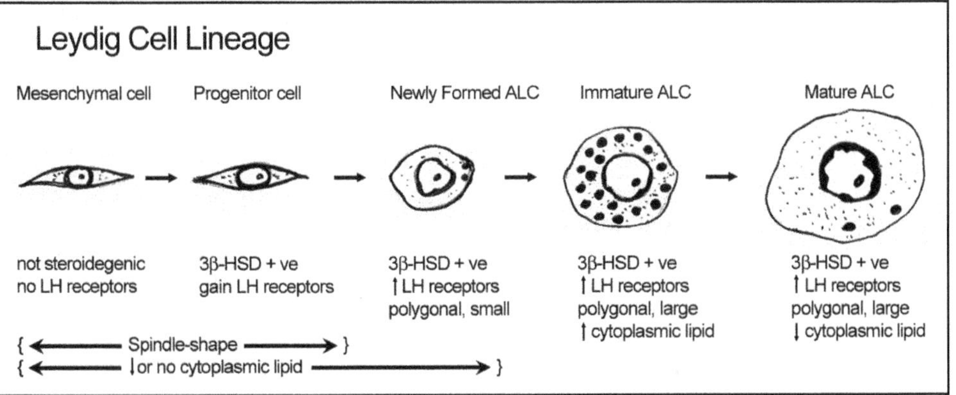

Fig. 6. Schematic diagram of Leydig cell lineage. (used with permission from the publisher, Mendis-Handagama and Ariyaratne, 2001, Biol.Reprod. 65:660-671). The stem cells for Leydig cells are the mesenchymal cells in the testis intersitium, which are spindle-shaped and non-steroidogenic. They first differentiate into progenitor cells, which are also spindle-shaped, but possess few steroidogenic enzymes (e.g. 3β-HSD) and LH receptors. Thyroid hormone is critical to stimulate the mesenchymal cells to differentiate into the progenitor cells (the first step in Leydig cell differentiation) to begin the process of Leydig cell differentiation. Progenitor cells differentiate into mature adult Leydig cells through stages of newly formed adult Leydig cells and immature adult Leydig cells, respectively. (Used with permisiion from the publisher, Mendis-Handagama and Ariyaratne, 2001, Biol. Reprod. 65:660-671.).

5. Thyroid hormone action on the neonatal-prepubertal testis

Until recent years, little was known about the effects of thyroid hormones on the neonatal-prepubertal testis development. In many investigations on the effect of neonatl-prepubertal hypothyroidism, the hypothyroid status was insduced in the experimental animals immediately after birth by feeding their lactating mothers the reversible goitrogen, 6-n-propyl-2-thiouracil (PTU), 0.1% (w/v; Cooke et al., 1991, 1992; Mendis-Handgama et al., 1998; Teerds et al., 1998; Ariyaratne et al., 2000a).) or 0.05%(w/v) methimazole (Antony et al., 1995; Maran et al., 1999) in their drinking water until the pups were weaned on day 21.

5.1 Leydig cells

In mammalian species studied to date, the adult Leydig cells are absent at birth. Therefore, the fetal Leydig cells are the only source of testicular androgens at this age, which is primarily testosterone. In control euthyroid (normal thyroid hormone levels) rats, adult type Leydig cells are observed as early as postnatal day 10 (Mendis-Handagama et al., 1987) and concomitantly increase in number (Mendis-Handagama et al., 1987). This is in addition to the fetal Leydig cells already present in the postnatal testis. From birth to 21days, fetal Leydig cell number in the normal rat testis do not change (Mendis-Handgama et al., 1987,1998; Ariyaratne and Mendis-Handagama, 2000). They could be differentially identified from the postnatally differentiated adult type Leydig cells using their morphology

(Mendis-Handgama et al., 1987,1998; Ariyaratne and Mendis-Handagama, 2000) and using 11β-HSD1 immunocytochemistry, as early as postnatal day 21 in the rat (Mendis-Handgama et al., 1998; Figure 8). These newly formed adult type Leydig cells primarily secrete androstenedione.

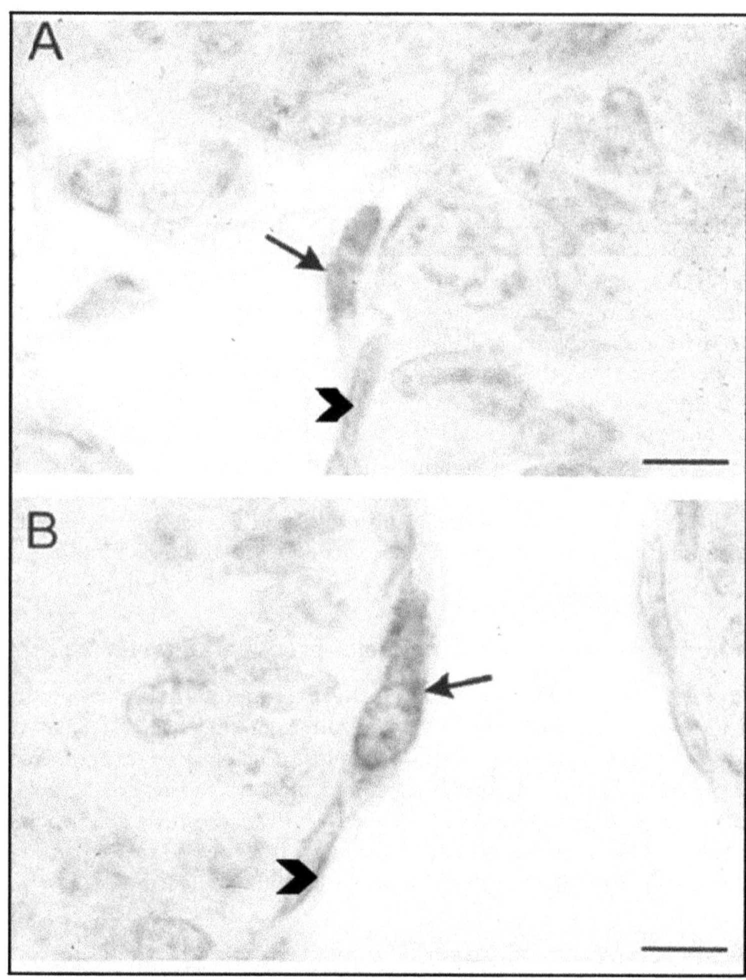

Fig. 7. Representative light micrographs from a 10 day old rat testis immunolabeled for 3β-HSD (shown in brown color) and demonstrate early steps in Leydig cell differentiation. With thyroid hormone stimulation, mesenchymal cells (arrow heads) in the periphery of the seminiferous tubules (S) differentiate into progenitor cells (arrows in Figures A,and B), which are still spindle-shaped; with the progression of their differentiation towards the newly formed adult Leydig cells, they become rounder in shape (compare cells depicted by arrows in Figures A and B, with A) and move gradually away from the peritubular region towards the central part of the testis interstitium. (used with permission from the publisher, Ariyaratne et al., 2000, Biol. 63:165-171., figure modified).

Postnatal Leydig cell differentiation in the neonatal-prepubertal testis is arrested with hypothyroidism (Mendis-Handgama et al., 1998; Teerds et al., 1998; Ariyaratne et al., 2000a) and therefore, these testes do not contain newly formed adult Leydig cells, evident by the absence of 11β-HSD1 labeled cells in their testes interstium (Figures 8c and f) in contrast to age-matching euthyroid rats (Figures 8a and d, respectively); they show 11β-HSD1 labeled Leydig from postnatal day 21 (Figure 8a).From birth to postnatal day 21, testes of hypothyroid rats contain only the fetal Leydig cells, which are fully functional, evident from their morphology and testosterone secretory capacity (Mendis-Handgama et al., 1998; Ariyaratne et al., 2000a) Additionally, an increased number of mesenchymal stem cells are also generated in the hypothyroid rat testes (Mendis-Handagama et al., 1998; Ariyaratne et al., 2000a). The fetal Leydig cells in control rats show cell atrophy on postnatal day 21 (Mendis-Handagama et al., 1987 and 1998; Ariyaratne and Mendis-Handagama, 2000), which is not seen in the 21day old hypothyroid rats (Mendis-Handagama et al., 1998), suggesting that the fetal Leydig cells in the neonatal-prepubertal testis do not regress under a hypothyroid status up to 21 postnatal day. Therefore, serum testosterone levels in these neonatal-prepubertal hypothyroid rats are maintained similar to the control rats up to this age, although the total number of Leydig cells in these rats are significantly lower compared to the age-matching control rats. This is because that the testosterone-producing capacity per fetal leydig cells at neonatal ages is significantly greater than the adult Leydig cells, even at day 90 (Tapanainenet al., 1984; Huhtaniemi et al., 1982). Control 21day old rats have shown greater serum androstenedione levels than their age-matching hypothyroid rats (Mendis-Handgama et al., 1998) indicating the greater numbers of newly formed adult Leydig cells in those testes. Absence of newly formed adult Leydig cells.

In testes of 21 day old hypothyroid rats agrees favorably with their lower levels of serum androstenedione (Mendis-Handgama et al., 1998).

When the hypothyroid status is extended beyond postnatal day 21 in the rat, fetal Leydig cells undergo cell atrophy together with the absence of newly formed adult Leydig cells in their testis interstitium, evident by the absence of cells labeled for 11β-HSD1 in the testis interstitium, the marker for adult Leydig cells (Figures 8c and f). By contrast, when hypothyroid status is stopped at postnatal day 21, newly formed adult Leydig cells are still absent on postnatal day 28, but present at day 40 (Figures 8b and c), greater in number compared to age-matching control/normal rats (Figures 8a and d). However, although these newly formed adult Leydig cells are greater in number (Figure 9a) they are smaller in size than their age-matching controls (Figure 9b). When prolonging the hypothyroid status from day 21 to day 40, testicular testosterone and androstenedione secretory capacity is also diminished (Mendis-Handagama and Ariyaratne, 2004; Figures 9c and d) and could be attributed to the fact that the regression of the fetal Leydig cells and arrest in the differentiation of adult Leydig cells with extended hypothyroidism in these rats.

When the hypothyroid status is discontinued at weaning of the pups at day 21 and raise them under euthyroid conditions until adult hood, which is referred to as transient neonatal hypothyroidism, the adult testis size of these rats become extremely larger (Cooke et al., 1991, 1992; Meisami et al., 1992; Mendis-Handagama and Sharma, 1994) and contain twice the number of Leydig cells per testis compared to the age-matching untreated controls (Mendis-Handagama and Sharma, 1994). However, these Leydig cells in the adult testes of the transiently hypothyroid rats are smaller in size and has 50% of testosterone secretory capacity (Mendis-Handagama and Sharma, 1994).Nevertheless, the testosterone secretory capacity per testis is maintained in these transiently hypothyroid rats at adulthood, because of doubling of the Leydig cell number per testis (Mendis-Handagama and Sharma, 1994). This is because, in rats subjected to neonatal hypothyroidism from birth to 21 days of postnatal age accumulate an abundance of mesenchymal stem cells in their testes due to their proliferation but undifferentian to Leydig cells during the hypothyroid period. Thus, when the hypothyroid status is withdrawn at postnatal day 21, the inhibition of these mesenchymal stem cell differentiation to Leydig cells is ceased and therefore, they begin to differentiate and first appear in these testes interstitium at day 40 as newly formed Leydig cells (Figure 8e; Figure 9a) in significantly greater numbers than their age-matching euthyroid rats and continue to increase in number up to adulthood (i.e. 90days; Figure 9a). However, as stated before, these Leydig cells cells are smaller in size and capable of producing only 50% of testosterone secretory capacity per cell. However, they maintain the serum testosterone levels at adulthood because they are greater in number (Mendis-Handagama and Sharma, 1994).

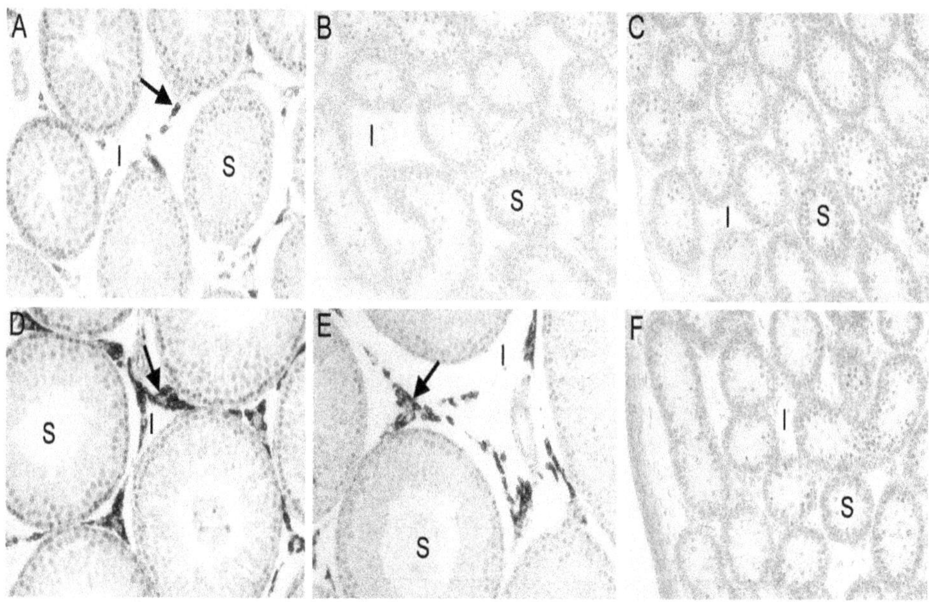

Fig. 8. Representative micrographs to show 11bHSD1 immunocytochemistry in testes interstitium of 28 and 40 day old control rats (A and D), PTU-water rats/transiently hypothyroid (B and E) and PTU/hypothyroid rats (C and F), respectively. 11bHSD1 positive cells (i.e. newly formed adult Leydig cells; arrow) were present in control rats in few numbers at day 28 (a)and more at day 40 (D), were absent at day 28 (B), but present at day 40 (e) in PTU-water/transiently hypothyroid rats, and were absent in PTU/hypothyroid rats at both days (C and F). Seminiferous tubule (S) diameter is much reduced in he PTU/hypothyroid rats compared to the other two groups. Interstitium of the testis. Bar=35 μm..(used with permission from the publisher, Mendis-Handagama and Ariyaratne 2004, Archives of Andrology 50:347-357)

Continuous exposure of lactating mothers to polychlorinated biphenyls results in significant effects on Leydig cells structure and function in the adult offspring males: Leydig cells hypotrophy and reduced capacity to produce testosterone *in vitro* in response to luteinizing hormone stimulation (Kim et al., 2000). It is reported that polychlorinated biphenyls disrupt the thyroid gland function in humans (Langer et al., 1998; Cheek et al., 1999; Nagayama et al., 1998) and in many other mammalian species, e.g. the rat (Collins, 1980; Saeed and Hansen 1985;

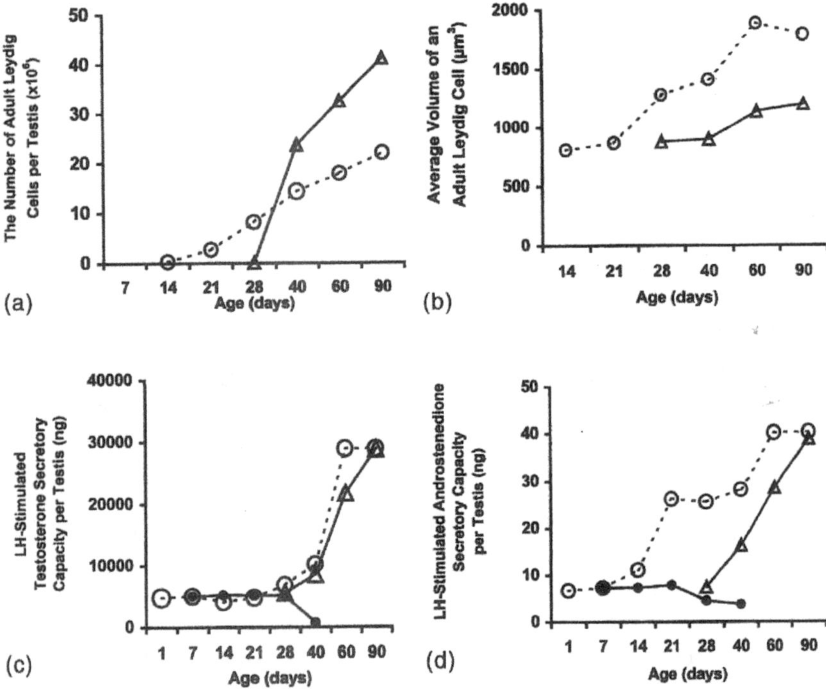

Fig. 9. Control rats—open circles, PTU-water rats/transiently hypothyroid—triangles, PTU/hypothyroid rats—filled circles. (a) The number of adult Leydig cells (ALC) per testis in control rats and PTU-water/transiently hypothyroid rats, ALC were first detected at day 14 in few numbers in control rats. In PTU/hypothyroid rats the ALC were absent, In PTU-water/transiently hypothyroid rats few were seen at day 28,but increase numbers were seen at day 40 onwards. (b) Average volume of an ALC. (c) LH-stimulated (LH, 100 ng per ml) testosterone production per testis in vitro for three hours. (d) LH-stimulated (LH, 100 ng per ml) androstenedione production per testis in vitro for three hours. (used with permission from the publisher, Mendis-Handagama and Ariyaratne, 2004, Archives of Andrology 50:347-357)

Ness et al., 1993; Cooke et al., 1996; Kato et al., 1998 and 1999; Desaulniers et al., 1999) and the grey seal (Wolstad and Jensen, 1999). Based on the observations of Cooke et. al (1996) and Kim et al. (2000), it appears that polychlorinated biphenyl exposure during the neonatal period has subjected these rats to undergo a transient hypothyroid status, which has caused an interference in the normal process of Leydig cell differentiation in the developing testis and produce a defect in the steroidogenic function of the Leydig cells in the adult. Moreover, it is important to note that in neonatal Syrian hamsters, Leydig cells differentiation is arrested with experimental exposure to extreme darkness (Hance at al., 2009), which causes low levels of thyroid hormones. This finding agrees favorably with the concept that mesenchymal stem cell differentiation into Leydig cells is arrested under low levels of thyroid hormones. Therefore, neonatal-prepubertal testes of these hamsters do not show peritubular mesenchymal stem cell differentiation into progenitor cells and newly formed adult Leydig cells in the prepubertal testes, in contrast to euthyroid control hamsters; they contain only the fetal Leydig cells (Figure 10).

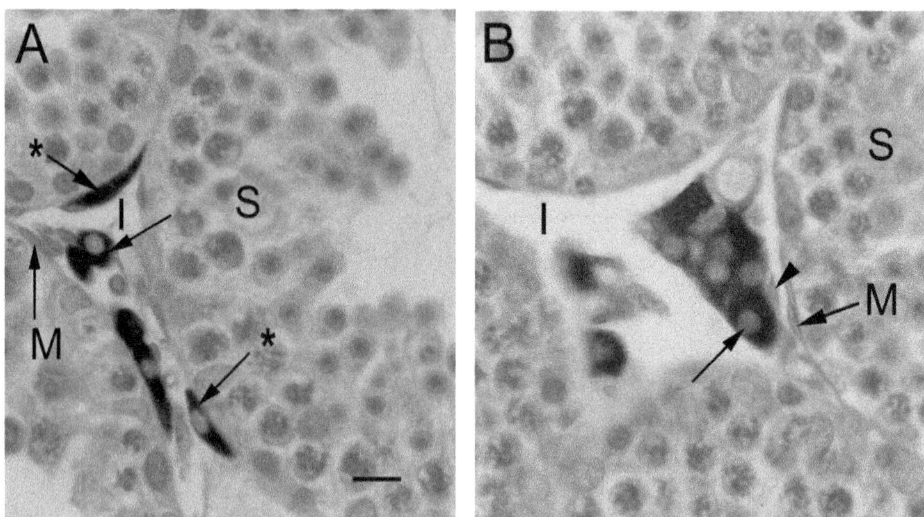

Fig. 10. Representative light micrographs of hamster testis of **(A)** 14hours of light and **(B)** 1 hour of light exposed hamsters, immunolabeled for 3ß-HSD. S=seminiferous tubules,I=testis interstitium, Bar=20µm for both A and B; same magnification).**A.** Single arrow depicts a newly formed adult Leydig cell positive for 3ß-HSD in a14 hours of light exposed hamster testis. Arrows with asterisks (*) depict Leydig progenitor cells, which are spindle-shaped cells located at the peritubular region and are positive for 3ß-HSD. Their presence indicates that Leydig cell differentiation is occurring in testes of these hamsters. Leydig stem cells / mesenchymal cells (M) are negative for 3ß-HSD. **B.** Single arrowdepicts fetal Leydig cells in a 1 hour of light exposed hamster testis. They are primarily observed in clusters surrounded by basement membrane components (arrow head).Leydig cell progenitors (Spindle-shaped cells located at the peritubularregion and positive for 3ß-HSD) were absent in 1L hamster testis.Leydig stem cells / mesenchymal cells (M) are negative for 3ß-HSD. (Hance et al., 2009, Histology and Histopathology,24: 1417-1424)

5.2 Seminiferous tubules

Hypothyroidism induced in new born male rats up to postnatal day 60 has shown reduced diameter of seminiferous tubules, arrest in proliferation and differentiation of germ cells, reduction in number of germ cells and plasma testosterone levels, estradiol and sex hormone binding globulins (Maran and Aruldhas, 2002), which are essential for normal testicular development. Transient neonatal-prepubertal hypothyroidism in rats causes significantly reduced body weight (Figure 11a) and significantly increased testis weight at adulthood, i.e. at 90days (Figure 11b; Mendis-Handagama and Ariyaratne, 2004; Lagu et al.,2005).

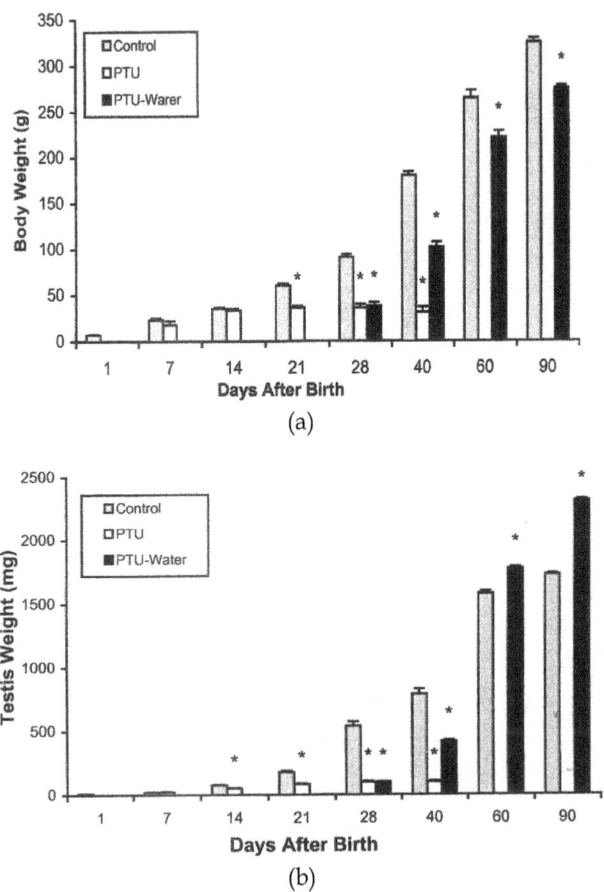

Fig. 11. (a) Body weights of control, PTU/hypothyroid and PTU-water treated/transiently hypothyroid rats. (b) Testis weights of control, PTU/hypothyroid and PTU-water treated/transiently hypothyroid rats. Mean±SE (n=5 rats per group). Asterisks (*) depict significant differences (P<0.05) from the control value at each age. (used with permission from the publisher, Mendis-Handagama and Ariyaratne, 2004, Archives of Andrology 50:347-357)

This increase in testis weight following transient neonatal hypothyroidism in these rats is due to the increase in number of Sertoli cells and germ cells (van Haaster et al., 1993; de Franca et al., 1995; Maran et al., 1999). van Haaster et al. (1993) showed that neonatal hypothyroidism in Wistar rats (from birth up to postnatal day 26) retards the morphological differentiation of Sertoli cells, prolongs their immature status and proliferation of these cells up to postnatal day 30. Sertoli cell numbers per testis in these hypothyroid rats determined at day 36, were increased compared to controls. These findings revealed that neonatal-prepubertal hypothyroidism delays maturation of Sertoli cells (van Haaster et al., 1993; de Franca et al., 1995) and extend their period of proliferation, which increase their numbers. Therefore, this increase in the number of Sertoli cells per testis in the transiently hypothyroid rats produces larger testes at adulthood (Meisami et al., 1992; Mendis-Handagama and Sharma, 1994). This increase in the number of Sertoli cells in the adult rats subjected to transient neonatal hypothyroidism is associated with increased daily production of sperm (Cooke et al.,1991, 1992).

It is also being reported that neonatal hyperthyroidism causes opposite effects on testis development. However, because 'hyperthyroidism' is not relevant to the title of this chapter, it is not discussed further.

6. Acknowledgements

Partially funded by The Center of Excellence of The University of Tennessee and Alliance of Women Philanthropists.

7. References

Antony, F.F., Aruldhas, M.M., Udhayakumar, R.C., Maran, R.R., Govindaraju, P. 1995. Antony, F.F., Aruldhas, M.M., Udhayakumar, R.C., Maran, R.R., Govindaraju, P. 1995. Inhibition of Leydig cell activity in-vivo and in-vitro in hypothyroid rats. J. Endocrinol. 144: 293-300.Inhibition of Leydig cell activity in-vivo and in-vitro in hypothyroid rats. J. Endocrinol. 144: 293-300.

Ariyaratne, H.B.S., Mendis-Handagama, S.L.M.C. 2000. Changes in structure and function of the testis interstitium in Sprague Dawley rats from birth to sexual maturity. Biol.Reprod. 62:680-690.

Ariyaratne, H.B.S., Mason, J.I., Mendis-Handagama, S.L.M.C. 2000a. Effects of thyroid and luteinizing hormone on the onset of precursor cell differentiation into Leydig progenitor cells in the prepubertal rat testis. Biol. Reprod. 63:898-904.

Ariyaratne, H.B.S., Mason, J.I., Mendis-Handagama, S.L.M.C. 2000b. Effects of thyroid hormone on Leydig cell regeneration in the adult rat following ethane dimethane sulphonate treatment. Biol. Reprod. 63:1115-1123.

Ariyaratne, H.B.S., Mason, J.I., Mendis-Handagama, S.L.M.C. 2000c. Effects of triiodothyronine on testicular interstitial cells and androgen secretory capacity of the prepubertal rat. Biol. Reprod. 63:493-502.

Ariyaratne, H.B.S., Mendis-Handagama, S.M.L.C, Hales, D.B., Mason, J.I. 2000d.Studies on the onset of Leydig precursor cell differentiation in the prepubertal rat testis. Biol. Reprod. 63:165-171.

Attal, J., Courot M. 1963. Development testiculaireet establishment de la spermatogenese chez le taureau. Ann. Biol. Anim. Biochem. Biophys. 3:219-241.

Baillie, A. H. 1964. Further observations on the growth and histochemistry of Leydig tissue in the postnatal prepubertal mouse testis. J. Anat. London 98:403-429.

Berndtson, W.E., Igboeli, G., Pickett, B.W. 1987. Relationship of absolute numbers of Sertoli cells to testicular size and spermatogenesis in young beef bulls. J Anim Sci., 64:241-246.

Banks, W.J. 1986. Male Reproductive System. In: Applied Veterinary Histology, Williams and Wilkins, pp 486-504.

Bishop, M.W.H., Walton, A. Spermatogenesis and structure of mammalian spermatozoa. In Marshall's Physiology of Reproduction. Vol. 1, London:Longmans Green1960, p1-29.

Bouin, P., Ancel, P. 1903. Recherches sur les cellules interstitielles dutesticule des mamiferes. Arch. d. zool. exper. et. gen. ; 1:437-523.

Brokelmann, J. 1963. Fine structure of germ cells and Sertoli cells during the cycle of the seminiferous epithelium in the rat. Z. Zellforsch.Mikroscopy.Anat. 58: 820-850.

Cheek, A.O., Kow, K., Chen, J., McLachlan, J.A. 1999. Potential mechanisms of thyroid disruption in humans: interaction of organochlorine compounds with thyroid receptor, transthyretin, and thyroid biding globulin. Environ. Health Perspect. 107:273-278.

Chemes, H.E. Leydig cell development in humans. In: The Leydig Cell. Payne AH, Hardy MP. Russell LD. (editors), 1996; pg 175-202, Cache River Press, Vienna, IL, U.S.A.

Christensen, A.K., Mason, V.R. 1965. Comparative ability of seminiferous tubules and interstitial tissue of rat testis to synthesize androgen from progesterone-4-^{14}C in vitro. Endocrinology 76:646-656.

Clermont, Y., 1963. The cycle of the seminiferou epithelium in man. Am.J. Anat. 112:35-45.

Clermont, Y., 1969. Two classes of spermatogonial stem cells in the monkey (*Cercopithercus aethiops*). Am. J. Anat. 126:57-72.

Collins, W.T. 1980. Fine structural lesions and hormonal alterations in thyroid glands of perinatal rats exposed *in utero* and by the milk to polychlorinated biphenyls. Am. J. Pathol. 99:125-142.

Cooke, P.S., Hess, R.A., Porcelli, J., Meisami, E. 1991. increased sperm production in adult rats after transient neonatal hypothyroidism. Endocrinology 129:244-248.

Cooke, P.S., Porcelli, J., Hess, R.A. 1992. Induction of increased testis growth and sperm production in adult rats by neonatal administration of the goitrogen propylthiouracil (PTU): the critical period. Biol Reprod. 46:146-154.

Cooke, P.S., Zhao, Y.D., Hansen, L.G. 1996. Neonatal polycholrinated biphenyl treatment increases adult testis size and sperm production in the rat. Toxicol. Appl. Pharmacol. 136:112-117.

Davis, J.R., Langford, G.A., Kirby, P.J. 1970. The testicular capsule. In: The Testis. Eds. A.D. Johnson, W.R. Gomes & N.L. Vandermark. Academic Press New York and London. 281-337.

De Franca, L.R., Hess, R.A., Cooke, P.S., Russell, L.D. 1995. Neonatal hypothyroidism causes delayed Sertoli cell maturation in rats treated with propylthiouracil: evidence that the Sertoli cell controls testis growth. Anat. Rec. 242: 57-69.

de Kretser, D.M., Hedger, M.P., Loveland, K.I., Phillips, D.J. 2002. Inhibins, activins and follistatin in reproduction. Hum Reprod Update. ;8:529-541. Review.

Desaulniers, D., Leingartner, K., Wade, M., Fintelman, E., Yagminas, A., Foster, W.G. 1999. Effects of acute exposure to PCBs 126 and 153 on anterior pituitary and thyroid hormones and FSH isoforms in adult Sprague Dawley male rats. Toxicol. Sci. 47:158-169.

Dym, M., Fawcett, D.W. 1970. The blood-testis barrier in the rat and the physiological compartmentation of the seminiferous epithelium. Biol. Reprod. 3:308-325.

Dym, M. 1973. The fine structure of the monkey (Macaca) Sertoli cell and its role in maintaining the blood-testis barrier. Anat. Rec.175:639-656.

Fawcett, D.W., Leak, L.V., Heidger, P.N. 1969. Electron micrographic observations on the structure of the bloodp-testis barrier. J.Rep.and Fert. Suppl.10: 105-122.

Fawcett, D.W., Phillips, D.M. 1969. Onservations on the release of spermatozoa and the changes in the head during passage through the epididymis. J. Reprod. Fert.; Suppl. 6: 405-418.

Fawcett, D.W., Neaves, W.B., Flores, M.N. 1973. Comparative observations on intertubular lymphatics and the organization of the interstitial tissue of the mammalian testis. Biol. Reprod.; 9:500-532.

Flickinger, C.J. Fawcett, D.W. 1967. The functional specialization of Sertoli cells in the seminiferous epithelium. Anat. Rec. 158:207-222.

French, F.S., Ritzen. E.N. 1979. Androgen binding protein in efferent duct fluid of rat testis. J. Reprod. Fert.; 32:479-483.

Gallagher, T.F., Koch, F.C. 1929. The testicular hormone. J. Biol. Chem. 84:495-500.

Hall, P.F. 1970. Endocrinology of the testis. In:The Testis. Eds. A.D.Johnson, W.R. Gomes and N.L. Vandermark. Acad. Press New York. 1-71.

Gudernatsch, J.F. 1912. Feeding experiments on tadpoles. 1. The influence of specific organs given as food on growth and differentiation. A contribution to the knowledge of organs with internal secretion. Wilhelm Roux Arch. Entwicklungsmech.Organismen 35:457-483.

Huhtaniemi, I.T., Nozu, K., Warren, D.W., Dufau, M.L., Catt, K.J. 1982. Acquisition of regulatory mechanisms for gonadotropin receptors and steroidogenesis in the maturing rat testis. Endocrinology ; 111:1711–1720.

Johnson, L. Neaves, W.B. 1981. Age related changes in the Leydig cell population, seminiferous tubules and sperm production in stallions. Biol. Reprod. 24:703-712.

Kaler, L.W., Neaves, W.B. 1978. Attrition of the human Leydig cell population with advancing age. Anat. Rec. 192: 513-518.

Kato, Y., Haraguchi, K., Shibahara, T., Masuda, Y., Kimura, R. 1998. Reduction of thyroid hormone levels by methylsulfonyl metabolites of polychlorinated biphenyl congeners in rats. Arch. Toxicol. 72:541-544.

Kato, Y., Haraguchi, K., Shibahara, T., Yumoto, S., Masuda, Y., Kimura, R. 1999. Reduction of thyroid hormone levels by methylsulfonyl metabolites of of tetra- and pentachlorinated biphenyls in male Sprague Dawley rats. Toxicol. Sci. 48:51-54.

Kerr, J.B., Knell, C.M. 1988. The fate of fetal Leydig cells during the development of the fetal and postnatal rat testis. Development **103**:535-544.

Kim, I., Ariyaratne, H.B.S., Mendis-Handagama, S.L.M.C. 2000. Effects of continuous and intermittent exposure of lactating mothers to Aroclor 1242 on testicular steroidogenic function in the adult offspring. Tissue Cell 33:169-177.

Lacy, D. 1967. The seminiferous tubules in mammala. Endevour; 26:100-109.

Langer, P., Tajtakova, M., Fodor, G., Kocan, A., Bohov, P.., Michalek, J., Kreze, A. 1998. Increased thyroid volume and prevalence of thyroid disorders in an area heavily polluted by polychlorinated biphenyls. Eur. J. Endocrinology 139:402-409.

Lagu, S.K., Bhavsar, N.G., Sharma, R.K., Ramachandran, A.V. 2005. Neonatal hypothyroidism-induced changes in rat testis size. Dependence on temperature. Neuro. Endocrinol. Lett. 26:780-788.

Leblond, C.F., Clermont, Y. 1952. Definition of the styages of the cycle of seminiferous epithelium in the rat. Ann. NY. Acad Sci. 55:545-573..

Levy, H., Deane, H., Rubin, B.I., 1959. Observations on steroid 3β-ol-dehydrogenase activity in tissues of intact and hypophysectomized rats. Endocrinology 65:932-943.

Leydig, F. 1850. Zur Anatomie der mannlichen Geschlechtsorgane und Analdrusen der Saugetgiere. Z. wiss. Zool. 2:1-57.

Lording, D.W., de Kretser, D.M. 1972. Comparative ultrastructural and histochemical studies of the interstitial cells of the rat testis during fetal and postnatal development. J. Reprod. Fert. 29:261-269.

Mancini, R.E., Vilar, O., Lavieri, J.C., Andrada, J.A., Heinrich, J.J. 1963. Development of Leydig cells in the normal human testis. A cytological, cytochemical and quantitative study. Am. J. Anat. 112:203-214.

Maran R.R., Sivakumar, R., Arunakaran, j., Ravisankar, B., Sidharthan, V., Jeyaraj, D.A., Arudhas, M.M. 1999. Duration-dependent effect of transient neonatal hypothyroidism on sertoli and germ cell number, and plasma and testicular interstitial fluid androgen binding protein concentration. Endocr. Res. 25:323-340.

Maran R.R., Arudhas, M.M. 2002. Adverse effects of neonatal hypothyroidism on Wistar rat spermatogenesis. Endocr. Res. 28: 141-154.

Mendis-Handagama, S.M.L.C., Risbridger, G.P., de Kretser, D.M. 1987. Morphometric analysis of the components of the neonatal and adult rat testis interstitium. Int. J. Androl. 10:525-534.

Mendis-Handagama, S.M.L.C., Zirkin, B.R., Ewing, L.L. 1988. Comparison of components of thetestis interstitium with testosterone secretion in hamster, rat and guinea pig testes perfused *invitro* Am.J.Anat. 181:12-22.

Mendis-Handagama, S.M.L.C., Kerr, J.B., de Kretser, D.M. 1990. Experimental cryptorchidism in the adult mouse I. Qualitative and quantitative light microscopic morphology. J.Andrology 11:539-547.

Mendis-Handagama, S.M.L.C., Ariyaratne, H.B.S., Teunissen van Manan, K.R., Haupt, R.L. 1998. Differentiation of adult Leydig cells in the neonatal rat testis is arrested by hypothyroidism. Biol.Reprod. 59: 351-357.

Mendis-Handagama, S.L.M.C., Sharma, O.P. 1994. Effects of neonatal administration of the reversible goitrogen propylthiouracil on the testis interstitium in adult rats. J. Reprod. Fert. 100:85-92.

Mendis-Handagama, S.L.M.C., Ariyaratne, H.B.S. 2001. Differentiation of the adult Leydig cell population in the postnatal testis. Biol. Reprod. 65:660-671.

Mendis-Handagama, S.L.M.C., Ariyaratne, H.B.S. 2004. Prolonged and transient neonatal hypothyroidism on Leydig cell differentiation in the postnatal rat testis. Arch Androl. 50:347-357.

Meisami, E., Sendera, T.J., Clay, L.B. 1992. Paradoxical hypertrophy and plasticity of the testis in rats recovering from early thyroid deficiency: growth study including effects of age and duration of hypothyroidism. J. Endocrinol. 135:495-505.

Mori, H., Christensen, A.K. 1980. Morphometric analysis of Leydig cells in the normal rat testis. J. Cell Biol. 84: 340-354.

Mori, H., Shimizu, D., Takeda, A., Takioka, Y., Fukunishi, R. 1980. Stereological analysis of Leydig cells in normal guinea pig testis. J. electr. Microsc. (Tokyo). 29:8-21.

Mori, H., Shimizu, D., Fukunishi, R., Christensen, A.K. 1982. Morphometeric analysis of testicular Leydig cells in normal adult mice. Anat. Rec. 204:333-339.

Moura, A.A., Souza, C.E., Erikson, B.H. 2011. Early prepubertal testis criteria, seminiferous epithelium and hormone concentrations as related to testicular development in beef bulls. Anim Reprod Sci., 124:39-47. Epub .

Nagano, T., Suzuki, F. 1976. he postnatal development of the junctional complexes of the mouse Sertoli cells as revealed by freeze fracture. Anat. Rec.; 185: 403-418.

Nagayama, J., Okamura, K., Iida, T., Hirakawa, H., Matsueds, T., Tsuji, H., Hasegawa, M., Sato, K., Ma, H.Y., Yanagawa, T., Igarashi, H., Fukushige, J., Watanabe, T. 1998.

Postnatal exposure to chlorinated dioxins and related chemicals on thyroid hormone status in Japanese breast-fed infants. Chemosphere 37:1789-1793.

Ness, D.K., Schantz, S.L., Moshtaghian, J., Hansen, L.G. 1993. Effects of perinatal exposure to specific PCB congeners on thyroid hormone concentrations and thyroid histology in the rat. Toxicol. Lett. 68:311-323.

Nicander, L. 1967. An electron microscopical study of cell contacts in the seminiferous tubules of some mammals. Z. Zellforsch. Mikroscopy. Anat. 83: 375-397.

Niemi, M., Kormano, M. 1964. Cell renewal in the interstitial tissue of postnatal prepubertal rat testis. Endocrinology 74:996-998.

O'Shaugnessy, P.J,, Willerton, L, Baker ,P.J. 2002. Changes in Leydig cell gene expression during development in the mouse.Biol Reprod. 66;966-75.

O'Shaughnessy, PJ., Fleming ,L.M., Jackson ,G,. Hochgeschwender, U., Reed ,P., Baker, P.J.. 2003. Adrenocorticotropic hormone directly stimulates testosterone production by the fetal and neonatal mouse testis. Endocrinology 144:3279-3284.

Ramos, A.S., Dym, M. 1979. Ultrastructural differentiation of rat Sertoli cells. Biol. Reprod.; 21:909-922.

Roosen-Runge, E.C., Anderson, A.D. 1959. The development of the interstitial cells in the testis of albino rat. Acta Anat. 37:125-137.

Rosas, M.H. 1970. The Sertoli cell and the blood-testis barrier, an electronmicroscopic study. Advan. Androl. 1: 83-86.

Saeed, A., Hansen, L.G. 1985. Morphometric changes in the prepubertal female rat thyroid gland following acute exposure to 2,2',4,4'-tetrachlorobiphenyl and Aroclor 1242. J. Toxicol. Environ. Heath. 51:503-513.

Sapsford, C.S. 1963. The development of the Sertoli cell of the rat and mouse: its existence as a mononucleate unit. J. Anat.; 97: 225-238.

Sapsford, C.S., Rae C.A. 1968. Sertoli cell-spermatids relationships: ultrastructural studies of the movements of the mature spermatids into the lumen of the seminiferous tubules. J. Anat.; 103: 214-215.

Setchell, B.P., Waites, G.M.H. 1975. The blood-testis barrier. In:Handbooh of physiology, sect.7, volume 5, Male Reproductive System. Eds. D.W. Hamilton and F.G. Greeps. American Physiological Society, Washington, D.C. 142-172.

Tapanainen J., Kuopio T., Pelliniemi L.J., Huhtaniemi, I. 1984. Rat testicular endogenous steroids and number of Leydig cells between the fetal period and sexual maturity. Biol. Reprod .31:1027–1035.

Teerds, KJ., de Rooij, D.G., de Jong, F.H., van Haaster, L.H. 1998. Development of the adult Leydig cell population in the rat testis is affected by neonatal thyroid hormone levels. Biol. Reprod. 59:344-350.

Vitale R., Fawcett, D.W., Dym, M. 1973. The normal development of the blood-testis barrier and the effects of clomiphene and estrogen treatment. Anat. Rec. 1973, 176:333-344.

Van Haster, L.H, De Jong , F.H, Docter, R., De Rooij, D.G. 1993. High neonatal triiodothyronine levels reduce the period of Sertoli cell proliferation and accelerate tubular lumen formation in the rat testis, and increase serum inhibin level. Endocrinology. 133: 755-760.

Wattenburg, L.W. 1958. Microscopic histological demonstration of steroid-3β-ol dehydrogenase in tissue sections. J. Histochem. Cytochem. 6:225-232.

Wolstad, S., Jensen, B.M. 1999. Thyroid hormones in grey seal pups (Halichoerus grypus). Comp. Biochem. Physiol. A. Mol. Integr-Physiol. 122:157-182.

12

Congenital Hypothyroidism and Thyroid Cancer

Minjing Zou and Yufei Shi
Dept. of Genetics King Faisal Specialist Hospital and Research Centre Riyadh, Saudi Arabia

1. Introduction

Congenital hypothyroidism (CH) is a condition of thyroid hormone deficiency present at birth and can result in severe neurodevelopmental impairment, growth failure and permanent mental retardation if treatment is delayed for several months after birth (1-3). Girls are more frequently affected than boys (female to male ratios ranging from 2:1 to 4:1)(4). The mental retardation and neurodevelopmental impairment include poor motor coordination, ataxia, spastic diplegia, muscular hypotonia, strabismus, learning disability and diminished attention span (5). Consequently, most countries operate neonatal screening programs to enable early detection of cases and therapeutic intervention. Treatment consists of a daily dose of thyroid hormone (thyroxine) by mouth (6, 7). Because the treatment is simple, effective, and inexpensive, nearly all of the developed world practices newborn screening to detect and treat CH in the first weeks of life. The diagnosis is based on the measurement of TSH on the second or third day of life. If the TSH is high, the infant's doctor and parents are called and a referral to a pediatric endocrinologist is recommended to confirm the diagnosis and initiate treatment (6). Often a technetium (Tc-99m pertechnetate) thyroid scan is performed to detect a structurally abnormal gland. The Tc-99m pertechnetate exam will help differentiate thyroid dysgenesis from thyroid dyshormonogenesis. Most children born with CH and correctly treated with thyroxine grow and develop normally in all respects. Even most of those with athyreosis and undetectable T_4 levels at birth develop with normal intelligence. However, in some cases mild learning problems, subtle neurological dysfunctions, and subnormal IQ have been reported (2, 5). In a 5 year follow-up study of children with CH, Arenz et al reported that children with an initial thyroid-stimulating hormone (TSH) value of >200 mU/L performed significantly worse in motor skills than children with TSH value of < or =200 mU/L although intellectual development was normal (8). Glorieux et al reported that 27 patients with congenital hypothyroidism diagnosed by neonatal screening were examined at the age of 12 years. The 12 patients with severe hypothyroidism at diagnosis (thyroxine < 26 nmol/L, and area-of-the-knee epiphyses < 0.05 cm2) had a lower IQ than the 15 patients with less severe hypothyroidism (9). Salerno et al evaluate the intellectual outcome in 40 12-year-old patients with CH detected by neonatal screening, 13 patients showed subnormal IQ score (72.4+/-4.9) compared with their siblings (86.7+/-9.6; P<0.0001) and with the other patients (96.1+/-9.6; P<0.0001). The low IQ score was associated with lower serum concentrations of thyroxine at diagnosis, poor treatment compliance during follow-up and lower familial IQ. Interviews with parents of CH children revealed that a refusal to acknowledge the disease was linked to poor attention to the child's emotional life and to poor treatment compliance in some cases (11%) (10). These data suggest that neurodevelopmental impairment may be associated with inadequate treatment in some of CH cases.

2. Congenital hypothyroidism in Saudi Arabia

Since CH is the most common preventable cause of mental retardation, the newborn screening program for CH was started in 1988 at the Ministry of Health Maternity Hospitals in Saudi Arabia to detect and treat this disorder (11, 12). The prevalence of CH in Riyadh is 1 in 3,450 live births with 279,482 newborn infants screened (11, 12), the most common etiology shown by thyroid scan being thyroid ectopy (50%), followed by dyshormonogenesis (26%) and athyrosis (24%) (11). Two other studies showed a different rate of CH and dyshormonogenesis (13, 14). The study by Henry et al showed the prevalence of 1 in 2759 live births with 121,404 newborn infants screened in the same Central region (Riyadh), the predominant cause of congenital hypothyroidism found in the study being athyreosis (45%), followed by thyroid ectopia (24%) and dyshormonogenesis (17%) (13). The study by Majeed-Saidan et al showed the prevalence of 1 in 2096 live births with 44,778 newborn infants screened and 8/17 (47%) CH had dyshormonogenesis (14). However, the number of the newborn infants screened is smaller in these two studies. The prevalence of CH in other regions of Saudi Arabia is about 1 in 2931 live births in the South region with 100,000 newborn infants screened (Najran province) (15) although 1 in 1400 live births was reported in a separate study with 30810 newborn infants screened (16), 1 in 4200 live births with 193,613 infants screened in the North-West region (Madina Al-Munawara region) (17), and 1 in 5061 live births in the Eastern region (18). The overall prevalence of CH in Saudi Arabia is similar to those reported in the literature from other countries although the prevalence of dyshormonogenesis appears to be higher than other parts of the world. The nationwide efforts to promote neonatal screening programs in recent years in the Kingdom have likely prevented severe mental and growth retardation in newborn infants and also sparked the interest of researchers in CH (12, 13, 17-19). However, molecular characterization of underlying genetic defects has not been systematically conducted yet among the patients. There is also a paucity of data on clinical treatment and follow-up of the patients. Major misconceptions are still very common among young parents in Saudi Arabia. First, many do not fully understand the seriousness of the disease, refuse to participate in the neonatal screening or otherwise show poor compliance in diagnosis, treatment and follow-up. Second, others believe that the treatment of CH implies a life-long dependency on drug administration and therefore feel highly distressed when confronted with their child's disease. Inadequate treatment can lead to poor academic performance and learning problems which tend to be overlooked by the child's parents (2)

3. The etiology of congenital hypothyroidism

The etiology of congenital hypothyroidism is heterogeneous and is caused by either thyroid dysgenesis (75-80%) or dyshormonogenesis (15-20%) (1, 20). The most common cause of CH is thyroid dysgenesis, a spectrum of defective thyroid gland development leading to athyrosis (without visible thyroid tissue in imaging studies) (35–40%), thyroid ectopy (frequently located in a sublingual position) (55–60%), and hypoplasia (a small-sized thyroid or remnants of thyroid tissue in the normal position) (5%) (21, 22). These forms represent 75-80% of all cases of CH (20). The pathogenesis of thyroid dysgenesis is largely unknown. The disorder is usually sporadic but up to 2% of familial cases have been reported (23-25). Genes associated with thyroid gland dysgenesis include the TSH receptor in non-syndromic congenital hypothyroidism, $G_s\alpha$, and the thyroid transcription factors (TTF-1, TTF-2, and Pax-8) (22, 24, 25). The extrathyroid genes involved in the control of migration of the median thyroid bud during embryogenesis, such as adhesion molecules, and vascular factors involved in the stabilization of the bi-lobed structure of the thyroid may also play a role (22). Thyroid dyshormonogenesis account for 15–20% of CH cases (20). In thyroid dyshormonogenesis (defects of thyroid hormone biosynthesis), patients have a normal sized or enlarged thyroid gland (goitre) in the normal position and are often recessively inherited (1). Thyroid dyshormonogenesis is a genetically heterogeneous group of inherited disorders in the enzymatic cascade of thyroid hormone synthesis. The underlining genetic defects causing dyshormonogenesis include gene mutations in the enzymatic cascade of thyroid hormone synthesis such as Na^+/I^- symporter (26), Tg (27), thyroperoxidase (TPO) (28), dual oxidase 2 (DUOX2 or THOX2)(29), dual oxidase maturation factor 2 (DUOXA2)(30), pendrin (SLC26A4/PDS/(31), and iodotyrosine dehalogenase1(DEHAL1) (32). Mutations in the TPO or Tg are the most frequent genetic defects in thyroid dyshormonogenesis.

4. Thyroid hormone synthesis and the genes involved in the process

Thyroid hormones, thyroxine (T_4) and triiodothyronine (T_3), are critical determinants of brain and somatic development in infants and of metabolic activity in adults; they also affect the function of virtually every organ system(33). They are tyrosine-based hormones produced by the thyroid gland. The synthetic process occurs in three major steps as shown in Figure 1(33, 34): production and accumulation of the raw materials, biosynthesis of the hormones on a backbone of Tg, release of the free hormones from Tg and secretion into blood. Tyrosines are provided from Tg, a large glycoprotein which is synthesized by thyroid epithelial cells and secreted into the lumen of the follicle forming colloid (essentially a pool of Tg). A molecule of Tg contains 134 tyrosines, although only a handful of these are actually used to synthesize T4 and T3. Another important component in the synthesis of thyroid hormones is iodine, which is taken up from blood by sodium-iodide symporters located on the outer plasma membrane of thyroid epithelial cells. Once inside the cell, iodide is transported into the follicular lumen presumably in part by the anion transporter pendrin, and oxidized by the membrane-bound enzyme TPO. This oxidation requires the presence of hydrogen peroxide, which is generated by DUOX2, an enzyme that requires a specific maturation factor dual oxidase 2A (DUOXA2). The biosynthesis of thyroid hormones is conducted by TPO, an integral membrane protein present in the apical (colloid-facing) plasma membrane of thyroid epithelial cells. TPO catalyzes two important reactions: the iodination of selected tyrosine residues (also known as organification of iodide) on Tg which serves as the matrix for thyroid hormone synthesis, producing monoiodotyrosine and diiodotyrosine, and the intramolecular coupling reaction of iodinated tyrosines from two monoiodotyrosine or diiodotyrosine, leading to the formation of either triiodothyronine (T_3) or thyroxine (T_4). Only a small fraction of iodotyrosines are used in this process. Through the action of TPO, thyroid hormones accumulate in colloid, on the surface of thyroid epithelial cells, but are still tied up with Tg. To release T_4 and T_3, thyroglobulin is engulfed by the thyrocytes through pinocytosis, digested in lysosomes, and then secreted into the bloodstream. In contrast, monoiodotyrosine and diiodotyrosine are found only in minute amounts in the bloodstream. The major form of thyroid hormone in the blood is thyroxine (T_4) (approximately 80%), which has a longer half life than T_3. The ratio of T_4 to T_3 released in the blood is roughly 20 to 1. T_4 is converted to the active T_3 (three to four times more potent than T_4) within cells by deiodinases (5'-iodinase).

The transportation and concentration of iodide within the thyroid gland are mediated through the sodium iodide symporter (NIS) located in the basolateral membrane of the thyroid follicular cell. NIS, a specialized plasma membrane glycoprotein with 13 transmembrane domains, belongs to the family of sodium-dependent cotransporters and has most sequence similarity with the human sodium/glucose cotransporter 1(26). NIS couples the inward translocation of two Na^+ down their electrochemical gradient to the simultaneous inward translocation of one I^- against its electrochemical gradient (35). The driving force for NIS activity is the Na^+ gradient generated by the Na^+/K^+ ATPase. Human *NIS* is located on chromosome 19, consists of 15 exons, and encodes a protein of 643 amino acids with a predicted molecular mass of 68.7 kDa (36, 37).Although NIS mutation is relatively rare, up to 12 mutations have been reported (V59E, G93R, R124H, ΔM143-Q323, Q267E, C272X, T354P, G395R, ΔA439-P443, frame-shift 515X, Y531X, and G543E) (38-40).

Tg is a large 660-kD glycoprotein synthesized by the thyroid gland. It functions as a matrix where thyroid hormones (T_4 and T_3) are produced from the coupling of iodotyrosyl residues, catalyzed by TPO (41). The human *TG* gene is 270 kb and contains an 8307 bp coding sequence divided into 48 exons. The preprotein is composed of a 19-amino acid signal peptide, followed by a 2749-residue polypeptide (42). To date, up to 50 different *TG* gene mutations have been identified (43). These mutations lead to varying degrees of hypothyroidism.

TPO is a thyroid-specific glycosylated hemoprotein of 110 kDa with a short trans-membrane domain that binds it to the apical membrane of the thyrocyte (44), with the catalytic part facing inside the follicle. It consists of 933 amino acids that are encoded by an mRNA of 3048 nucleotides (44). The *TPO* gene spans over 150 kb on the short arm of chromosome 2, locus 2p25, and consists of 17 exons (45). *TPO* gene mutations are one of the most common causes of thyroid dyshormonogenesis, with several different inactivating mutations being identified in patients with total iodide organification defects (46-49).

The thyroid oxidase 2 (THOX) gene, known as dual oxidase 2 (DUOX2) is located at the apical membrane of thyrocytes and is involved in the Ca^{2+}/reduced nicotinamide adenine dinucleotide phosphate-dependent generation of H_2O_2 (50, 51). In thyroid hormone synthesis, H_2O_2 is used as a substrate by TPO to catalyze both the iodination of tyrosine residues and incorporation of iodine into TG (52). *DUOX2* is located on chromosome 15 and consists of 33 exons encoding a mRNA of 6376 nucleotides long. The DUOX2 protein is a 1548-amino-acid polypeptide, including a 26-amino-acid signal peptide. Because defects in DUOX2 result in lack of H_2O_2, this protein is essential for thyroid hormone synthesis. Evidence for the involvement of DUOX2 in thyroid hormonogenesis came from the identification of naturally occurring mutations; biallelic homozygous or compound heterozygous *DUOX2* mutations lead to goitrous CH (29, 53, 54), whereas monoallelic nonsense defects cause transient CH (29, 31) although biallelic *DUOX2* mutations have also been reported recently in transient CH (55). Up to 23 DUOX2 mutations have been identified in patients with congenital hypothyroidism (29, 55-57). Recently, two novel genes, called DUOX maturation factors (*DUOXA1* and *DUOXA2*) were cloned (58). These genes are oriented head-to-head to the *DUOX* genes in the *DUOX1/DUOX2* intergenic region(58). The *DUOXA2* gene encodes an endoplasmic reticulum (ER) resident protein comprising five membrane-integral regions. *DUOXA2* mRNA is predominantly expressed in thyroid gland with lower levels in gastrointestinal epithelia, reminiscent of the expression profile of *DUOX2*. Whereas DUOX2 expressed in nonthyroidal cells is completely retained in the ER (59), coexpression of DUOXA2 rescues ER-to-Golgi transition, maturation, and translocation to the plasma membrane of functional DUOX2 (58). A genetic defect in DUOXA2 impairs expression of DUOX2, resulting in decreased H_2O_2 production by thyrocytes, and CH (30).

Pendred's syndrome (PS) is an autosomal recessive disease characterized by goitre without or with hypothyroidism, impaired iodide organification, and congenital sensorineural deafness(60), although studies on CH patients also show that a direct relation exists between the extent of hearing loss and the age at which treatment for CH was initiated (61). It is caused by biallelic mutations in the *SLC26A4* (solute carrier family 26, member 4), the PS gene (62), which contains an open reading frame of 2343 bp and encompasses 21 exons. The 780 amino acid transmembrane protein (pendrin) expressed in the thyroid gland, inner ear, endometrium, and kidney, where it is involved in iodide, chloride, formate, and nitrate transport (63). In the thyroid gland, pendrin acts at the apical pole of thyrocytes to transport intracellular iodide into the follicular lumen (64). Loss of pendrin function causes a failure in iodine supply and an organification defect often leading to euthyroid goitres (65). Because both TPO defects and PS may present with goitre, hypothyroidism, partial iodide organification defects, and a positive perchlorate test (31, 66), a definite etiologic diagnosis is impossible without molecular diagnosis.

Iodine is an essential component of thyroid hormone. To ensure that iodine is available for thyroid hormone biosynthesis, two highly specialized systems evolved in the thyroid gland. One accumulates iodide in thyroid cells by active membrane transport via the sodium-iodide symporter (67). The other recycles iodide through the deiodination of monoiodotyrosine and diiodotyrosine (but not T_4), the main iodinated by-products of thyroid hormone synthesis by thyroidal iodotyrosine dehalogenase (DEHAL1), a flavin mononucleotide-dependent enzyme(68). The gene is 36 kb and contains an 867 bp coding sequence divided into 5 exons and is located on chromosome 6 (6q24-25)(69-71). Mutation of the gene has been recently reported in patients with severe hypothyroidism (32).

5. Thyroid dysgenesis and the genes involved in the process

Thyroid dysgenesis is a defect in the organogenesis of the gland resulting in hypoplastic, ectopic or absent-thyroid gland and the underlying pathogenesis is largely unknown. Although the disorder is usually sporadic, a minority of cases are transmitted as Mendelian diseases (21-25, 72). Genes associated with thyroid gland dysgenesis include the TSH receptor in non-syndromic congenital hypothyroidism, $G_s\alpha$, and the thyroid transcription factors (TTF-1, TTF-2 or FOXE1, Pax-8, NKX2.1 and NKX2.5) (22, 24, 25, 73-75). The extrathyroid genes involved in the control of migration of the median thyroid bud during embryogenesis, such as adhesion molecules, and vascular factors involved in the stabilization of the bi-lobed structure of thyroid may also play a role (22).

6. Congenital hypothyroidism and thyroid cancer

Although rarely reported in the literature, malignant transformation from dyshormonogenic goitres is one of the most serious complications of CH. More than 20 cases of thyroid cancer have been reported in the literature with similar frequency of either papillary or follicular cancer type (Table1) (27). The most common genetic defects are *TG* mutation, resulting in dyshormonogenesis and CH. All the reported cases of thyroid carcinoma have long-standing congenital goitres and elevated thyroid stimulating hormone (TSH) (27, 76, 77), indicating that TSH plays a central role in the development and/or progression of thyroid carcinoma.

TSH is a well-known growth factor for thyroid epithelial cells, and can promote thyroid nodule formation and cancer progression (78). It has been suggested that constant and prolonged stimulation by TSH may result in the malignant transformation of thyroid follicular cells (76, 79), although a causal role for TSH in thyroid cancer initiation has not been conclusively demonstrated. In experimental studies, Morris *et al* found that prolonged exposure of transplanted thyroid tissue to excessive amounts of TSH in mice led to the development of malignant thyroid neoplasms with pulmonary metastases (79). Induction of papillary thyroid carcinoma following subtotal thyroidectomy has also been reported in rats (80). These data indicate that chronic TSH stimulation may be associated with thyroid cancer development. The significance of TSH in thyroid cancer initiation has recently been demonstrated in mice with a thyroid-specific knock-in of oncogenic $BRAF^{V600E}$, mutations of which are found in about 45% of papillary thyroid carcinomas (81). $BRAF^{V600E}$ -expressing thyroid follicular cells become transformed and progress to invasive carcinomas with a very short latency. These mice also develop hypothyroidism with high TSH levels due to deregulation of genes involved in thyroid hormone biosynthesis. However, $BRAF^{V600E}$ induced oncogenic transformation of thyroid follicular cells is lost when TSH receptor is knockout, indicating the dependence of TSH mediated cAMP signaling in $BRAF^{V600E}$ induced papillary thyroid carcinoma initiation (81). Although the study by Franco et al (81) provides experimental support for a strong association between TSH levels and thyroid cancer incidence, it remains to be determined whether long-term TSH stimulation alone can induce thyroid cancer. It is likely that mutations in oncogenes or tumor suppressor genes may be needed for tumor initiation apart from long-term TSH stimulation.

Brewer et al have demonstrated that the mammalian target of rapamycin (mTOR/S6K1) signaling pathway is also involved in the TSH mediated proliferative signals (82). mTOR/S6K1 signaling pathway is the key effector of phosphoinositide 3-kinase (PI3K) initiated proliferative signals in the thyroid follicular cells (83).Constitutive activation of PI3K signaling has been frequently found in thyroid cancers including those with aggressive clinical behaviors (84). However, genetic defect in the genes involved in this signalling pathway has not been investigated in thyroid cancers derived from dyshormonogenic goitres. Although less frequently, genetic defects in the MAPK/ERK signaling pathway have been reported, for example, *BRAF*V600E and K601E mutations in one PTC and one FTC cases, respectively (85) as well as abnormal p53 expression in one case of follicular carcinoma with anaplastic transformation (77).

For CH caused by thyroid dyshormonogenesis, thyroid goitre can develop and, in rare cases, thyroid cancer occurs from dyshormonogenic goitre. In our previous studies, we have reported two cases of metastatic thyroid carcinoma derived from congenital dyshormonogenic goitres (Figure 2) from two consanguineal families (27, 86). They presented with large recurrent goitres and hypothyroidism since childhood. They were non-compliant with L-thyroxine treatment and had multiple surgeries since childhood due to recurrence of dyshormonogenic goitres and pressure problems. One of them eventually developed a metastatic FTC and the other metastatic FVPTC. The underlying genetic defects in these two cases are germline *TG* mutation. Other genes involved in the different signalling pathways are investigated such as mutations in the *RAS, BRAF* or *P53,* and *PAX8/PPAR-γ* rearrangement. All come negative and it remains to be seen whether other genetic defects leading to malignant transformation can be detected such as mutations in the genes involved in the PI3K/Akt and mTOR/S6K1 pathways. These findings suggest that many CH cases in remote areas may not be adequately treated. It is unfortunate to see goitres and cancer development in these patients given that these complications can be easily prevented if proper L-thyroxine treatment is given. The health care cost for treating these complications, and physical and mental sufferings for the patients are huge as compared to L-thyroxine replacement therapy.

In summary, the serious detrimental effect of CH on the child's cognitive and motor development, which used to be a major feature of the disease, is now mostly prevented since the introduction of newborn screening program. However, inadequate treatment or poor compliant with treatment can lead to poor academic performance, and in severe cases, thyroid goitre and cancer. Education and close follow-up are warranted for patients with poor response to L-thyroxine replacement therapy. Adequate amounts of L-thyroxine treatment are essential to prevent cancer development.

Cases	Tumor	Major Genetic defects	Functional consequence	Other genetic defects
1.	FTC	g.279 del T in *PDS* (77)	Truncated pendrin	abnormal p53 expression
2.	FTC	g.2505_2506 ins C in *TPO* (87)	Truncated TPO	
3.	FTC	g.IVS5+1G>A in *TG*(27)	Truncated Tg	
4.	PTC	p.C1245R in *TG* (85)	Impaired intracellular Tg transport	
5.	PTC	p.C1245R in *TG* (85)	Impaired intracellular Tg transport	

Cases	Tumor	Major Genetic defects	Functional consequence	Other genetic defects
6.	PTC	p.C1245R/G2356R in *TG* (85)	Impaired intracellular Tg transport	
7.	FTC	p.C1977S in *TG* (85)	Impaired intracellular Tg transport	BRAF K601E mutation
8.	PTC	p.C1977S in *TG* (85)	Impaired intracellular Tg transport	
9.	PTC	p.C1958S in *TG* (85)	unknown	BRAF V600E mutation
10.	PTC	p.C1958S in *TG* (85)	unknown	
11.	FVPTC	p.R2223H in *TG* (88)	Impaired intracellular Tg transport	
12.	FTC	unknown (76)	unknown	
13.	FTC	unknown(76)	unknown	
14.	PTC	unknown(89)	unknown	
15.	PTC	unknown(90)	unknown	
16.	PTC	unknown(91)	unknown	

Note:

1. Cooper et al reported a large kindred of patients with congenital goitre, in which two siblings developed metastatic follicular thyroid carcinoma and a leak of nonhormonal iodide from the thyroid. However, the underlyning genetic defect is unknown (76).
2. Medeiros-Neto and Stanbury reviewed 109 patients with dyshormonogenesis, 15 patients had thyroid follicular cancer with unknown genetic defects (92). Based on rigid criteria of malignancy such as vascular invasion, 8 of the 15 reported cases in the literature appear to be clear examples of thyroid malignancy. Five of them had bone or lung metastases (87).

PDS: Pendred's syndrome; PTC: papillary thyroid carcinoma; FTC: follicular thyroid carcinoma; FVPTC: follicular variant of papillary thyroid carcinoma

Table 1. Thyroid cancer cases developing from dyshormonogenic goitre.

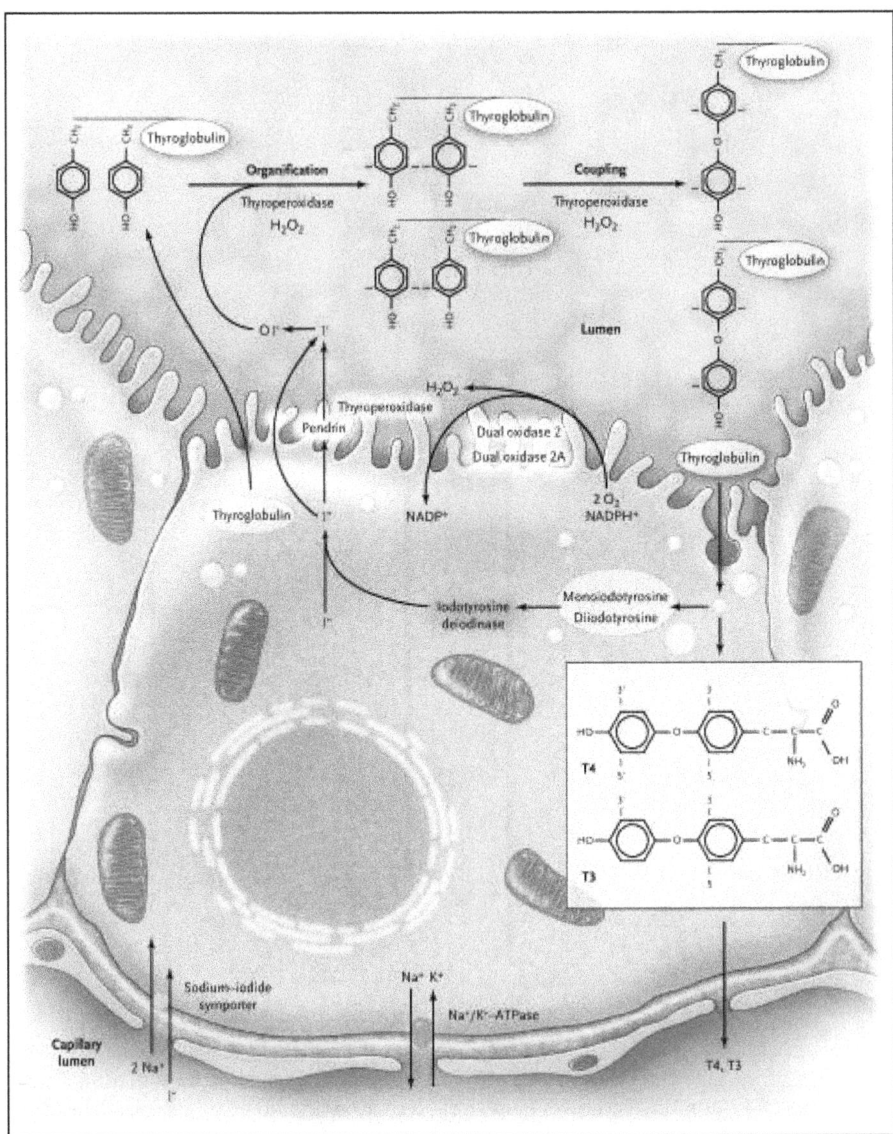

Fig. 1. **Key Steps in Thyroid Hormone Synthesis.** Monoiodotyrosine and diiodotyrosine are synthesized from the iodination of tyrosyl residues within thyroglobulin. After organification, iodinated donor and acceptor iodotyrosines are fused in the coupling reaction to form either triiodothyronine (T_3) or thyroxine (T_4), a process that involves only a small fraction of iodotyrosines. Thyroglobulin is then engulfed by thyrocytes through pinocytosis and digested in lysosomes, and T_4 and T_3 are secreted into the bloodstream. Monoiodotyrosine and diiodotyrosine are deiodinated by iodotyrosine deiodinase, and the released iodide is recycled (68).

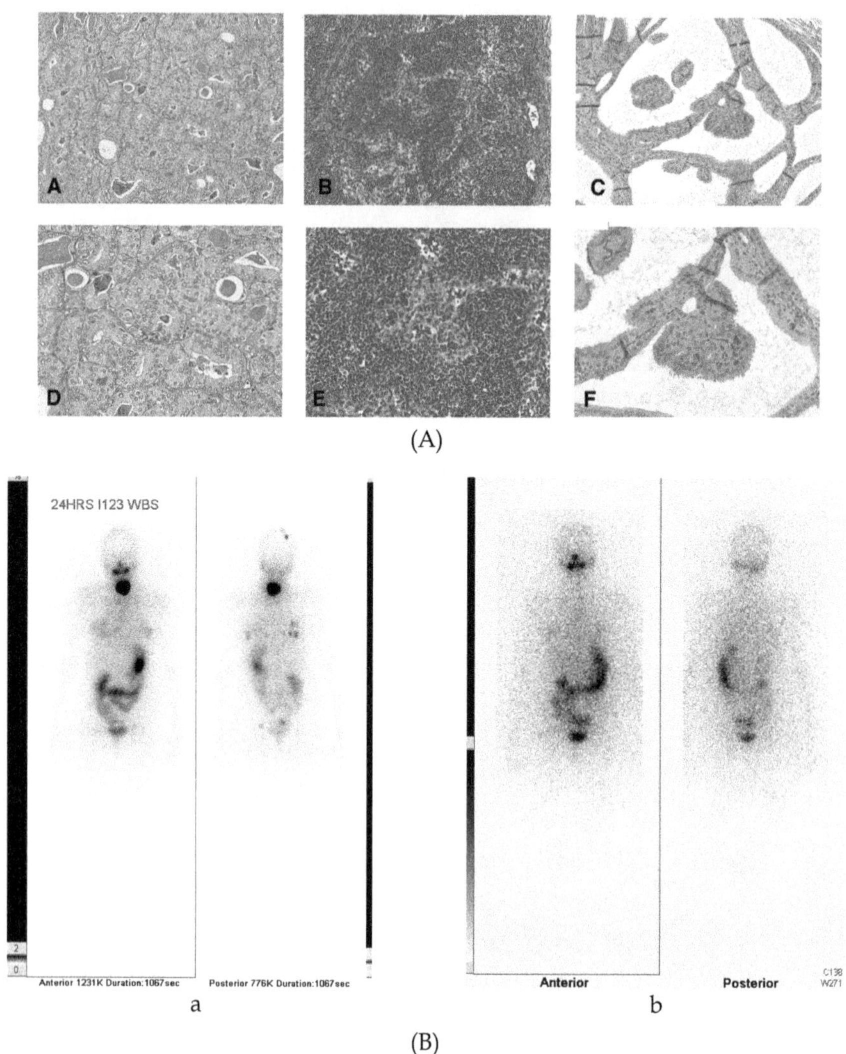

Fig. 2. Follicular variant of PTC (FVPTC) derived from thyroid dyshormonogenesis due to biallelic p.R2223H mutation in the *TG* gene. (A) Hematoxylin and eosin staining shows FVPTC with oncocytic features (A, x20; D, x40); Lymph note metastases were also observed (B, x 20; E, x 40). The non-tumor area shows hyperplastic thyroid micro-and macro-follicles without colloid, and cytological atypia, which are consistent with dyshormonogenesis (C, x20; F, x40). (B) Diagnostic 24 h I ^{123} whole body scan. The scan was performed 24 h following the oral administration of 74 MBq (2 mCi) of I ^{123}. Whole body images were acquired in anterior and posterior projections before I ^{131} ablation. The scan showed large neck uptake and multiple foci in the chest, skull, and pelvis suggestive of lung and bone metastasis (a). The patient received a therapeutic dose of radioactive iodine I ^{131} of 3,831.35 MBq (103.55 mCi). Six month later, a follow-up scan showed complete resolution of the neck, lung and bone uptakes (b).

7. References

[1] Kopp P 2002 Perspective: genetic defects in the etiology of congenital hypothyroidism. Endocrinology 143:2019-24.
[2] Moltz KC, Postellon DC 1994 Congenital hypothyroidism and mental development. Compr Ther 20:342-6
[3] Peter F, Muzsnai A 2009 Congenital disorders of the thyroid: hypo/hyper. Endocrinol Metab Clin North Am 38:491-507
[4] Lorey FW, Cunningham GC 1992 Birth prevalence of primary congenital hypothyroidism by sex and ethnicity. Hum Biol 64:531-8
[5] Buyukgebiz A 2003 Congenital hypothyroidism clinical aspects and late consequences. Pediatr Endocrinol Rev 1 Suppl 2:185-90; discussion 190
[6] LaFranchi SH, Austin J 2007 How should we be treating children with congenital hypothyroidism? J Pediatr Endocrinol Metab 20:559-78
[7] Gruters A, Krude H 2007 Update on the management of congenital hypothyroidism. Horm Res 68 Suppl 5:107-11
[8] Arenz S, Nennstiel-Ratzel U, Wildner M, Dorr HG, von Kries R 2008 Intellectual outcome, motor skills and BMI of children with congenital hypothyroidism: a population-based study. Acta Paediatr 97:447-50
[9] Glorieux J, Dussault J, Van Vliet G 1992 Intellectual development at age 12 years of children with congenital hypothyroidism diagnosed by neonatal screening. J Pediatr 121:581-4
[10] Salerno M, Militerni R, Di Maio S, Bravaccio C, Gasparini N, Tenore A 1999 Intellectual outcome at 12 years of age in congenital hypothyroidism. Eur J Endocrinol 141:105-10
[11] Al-Jurayyan NA, Al-Nuaim AA, Redha MA, El-Desouki MI, Al Herbish AS, Abo Bakr AM, Al Swailem AA, Al Mazrou YY, Al Deress A 1996 Neonatal screening for congenital hypothyroidism in Riyadh: Analysis of six year's experience. Ann Saudi Med 16:20-3
[12] Al-Jurayyan NA, Al-Herbish AS, El-Desouki MI, Al-Nuaim AA, Abo-Bakr AM, Al-Husain MA 1997 Congenital anomalies in infants with congenital hypothyroidism: is it a coincidental or an associated finding? Hum Hered 47:33-7
[13] Henry G, Sobki SH, Othman JM 2002 Screening for congenital hypothyroidism. Saudi Med J 23:529-35
[14] Majeed-Saidan MA, Joyce B, Khan M, Hamam HD 1993 Congenital hypothyroidism: the Riyadh Military Hospital experience. Clin Endocrinol (Oxf) 38:191-5
[15] Ogunkeye OO, Roluga AI, Khan FA 2008 Resetting the detection level of cord blood thyroid stimulating hormone (TSH) for the diagnosis of congenital hypothyroidism. J Trop Pediatr 54:74-7
[16] al-Jurayyan NA, Shaheen FI, al-Nuaim AA, el-Desouki MI, Faiz A, al Herbish AS, Bakr AM, al-Swailem AA, al Mazrou YY 1996 Congenital hypothyroidism: increased incidence in Najran province, Saudi Arabia. J Trop Pediatr 42:348-51
[17] Al-Maghamsi MS, Al-Hawsawi ZM, Ghulam GN, Okasha AM 2002 Screening for congenital hypothyroidism in North-West region of Saudi Arabia. Saudi Med J 23:1518-21
[18] Narchi HH, Kulaylat NA 1996 Congenital hypothyroidism screening program: A five-year experience at Saudi ARAMCO Al Hasa Health Center. Ann Saudi Med 16:47-9

[19] Afifi AM, Abdul-Jabbar MA 2007 Saudi newborn screening. A national public health program: needs, costs, and challenges. Saudi Med J 28:1167-70
[20] De Felice M, Di Lauro R 2004 Thyroid development and its disorders: genetics and molecular mechanisms. Endocr Rev 25:722-46
[21] Topaloglu AK 2006 Athyreosis, dysgenesis, and dyshormonogenesis in congenital hypothyroidism. Pediatr Endocrinol Rev 3 Suppl 3:498-502
[22] Deladoey J, Vassart G, Van Vliet G 2007 Possible non-Mendelian mechanisms of thyroid dysgenesis. Endocr Dev 10:29-42
[23] Castanet M, Lyonnet S, Bonaiti-Pellie C, Polak M, Czernichow P, Leger J 2000 Familial forms of thyroid dysgenesis among infants with congenital hypothyroidism. N Engl J Med 343:441-2
[24] Castanet M, Polak M, Leger J 2007 Familial forms of thyroid dysgenesis. Endocr Dev 10:15-28
[25] Park SM, Chatterjee VK 2005 Genetics of congenital hypothyroidism. J Med Genet 42:379-89
[26] Pohlenz J, Rosenthal IM, Weiss RE, Jhiang SM, Burant C, Refetoff S 1998 Congenital hypothyroidism due to mutations in the sodium/iodide symporter. Identification of a nonsense mutation producing a downstream cryptic 3' splice site. J Clin Invest 101:1028-35.
[27] Alzahrani AS, Baitei EY, Zou M, Shi Y 2006 Clinical case seminar: metastatic follicular thyroid carcinoma arising from congenital goiter as a result of a novel splice donor site mutation in the thyroglobulin gene. J Clin Endocrinol Metab 91:740-6
[28] Bikker H, den Hartog MT, Baas F, Gons MH, Vulsma T, de Vijlder JJ 1994 A 20-basepair duplication in the human thyroid peroxidase gene results in a total iodide organification defect and congenital hypothyroidism. J Clin Endocrinol Metab 79:248-52.
[29] Moreno JC, Bikker H, Kempers MJ, van Trotsenburg AS, Baas F, de Vijlder JJ, Vulsma T, Ris-Stalpers C 2002 Inactivating mutations in the gene for thyroid oxidase 2 (THOX2) and congenital hypothyroidism. N Engl J Med 347:95-102.
[30] Zamproni I, Grasberger H, Cortinovis F, Vigone MC, Chiumello G, Mora S, Onigata K, Fugazzola L, Refetoff S, Persani L, Weber G 2008 Biallelic inactivation of the dual oxidase maturation factor 2 (DUOXA2) gene as a novel cause of congenital hypothyroidism. J Clin Endocrinol Metab 93:605-10
[31] Pfarr N, Borck G, Turk A, Napiontek U, Keilmann A, Muller-Forell W, Kopp P, Pohlenz J 2006 Goitrous congenital hypothyroidism and hearing impairment associated with mutations in the TPO and SLC26A4/PDS genes. J Clin Endocrinol Metab 91:2678-81
[32] Moreno JC, Klootwijk W, van Toor H, Pinto G, D'Alessandro M, Leger A, Goudie D, Polak M, Gruters A, Visser TJ 2008 Mutations in the iodotyrosine deiodinase gene and hypothyroidism. N Engl J Med 358:1811-8
[33] Van Herle AJ, Vassart G, Dumont JE 1979 Control of thyroglobulin synthesis and secretion. (First of two parts). N Engl J Med 301:239-49
[34] Van Herle AJ, Vassart G, Dumont JE 1979 Control of thyroglobulin synthesis and secretion (second of two parts). N Engl J Med 301:307-14
[35] Eskandari S, Loo DD, Dai G, Levy O, Wright EM, Carrasco N 1997 Thyroid Na+/I- symporter. Mechanism, stoichiometry, and specificity. J Biol Chem 272:27230-8

[36] Smanik PA, Liu Q, Furminger TL, Ryu K, Xing S, Mazzaferri EL, Jhiang SM 1996 Cloning of the human sodium lodide symporter. Biochem Biophys Res Commun 226:339-45

[37] Smanik PA, Ryu KY, Theil KS, Mazzaferri EL, Jhiang SM 1997 Expression, exon-intron organization, and chromosome mapping of the human sodium iodide symporter. Endocrinology 138:3555-8

[38] Pohlenz J, Refetoff S 1999 Mutations in the sodium/iodide symporter (NIS) gene as a cause for iodide transport defects and congenital hypothyroidism. Biochimie 81:469-76

[39] Szinnai G, Kosugi S, Derrien C, Lucidarme N, David V, Czernichow P, Polak M 2006 Extending the clinical heterogeneity of iodide transport defect (ITD): a novel mutation R124H of the sodium/iodide symporter gene and review of genotype-phenotype correlations in ITD. J Clin Endocrinol Metab 91:1199-204

[40] Reed-Tsur MD, De la Vieja A, Ginter CS, Carrasco N 2008 Molecular characterization of V59E NIS, a Na+/I- symporter mutant that causes congenital I- transport defect. Endocrinology 149:3077-84

[41] Medeiros-Neto G, Targovnik HM, Vassart G 1993 Defective thyroglobulin synthesis and secretion causing goiter and hypothyroidism. Endocr Rev 14:165-83.

[42] van de Graaf SA, Ris-Stalpers C, Pauws E, Mendive FM, Targovnik HM, de Vijlder JJ 2001 Up to date with human thyroglobulin. J Endocrinol 170:307-21.

[43] Niu DM, Hsu JH, Chong KW, Huang CH, Lu YH, Kao CH, Yu HC, Lo MY, Jap TS 2009 Six New Mutations of the Thyroglobulin Gene Discovered in Taiwanese Children Presenting with Thyroid Dyshormonogenesis. J Clin Endocrinol Metab

[44] Kimura S, Kotani T, McBride OW, Umeki K, Hirai K, Nakayama T, Ohtaki S 1987 Human thyroid peroxidase: complete cDNA and protein sequence, chromosome mapping, and identification of two alternately spliced mRNAs. Proc Natl Acad Sci U S A 84:5555-9

[45] Kimura S, Hong YS, Kotani T, Ohtaki S, Kikkawa F 1989 Structure of the human thyroid peroxidase gene: comparison and relationship to the human myeloperoxidase gene. Biochemistry 28:4481-9

[46] Bakker B, Bikker H, Vulsma T, de Randamie JS, Wiedijk BM, De Vijlder JJ 2000 Two decades of screening for congenital hypothyroidism in The Netherlands: TPO gene mutations in total iodide organification defects (an update). J Clin Endocrinol Metab 85:3708-12

[47] Niu DM, Hwang B, Chu YK, Liao CJ, Wang PL, Lin CY 2002 High prevalence of a novel mutation (2268 insT) of the thyroid peroxidase gene in Taiwanese patients with total iodide organification defect, and evidence for a founder effect. J Clin Endocrinol Metab 87:4208-12

[48] Pannain S, Weiss RE, Jackson CE, Dian D, Beck JC, Sheffield VC, Cox N, Refetoff S 1999 Two different mutations in the thyroid peroxidase gene of a large inbred Amish kindred: power and limits of homozygosity mapping. J Clin Endocrinol Metab 84:1061-71

[49] Avbelj M, Tahirovic H, Debeljak M, Kusekova M, Toromanovic A, Krzisnik C, Battelino T 2007 High prevalence of thyroid peroxidase gene mutations in patients with thyroid dyshormonogenesis. Eur J Endocrinol 156:511-9

[50] Dupuy C, Ohayon R, Valent A, Noel-Hudson MS, Deme D, Virion A 1999 Purification of a novel flavoprotein involved in the thyroid NADPH oxidase. Cloning of the porcine and human cdnas. J Biol Chem 274:37265-9

[51] De Deken X, Wang D, Many MC, Costagliola S, Libert F, Vassart G, Dumont JE, Miot F 2000 Cloning of two human thyroid cDNAs encoding new members of the NADPH oxidase family. J Biol Chem 275:23227-33

[52] Corvilain B, van Sande J, Laurent E, Dumont JE 1991 The H2O2-generating system modulates protein iodination and the activity of the pentose phosphate pathway in dog thyroid. Endocrinology 128:779-85

[53] Vigone MC, Fugazzola L, Zamproni I, Passoni A, Di Candia S, Chiumello G, Persani L, Weber G 2005 Persistent mild hypothyroidism associated with novel sequence variants of the DUOX2 gene in two siblings. Hum Mutat 26:395

[54] Varela V, Rivolta CM, Esperante SA, Gruneiro-Papendieck L, Chiesa A, Targovnik HM 2006 Three mutations (p.Q36H, p.G418fsX482, and g.IVS19-2A>C) in the dual oxidase 2 gene responsible for congenital goiter and iodide organification defect. Clin Chem 52:182-91

[55] Maruo Y, Takahashi H, Soeda I, Nishikura N, Matsui K, Ota Y, Mimura Y, Mori A, Sato H, Takeuchi Y 2008 Transient congenital hypothyroidism caused by biallelic mutations of the dual oxidase 2 gene in Japanese patients detected by a neonatal screening program. J Clin Endocrinol Metab 93:4261-7

[56] Moreno JC, Visser TJ 2007 New phenotypes in thyroid dyshormonogenesis: hypothyroidism due to DUOX2 mutations. Endocr Dev 10:99-117

[57] Pfarr N, Korsch E, Kaspers S, Herbst A, Stach A, Zimmer C, Pohlenz J 2006 Congenital hypothyroidism caused by new mutations in the thyroid oxidase 2 (THOX2) gene. Clin Endocrinol (Oxf) 65:810-5

[58] Grasberger H, Refetoff S 2006 Identification of the maturation factor for dual oxidase. Evolution of an eukaryotic operon equivalent. J Biol Chem 281:18269-72

[59] De Deken X, Wang D, Dumont JE, Miot F 2002 Characterization of ThOX proteins as components of the thyroid H(2)O(2)-generating system. Exp Cell Res 273:187-96

[60] Kopp P 2000 Pendred's syndrome and genetic defects in thyroid hormone synthesis. Rev Endocr Metab Disord 1:109-21

[61] Wasniewska M, De Luca F, Siclari S, Salzano G, Messina MF, Lombardo F, Valenzise M, Ruggeri C, Arrigo T 2002 Hearing loss in congenital hypothalamic hypothyroidism: a wide therapeutic window. Hear Res 172:87-91

[62] Everett LA, Glaser B, Beck JC, Idol JR, Buchs A, Heyman M, Adawi F, Hazani E, Nassir E, Baxevanis AD, Sheffield VC, Green ED 1997 Pendred syndrome is caused by mutations in a putative sulphate transporter gene (PDS). Nat Genet 17:411-22

[63] Everett LA, Belyantseva IA, Noben-Trauth K, Cantos R, Chen A, Thakkar SI, Hoogstraten-Miller SL, Kachar B, Wu DK, Green ED 2001 Targeted disruption of mouse Pds provides insight about the inner-ear defects encountered in Pendred syndrome. Hum Mol Genet 10:153-61

[64] Royaux IE, Suzuki K, Mori A, Katoh R, Everett LA, Kohn LD, Green ED 2000 Pendrin, the protein encoded by the Pendred syndrome gene (PDS), is an apical porter of iodide in the thyroid and is regulated by thyroglobulin in FRTL-5 cells. Endocrinology 141:839-45

[65] Blons H, Feldmann D, Duval V, Messaz O, Denoyelle F, Loundon N, Sergout-Allaoui A, Houang M, Duriez F, Lacombe D, Delobel B, Leman J, Catros H, Journel H, Drouin-Garraud V, Obstoy MF, Toutain A, Oden S, Toublanc JE, Couderc R, Petit C, Garabedian EN, Marlin S 2004 Screening of SLC26A4 (PDS) gene in Pendred's syndrome: a large spectrum of mutations in France and phenotypic heterogeneity. Clin Genet 66:333-40

[66] Gausden E, Armour JA, Coyle B, Coffey R, Hochberg Z, Pembrey M, Britton KE, Grossman A, Reardon W, Trembath R 1996 Thyroid peroxidase: evidence for disease gene exclusion in Pendred's syndrome. Clin Endocrinol (Oxf) 44:441-6

[67] Dai G, Levy O, Carrasco N 1996 Cloning and characterization of the thyroid iodide transporter. Nature 379:458-60

[68] Kopp PA 2008 Reduce, recycle, reuse--iodotyrosine deiodinase in thyroid iodide metabolism. N Engl J Med 358:1856-9

[69] Moreno JC, Pauws E, van Kampen AH, Jedlickova M, de Vijlder JJ, Ris-Stalpers C 2001 Cloning of tissue-specific genes using serial analysis of gene expression and a novel computational substraction approach. Genomics 75:70-6

[70] Gnidehou S, Caillou B, Talbot M, Ohayon R, Kaniewski J, Noel-Hudson MS, Morand S, Agnangji D, Sezan A, Courtin F, Virion A, Dupuy C 2004 Iodotyrosine dehalogenase 1 (DEHAL1) is a transmembrane protein involved in the recycling of iodide close to the thyroglobulin iodination site. Faseb J 18:1574-6

[71] Moreno JC 2003 Identification of novel genes involved in congenital hypothyroidism using serial analysis of gene expression. Horm Res 60 Suppl 3:96-102

[72] Montanelli L, Tonacchera M 2010 Genetics and phenomics of hypothyroidism and thyroid dys- and agenesis due to PAX8 and TTF1 mutations. Mol Cell Endocrinol 322:64-71

[73] Vilain C, Rydlewski C, Duprez L, Heinrichs C, Abramowicz M, Malvaux P, Renneboog B, Parma J, Costagliola S, Vassart G 2001 Autosomal dominant transmission of congenital thyroid hypoplasia due to loss-of-function mutation of PAX8. J Clin Endocrinol Metab 86:234-8

[74] Meeus L, Gilbert B, Rydlewski C, Parma J, Roussie AL, Abramowicz M, Vilain C, Christophe D, Costagliola S, Vassart G 2004 Characterization of a novel loss of function mutation of PAX8 in a familial case of congenital hypothyroidism with in-place, normal-sized thyroid. J Clin Endocrinol Metab 89:4285-91

[75] Moya CM, Perez de Nanclares G, Castano L, Potau N, Bilbao JR, Carrascosa A, Bargada M, Coya R, Martul P, Vicens-Calvet E, Santisteban P 2006 Functional study of a novel single deletion in the TITF1/NKX2.1 homeobox gene that produces congenital hypothyroidism and benign chorea but not pulmonary distress. J Clin Endocrinol Metab 91:1832-41

[76] Cooper DS, Axelrod L, DeGroot LJ, Vickery AL, Jr., Maloof F 1981 Congenital goiter and the development of metastatic follicular carcinoma with evidence for a leak of nonhormonal iodide: clinical, pathological, kinetic, and biochemical studies and a review of the literature. J Clin Endocrinol Metab 52:294-306.

[77] Camargo R, Limbert E, Gillam M, Henriques MM, Fernandes C, Catarino AL, Soares J, Alves VA, Kopp P, Medeiros-Neto G 2001 Aggressive metastatic follicular thyroid carcinoma with anaplastic transformation arising from a long-standing goiter in a patient with Pendred's syndrome. Thyroid 11:981-8.

[78] Boelaert K 2009 The association between serum TSH concentration and thyroid cancer. Endocr Relat Cancer

[79] Morris HP, Dalton AJ, Green CD 1951 Malignant thyroid tumors occurring in the mouse after prolonged hormonal imbalance during the ingestion of thiouracil. J Clin Endocrinol Metab 11:1281-95.

[80] Goldberg RC, Lindsay S, Nichols CW, Jr., Chaikoff IL 1964 Induction of Neoplasms in Thyroid Glands of Rats by Subtotal Thyroidectomy and by the Injection of One Microcurie of I-131. Cancer Res 24:35-43

[81] Franco AT, Malaguarnera R, Refetoff S, Liao XH, Lundsmith E, Kimura S, Pritchard C, Marais R, Davies TF, Weinstein LS, Chen M, Rosen N, Ghossein R, Knauf JA, Fagin JA 2011 Thyrotrophin receptor signaling dependence of Braf-induced thyroid tumor initiation in mice. Proc Natl Acad Sci U S A 108:1615-20

[82] Brewer C, Yeager N, Di Cristofano A 2007 Thyroid-stimulating hormone initiated proliferative signals converge in vivo on the mTOR kinase without activating AKT. Cancer Res 67:8002-6

[83] Yeager N, Brewer C, Cai KQ, Xu XX, Di Cristofano A 2008 Mammalian target of rapamycin is the key effector of phosphatidylinositol-3-OH-initiated proliferative signals in the thyroid follicular epithelium. Cancer Res 68:444-9

[84] Saji M, Ringel MD 2010 The PI3K-Akt-mTOR pathway in initiation and progression of thyroid tumors. Mol Cell Endocrinol 321:20-8

[85] Hishinuma A, Fukata S, Kakudo K, Murata Y, Ieiri T 2005 High incidence of thyroid cancer in long-standing goiters with thyroglobulin mutations. Thyroid 15:1079-84.

[86] Raef H, Al-Rijjal R, Al-Shehri S, Zou M, Al-Mana H, Baitei EY, Parhar RS, Al-Mohanna FA, Shi Y 2010 Biallelic p.R2223H Mutation in the Thyroglobulin Gene Causes Thyroglobulin Retention and Severe Hypothyroidism with Subsequent Development of Thyroid Carcinoma. J Clin Endocrinol Metab 95:1000-6

[87] Medeiros-Neto G, Gil-Da-Costa MJ, Santos CL, Medina AM, Silva JC, Tsou RM, Sobrinho-Simoes M 1998 Metastatic thyroid carcinoma arising from congenital goiter due to mutation in the thyroperoxidase gene. J Clin Endocrinol Metab 83:4162-6.

[88] Raef H, Al-Rijjal R, Al-Shehri S, Zou M, Al-Mana H, Baitei EY, Parhar RS, Al-Mohanna FA, Shi Y 2010 Biallelic p.R2223H Mutation in the Thyroglobulin Gene Causes Thyroglobulin Retention and Severe Hypothyroidism with Subsequent Development of Thyroid Carcinoma. J Clin Endocrinol Metab

[89] Kallel R, Mnif Hachicha L, Mnif M, Hammami B, Ayadi L, Bahri I, Ghorbel A, Abid M, Makni S, Boudawara T 2009 [Papillary carcinoma arising from dyshormonogenetic goiter]. Ann Endocrinol (Paris) 70:485-8

[90] Drut R, Moreno A 2009 Papillary carcinoma of the thyroid developed in congenital dyshormonogenetic hypothyroidism without goiter: Diagnosis by FNAB. Diagn Cytopathol 37:707-9

[91] Yashiro T, Ito K, Akiba M, Kanaji Y, Obara T, Fujimoto Y, Hirayama A, Nakajima H 1987 Papillary carcinoma of the thyroid arising from dyshormonogenetic goiter. Endocrinol Jpn 34:955-64

[92] Medeiros-Neto G SJ 1994 Thyroid malignancy and dyshormonogenetic goiter. CRC Press, Boca Raton

13

Congenital Hypothyroidism due to Thyroid Dysgenesis: From Epidemiology to Molecular Mechanisms

Johnny Deladoey
CHU Sainte-Justine, University of Montreal
Canada

1. Introduction

1.1 Etiology of CH (Dyshormonogenesis / Dysgenesis)

1.1.1 Dyshormonogenesis

Thyroid dyshormonogenesis results from a defect in any one of the steps involved in the biosynthesis of thyroid hormone, from the transport of iodine across the apical membrane to its intracellular recycling from mono- and di-iodotyrosines. These defects are inherited as autosomal recessive traits and occur at higher frequency in consanguineous families. In population-based studies, mutations inactivating the thyroperoxidase gene (*TPO*)[1-4] and the dual oxidase-like domains 2 gene (*DUOX2*; see www.endocrine-abstracts.org/ea/0020/ea0020s14.2.htm) seem to be the most commonly involved.

1.1.2 Congenital Hypothyroidism from Thyroid Dysgenesis (CHTD) – The most frequent form

Congenital hypothyroidism from thyroid dysgenesis (CHTD) is a common disorder with a birth prevalence of 1 case in 4,000 live births [5]. CHTD is the consequence of a failure of the thyroid to migrate to its anatomical location (anterior part of the neck), which results in thyroid ectopy (lingual or sub-lingual) or of a complete absence of thyroid (athyreosis). The most common diagnostic category is thyroid ectopy (up to 80%). The majority of CHTD cases has no known cause, but is associated with a severe deficiency in thyroid hormones (hypothyroidism), which can lead to severe mental retardation if left untreated. Therefore, CHTD is detected by biochemical screening at 2 days of life, which enables initiation of thyroid hormone therapy during the second week of life. Even with early treatment (on average at 9 d), developmental delay may still be observed in severe cases (i.e., IQ loss of 10 points)[6].

CHTD is predominantly non-syndromic and sporadic (i.e. 98% of cases are non-familial), has a discordance rate of 92% in MZ twins, and has a female and ethnic (i.e., Caucasian) predominance [7, 8]. Moreover, germinal mutations in thyroid related transcription factors NKX2.1, FOXE1, PAX-8, and NKX2.5 have been identified in only 3% of patients with sporadic CHTD [9] and linkage analysis excluded these genes in some multiplex families with

CHTD [9]. Recent works have shown that (i) ectopic thyroids show a differential gene expression compared to that of normal thyroids (with enrichment for the Wnt signaling pathway)[10] and (ii) cases of CHTD are associated with rare CNVs [11].

1.2 Thyroid embryology

In all vertebrates, the developing thyroid is first visible as a thickening of the endodermal epithelium emerging at the most anterior part of the foregut, named *foramen caecum* in humans. This structure, the median thyroid anlage, is evident by E8-8.5 day in mice, 24 hpf in zebrafish and by E20-22 day in humans [12]. At this time, primitive thyroid cells already have a distinct molecular signature, with co-expression of four transcription factors *Hhex, Tift1, Pax8* and *Foxe1* [12]. Thereafter, the primitive thyroid moves progressively to reach its final location by the seventh week in humans (see **Table 1** below for comparison between species).

Species	Specification	Budding	Migration	Follicle formation
Human [12]	E20-22	E24	E25-50	E70
Mouse [13]	E8.5	E10	E10.5-13.5	E15.5
Zebrafish [14, 15]	24 hpf	36-46 hpf	48-55 hpf	55 hpf

E, embryonic day; **hpf**, hours post-fertilization.

Table 1. Timing of key morphogenic events during thyroid development in different species (adapted from [13]).

2. Epidemiology of CH

2.1 Basics

Permanent primary congenital hypothyroidism is the most common form of congenital hypothyroidism, and is in fact the most common congenital endocrine disorder: estimates of its prevalence depend on the screening methods, algorithms and cut-offs used but average 1 in 2,500 newborn infants [16-18]. Two thirds of the cases are due to thyroid dysgenesis (thyroid ectopy, athyreosis and thyroid hypoplasia) with a prevalence of 1 in 4,000 newborn infants, which has remained stable over the last 20 years in our jurisdiction[17] and which is not influenced by seasonal factors [5]. Ten to fifteen percent are due to recessively inherited defects in hormone synthesis resulting in goiter (birth prevalence of 1:30,000), while a growing number of cases, as a consequence of lower TSH cut-offs, are due to mild functional disorders with a normal thyroid gland *in situ* (15-20%, birth prevalence of 1:20,000 to 1:15,000)[17].

2.2 Controversies about neonatal screening program for CH

While screening for CH is an unqualified public-health success [19], a number of controversies mark the almost four decades since it was first implemented. All these controversies have three points in common: (a) the biochemical identification of CH and the lack of agreement on the cutoffs used to detect CH [16], (b) whether there is a correlation between neonatal TSH and T_4 values and later mental development [20, 21], and (c) the fact that CH encompasses a variety of different thyroid etiologies (dysgenesis, dyshormogenesis with goiter, normal-size gland *in situ*) [12]. Consequently, a uniform definition of CH is difficult considering the spectrum of pathologies and the continuous nature of the distribution of TSH levels [22, 23].

2.2.1 Which biochemical test to use for neonatal CH screening?

The first controversy was about the nature of the biochemical test to use for neonatal CH screening. For technical reasons related to the precision of the measurements around the cutoff values, Dussault and Laberge had initially developed a screening program based on total T_4 as the primary measurement [24]. However, because primary CH is at least 10-fold more common than central hypothyroidism, TSH is the most logical analyte to measure [25]. Technical improvements leading to accurate TSH measurements on eluates of blood collected on dried spots have led to the adoption of TSH-based screening by an increasing number of jurisdictions, including Québec since 1987.

2.2.2 Should there be specific guidelines for screening for CH in premature and/or (very) low birth weight newborns?

A second controversy relates to whether there should be specific guidelines for screening for CH in premature and/or (very) low birth weight ((V)LBW) newborns. These newborns generally have low T_4 with normal TSH, a condition that has been named hypothyroxinemia of prematurity for which there is at present no evidence that it should be screened for or treated [26]. By contrast, transient primary CH has been convincingly shown to be more frequent in premature newborns only in areas with a borderline low iodine intake [27] and attributed in large part to the use of iodine-containing disinfectants [28]. However, permanent CH from dysgenesis or dyshormonogenesis is not more frequent in premature newborns. On the contrary, it tends to be associated with prolonged gestation [29] and with a skewing of the birth weight distribution to the right [30]. Nevertheless, the New England CH Cooperative reported in 2003 that a 'delayed TSH rise' occurred more often in VLBW newborns and suggested that a second sample be systematically obtained; scintigraphic scans to determine the possible cause of this delayed-onset hyperthyrotropinemia were not performed [31] and a recent update on a subset of these VLBW newborns has shown that the problem was transient, with no evidence of benefit from treatment [32]. Other studies showed that lowering the TSH cutoff on the first blood sample increased the number of preterm infants labeled as having CH [33-35]. Our previous study did not support the need for a specific protocol for low birth weight infants [36] and our more recent one confirms that the incidence of CH in LBW newborns has remained stable in spite of the decreased cutoff on the repeat screening specimen [17]. Additionally, we have not identified a single patient with trisomy 21 and CH at screening. This is consistent with the observations of van Trotsenburg *et al.* [37] that the rightward shift of the distribution of neonatal screening TSH is minimal (95% confidence intervals: 4.8-7.6 *vs* 3-3.1 mU/L in controls) and insufficient to result in these patients being identified as having CH with our screening algorithm.

2.2.3 Is CH incidence increasing?

The last controversy arose from the reported increase in global incidence of CH in the United States [38]. The cause of this increase is difficult to ascertain for the following reasons: (a) CH is a spectrum of different disorders which have only an elevated TSH in common, (b) newborn screening practices vary between jurisdictions, even within the same country, as does the documentation of the etiology or of the transient or permanent nature of CH, (c) most studies reporting an increased incidence of CH did not classify cases through the systematic use of thyroid scintigraphy [38-40].

In a recent study, we were able to assess the impact of a change (made in 2001) in screening practice on the incidence of CH, globally and by diagnostic sub-groups over a period of 20 years. Had the TSH cutoff remained unchanged in 2001, the incidence of CH (global and by diagnostic sub-groups) would have remained stable [17]. Moreover, our lowering of the TSH cutoff at re-testing did not significantly increase the incidence of the most severe types of CH (athyreosis, ectopy and dyshormonogenesis with goiter). Rather, the additional cases identified predominantly had functional disorders with a normal-size gland *in situ* and a normal or low isotope uptake. Of note, even though these cases were associated with mild primary hypothyroidism, 86% were permanent. This finding is consistent with previous studies showing that even mild CH diagnosed after lowering the TSH cutoff was permanent in 75 to 89% of cases [33, 34, 41].

The next question is whether these cases of mild CH require L-T_4 treatment to attain their full intellectual potential. The original purpose of screening for CH was to identify severe cases in which a benefit was clear (i.e., prevention of intellectual disability) [42]. Over the last two decades, this original paradigm progressively shifted to the detection and treatment of all CH cases, including isolated hyperthyrotropinemias. With lower TSH cutoffs, additional cases are detected and treated but without evidence of benefit of this intervention on intellectual outcome. This lack of obvious benefit might be the reason why, in the United States, more than a third of children labeled as having CH on the basis of neonatal screening no longer receive treatment after age 4 years [43]. If we are to treat patients and not numbers, there is an urgent need to come back to the original intent of screening for CH and, consequently, to evaluate whether newborns with mildly elevated TSH benefit from early diagnosis and treatment [26, 44, 45]. Given that pediatric endocrinologists tend to recommend treatment, a controlled study to answer that question is unlikely to be performed. An alternative could be to track children with TSH levels in the upper 10 % of the distribution of screening results but lower than the cutoff and to evaluate whether they have any evidence of intellectual disability. Such a 'retrospective screening study' was reported in 1984 by Alm and colleagues[46] and did not suggest any harm from transient and untreated neonatal hyperthyrotropinemia. Whether the same would be true of persistent infantile hyperthyrotropinemia remains to be determined.

2.3 CH and its impact on neurocognitive development

Before biochemical screening of newborn infants for hypothyroidism was introduced, the mean IQ of children with congenital hypothyroidism was 85 [19], mainly because less than 20% of affected infants were diagnosed within three months after birth; even those with a normal IQ had deficits in fine motor control and learning disabilities [47]. When biochemical screening was implemented, it was rapidly shown that most infants with hypothyroidism treated soon after birth have normal psychomotor development [48]. However, some controversy remains as to whether the consequences of very severe congenital hypothyroidism can be entirely avoided [6, 49]. Indeed, with early treatment, normalization of neurocognitive development is generally achieved [50, 51], but a relative developmental delay is still observed in the most severely affected (i.e., IQ of 101 *vs* 111 in controls, loss of 10 points)[6].

2.4 From epidemiology to molecular mechanisms

CHTD is predominantly not inherited (98% of cases are non-familial[52]), it has a high discordance rate of 92% in monozygotic (MZ) twins, and it has a female and ethnic (*i.e.*, Caucasian) predominance [7, 53]. Germinal mutations in thyroid-related transcription factors NKX2.1, FOXE1, PAX-8, and NKX2.5 have been identified by candidate gene screening in a small subset (3%) of patients with sporadic CHTD [9]. Linkage analysis has excluded these genes in rare multiplex families with CHTD [54]. Moreover, evidence of non-penetrance of mutations in close relatives of patients (e.g. NKX2.5 [55]) suggests that modifiers, possibly additional *de novo* germline mutations such as copy number variants (CNVs) and/or somatic mutations, are associated with CHTD. Therefore, we hypothesize that the lack of clear familial transmission of CTHD may result from a requirement for two different genetic hits in genes involved in thyroid development [56]. The first hit could be a rare inherited or *de novo* mutation in the germline, while the second mutation, in a different gene, could be germinal or somatic .

3. Genetic determinants of CHTD

3.1 Thyroid dysgenesis and genes, a complex duet

Currently, 26 genes (see **Table 2**) have been directly implicated in thyroid development, based on animal models and/or on their role in known human syndromes including CHTD. At the present time, sytematic sequencing of four candidate genes (i.e., thyroid related transcription factors *TITF-1/NKX2.1, FOXE1, PAX-8,* and *NKX2.5*) identified mutations in only 3% of human CHTD [9, 55, 57-61].

Evidence from animal models to date suggests that the embryonic development of the gland and its normal migration are dependent on the interplay among several transcription factors. In mice, the simultaneous expression of *Titf1, Foxe1* and *Pax8* is required for thyroid survival and migration, and all knockouts present with athyreosis at birth, although *Foxe1 -/-* mouse embryos at E11.5 have either thyroid ectopy (50%) or athyreosis (50%) [12]. *Titf1, Foxe1* and *Pax8* expression in thyroid follicular cells persist into adulthood [62]. A multigenic model has been proposed based on studies of different strains of mice heterozygous for *Pax8* and *Titf1* genetic ablation. The two strains showed a differential predisposition to CHTD depending on several single-nucleotide polymorphisms in a third locus [63, 64]. Furthermore, inactivation of endodermic genes implicated in thyroid bud formation (i.e *Hoxa5, Hoxa3, Hoxb3, Hoxd3, Shh* and *Hes1*) [65-67] or of genes implicated in cardiac (i.e. *Nkx2.5, Nkx2.6, Hhex, Tbx1, Fibulin-1, Isl1 and Chordin*)[55, 68-71] or musculoskeletal malformations (*Shh* inversion in *short digits* mice, *Fgf10*) [72] point to new candidate genes in humans with CHTD. Genes implicated in congenital heart malformations or in musculoskeletal malformations are of particular interest, as these conditions occur in up to 8% of CHTD cases [73, 74]. Another animal model, the zebrafish, has recently been used to study the origin of the thyroid by fate-mapping. Embryonic progenitor of thyroid cells stem from the definitive endoderm [75] and inactivation of genes implicated in endoderm formation (e.g. *bon, cas,* and *oep*) subsequently impair thyroid gland formation in zebrafish [76]. In contrast to human and mice, TSH-TSHR axis seem to be necessary at early steps of thyroid morphogenesis [15]. Moreover, work in zebrafish also highlights the role of tissue-tissue interactions in normal thyroid development. For example, impaired activity of the transcription factor *hand2* in cardiac mesoderm has been shown to result in defective thyroid development [77].

In humans, mutations have been found in leukocyte DNA of CHTD patients in the genes encoding transcription factors *TITF-1/NKX2.1* [57, 58, 78, 79], *FOXE1* [59, 60], *PAX8* [61], and *NKX2.5* [55]. In these genes, all reported mutations so far were heterozygous and patients presented with thyroid gland hypoplasia; *except* for *FOXE1* mutations which have been found exclusively in the homozygous state in patients presenting with athyreosis, cleft palate and spiky hair [59]. *TITF-1/NKX2.1* mutations are almost always *de novo,* whereas *PAX8* and *NKX2.5* mutations are often inherited with incomplete penetrance (*i.e.* a mutation-carrier parent is unaffected) [55, 57-61]. Other genes (*GLIS3, URB1, SALL1* and *TBX1*) are mutated in syndromes where thyroid dysfunction is associated with other dysmorphisms and is generally mild, except for *GLIS3* patients, which can have severe CH [80, 81].

Current knowledge on possible causes of CHTD suggests multiple loci that interact with modifiers such as sex and genetic background whereas environmental factors seem to have little impact. CHTD is sporadic in 98% of cases (i.e. nonetheless, 2% of cases are familial) [82]. A systematic survey of monozygotic (MZ) twins, which yielded a discordance rate of 92% [7], as well as the documented ethnic (Caucasian) [53] and female predominance in CHTD (i.e. 2:1 female:male) [73] suggest that the genetic predisposition to CHTD is complex. Our published studies, showing no temporal or seasonal trends for CHTD and no effect of maternal folate supplementation on CHTD incidence, suggest that major environmental co-factors are unlikely [5, 17].

3.2 Rationale to study genetic determinants of thyroid dysgenesis

Another sporadic congenital endocrine disorder that is much less common than thyroid dysgenesis, focal hyperinsulinism, has been shown to result from a two-hit model combining a germinal mutational hit (consistent with the rare occurrence of familial cases [83]) with a somatic loss of genomic imprinting [84]: in the pancreatic lesions found in these patients, a paternally inherited mutation in the SUR1 or KIR6.2 gene is found together with loss of the maternal 11p15 allele (loss of heterozygosity), a locus which contains many imprinted genes. The loss of heterozygosity is a somatic event restricted to the pancreatic lesion, which explains why focal congenital hyperinsulinism is a sporadic disease with a genetic etiology. A two-hit model combining inherited susceptibility polymorphisms with germ line or somatic mutation at a second locus in threshold-sensitive genes has recently been shown to be relevant for a severe form of mental retardation [85].

Gene	Features	Species	Thyroid phenotype	Additional phenotype
▼ zebrafish				
ace	growth factor, fgf8	zebrafish	Hypoplasia	Lack of cerebellum and mid-hindbrain-boundary
bon	mixer TF	zebrafish	Athyreosis	Overall reduction of the endoderm
cas	sox TF	zebrafish	Athyreosis	Absence of endoderm
cyc	nodal ligand	zebrafish	Hypoplasia	Overall reduction of the endoderm, neural tubes defects, cyclopia
fau	GATA5 TF	zebrafish	Athyreosis	Aplasia of liver, pancreas, thymus
hand2	bHLH TF	zebrafish	Athyreosis or hypoplasia	Heart, pharynx, pectoral defects
hhex	Homeobox TF	zebrafish	Athyreosis or hypoplasia	Liver aplasia
nkx2.1a	Homeodomain TF	zebrafish	Athyreosis	Forebrain defect
noi (pax2.1)	Paired-box TF	zebrafish	Athyreosis	Lack of pronephric duct and
oep	Nodal cofactor	zebrafish	Athyreosis	Absence of endoderm
▼ mouse				
Chordin	Extracellular BMP antagonist	mouse	Hypoplasia	Cardiac outflow tract defects, aplasia of thymus, parathyroid
Edn1	Endothelin signalin peptide	mouse	Hypoplasia, absent isthmus	Craniofacial, cardiac and thymus defects
Eya1	Eya TF	mouse	Hypoplasia	Aplasia of kidneys, thyrmu, parathyroid
Fgf10	Growth factor	mouse	Athyreosis	Aplasia of limbs, lungs, pituitary, salivary glands
Fibulin-1	ECM protein	mouse	Hypoplasia	Craniofacial, cardiac and thymus defects
Foxe1	Forkhead TF	mouse	Ectopy or athyreosis	Cleft palate
Frs2	Transducer of FGF signalling	mouse	hypoplasia, bilobation defect	Thymus and parathyroid defects
Hes1	basic helix-loop-helix TF	mouse	Hypoplasia	Hypoplastic UBB
Hhex	Homeobox TF	mouse	Athyreosis	Forebrain truncations, liver aplasia, complex heart malformations
Hoxa3	Homeobox TF	mouse	Hypoplasia, bilobation defects	Cardiovascular and skeletal defects
Hoxa5	Homeobox TF	mouse	Empty thyroid follicle	
Hoxb3	Homeobox TF	mouse	Ectopy in Hoxa3,Hoxb3 double mutants	Cardiovascular and skeletal defects
Hoxd3	Homeobox TF	mouse	Ectopy in Hoxa3,Hoxd3 double mutants	Thymus and parathyroids agenesis
Isl1	LIM homeodomain TF	mouse	hypoplasia of thyroid placode	Heart, pancreas and neural defects
Nkx2.1	Homeodomain TF	mouse	Athyreosis	Pulmonary aplasia, neural defects.
Nkx2.5	Homeodomain TF	mouse	Hypoplasia	Congenital heart malformations only in the Nkx2.5, Nkx2.6 double heterozygous mice
Pax3	Paired-box TF	mouse	Hypoplasia, bilobation defects	Thymus and parathyroid defects
Pax8	Paired-box TF	mouse	Athyreosis	Reproductive tract defects
Shh	Secreted morphogen	mouse	Hemiagenesis	Holoprosencephaly, midline defect, aberrant carotid arteries and short digits
Tbx1	T-box TF	mouse	Hypoplasia, bilobation defects	Cardiac outflow tract defects, aplasia of thymus, parathyroid
Twisted	modulator of BMP signalling	mouse	Loss of Hhex expreesion at bud-stage	Vertebral defects, spectrum of midline defect, agnathia
▼ human				
FOXE1 (TITF2)	Forkhead TF	human	Athyreosis	Cleft palate, choanal atresia, Spiky hair
GLIS3		human	Hypoplasia	Neonatal diabetes, cystic kidneys, cholestasis,
NKX2.5	Homeodomain TF	human	Thyroid in situ with primary hypothyroidism	Congenital heart malformations
PAX8	Paired-box TF	human	Hypoplasia	Unilateral renal agenesis
SALL1	Zinc finger TF	human	Thyroid in situ with primary hypothyroidism	Townes-Brocks syndrome
TBX1	T-box TF	human	Thyroid in situ with primary hypothyroidism	DiGeorge with congenital heart malformations
TITF1 (NKX2.1)	Homeodomain TF	human	Thyroid in situ with mild primary hypothyroidism	Respiratory failure, choreoathetosis
URB1	E3 ubiquitin ligases of the N-end rule pathway	human	Thyroid in situ with primary hypothyroidism	Johanson-Blizzard Syndrome

Table 2. Human genes and animal models of thyroid dysgenesis (adapted from [13]).

3.3 Discordance between MZ twins for CHTD argues for association of somatic mutations with CHTD

Discordance between MZ twins argues against a germline mutation of high penetrance. However, the occurrence of familial cases (2%, 15 times more than expected by chance alone [52]) and evidence of non-penetrance of mutations in close relatives of patients (e.g. NKX2.5, [55]) suggests that modifiers, possibly additional *de novo* germline mutations such as copy number variants (CNVs) and/or somatic mutations are associated with CHTD. Postzygotic (somatic) mutations, resulting in mosaicism, has been associated with discordance in MZ pairs for genetic conditions such as otopalatodigital syndrome spectrum disorders [86] or Dravet's syndrome [87]. Classical twin studies (i.e., studies of affected *vs* unaffected MZ pairs) have limitations because: (i) the process of twining might itself be a risk factor for congenital birth defects (CHTD included) and (ii) a differential extent of chimerism in blood versus other tissues could interfere with detection of clear genetic differences between MZ twins using leukocyte-derived DNA [88, 89]. These limitations are potentially overcome by studying the genomes in somatic tissue of MZ twins discordant for CHTD.

4. Conclusion: Thyroid dysgenesis is a model disorder for congenital malformations and neurocognitive development

CHTD is a common disorder with a birth prevalence of 1 case in 4,000 live births[5]. Even with early treatment (on average at 9 d), developmental delay is still observed in some patients (with an average IQ reduction of 10 points)[6]. The severity of the hypothyroidism is not solely responsible for this. Therefore, molecular markers are necessary to identify patients with possible susceptibility for mental retardation (*i.e.* genes involved both in neuronal and thyroid migration during development, such as *NKX2.1*). Patients in this category will benefit from earlier intervention to stimulate their neurocognitive development. The next logical goals will be (i) to determine whether mutations of discovered genes are associated with poor neurocognitive outcome, by sequencing these genes in CHTD patients with significant intellectual disabilities (need of special educational support) and (ii) to assess if patients in this category will benefit from earlier intervention to stimulate their neurocognitive development.

More generally, unraveling the etiology of CHTD may shed light on other more complex and less easily treatable congenital malformations (e.g. of the brain and heart) and provides a prototype approach for the study of congenital disorders currently unexplained by classical genetics.

5. Acknowledgments

I thank Dr Guy Van Vliet (CHU Sainte-Justine, University of Montreal) for his continuous support and helpful comments about this chapter.

6. References

[1] Bakker B, Bikker H, Vulsma T, de Randamie JS, Wiedijk BM, De Vijlder JJ. Two decades of screening for congenital hypothyroidism in The Netherlands: TPO gene mutations in total iodide organification defects (an update). *J Clin Endocrinol Metab.* 2000;85(10):3708-3712.

[2] Avbelj M, Tahirovic H, Debeljak M, Kusekova M, Toromanovic A, Krzisnik C, et al. High prevalence of thyroid peroxidase gene mutations in patients with thyroid dyshormonogenesis. *Eur J Endocrinol.* 2007;156(5):511-519.

[3] Tenenbaum-Rakover Y, Mamanasiri S, Ris-Stalpers C, German A, Sack J, Allon-Shalev S, et al. Clinical and genetic characteristics of congenital hypothyroidism due to mutations in the thyroid peroxidase (TPO) gene in Israelis. *Clin Endocrinol (Oxf).* 2007;66(5):695-702.

[4] Rodrigues C, Jorge P, Soares JP, Santos I, Salomao R, Madeira M, et al. Mutation screening of the thyroid peroxidase gene in a cohort of 55 Portuguese patients with congenital hypothyroidism. *Eur J Endocrinol.* 2005;152(2):193-198.

[5] Deladoey J, Belanger N, Van Vliet G. Random Variability in Congenital Hypothyroidism from Thyroid Dysgenesis over 16 Years in Quebec. *J Clin Endocrinol Metab.* 2007;92(8):3158-3161.

[6] Dimitropoulos A, Molinari L, Etter K, Torresani T, Lang-Muritano M, Jenni OG, et al. Children with congenital hypothyroidism: long-term intellectual outcome after early high-dose treatment. *Pediatr Res.* 2009;65(2):242-248.

[7] Perry R, Heinrichs C, Bourdoux P, Khoury K, Szots F, Dussault JH, et al. Discordance of monozygotic twins for thyroid dysgenesis: implications for screening and for molecular pathophysiology. *J Clin Endocrinol Metab.* 2002;87(9):4072-4077.

[8] Stoppa-Vaucher S, Van Vliet G, Deladoey J. Variation by ethnicity in the prevalence of congenital hypothyroidism due to thyroid dysgenesis. *Thyroid.* 2010;21(1):13-18.

[9] Narumi S, Muroya K, Asakura Y, Adachi M, Hasegawa T. Transcription factor mutations and congenital hypothyroidism: systematic genetic screening of a population-based cohort of Japanese patients. *J Clin Endocrinol Metab.* 2010;95(4):1981-1985.

[10] Abu-Khudir R, Paquette J, Lefort A, Libert F, Chanoine JP, Vassart G, et al. Transcriptome, methylome and genomic variations analysis of ectopic thyroid glands. *PLoS One.* 2010;5(10):e13420.

[11] Thorwarth A, Mueller I, Biebermann H, Ropers HH, Grueters A, Krude H, et al. Screening chromosomal aberrations by array comparative genomic hybridization in 80 patients with congenital hypothyroidism and thyroid dysgenesis. *J Clin Endocrinol Metab.* 2010;95(7):3446-3452.

[12] De Felice M, Di Lauro R. Thyroid Development and Its Disorders: Genetics and Molecular Mechanisms. *Endocr Rev.* 2004;25(5):722-746.

[13] Fagman H, Nilsson M. Morphogenesis of the thyroid gland. *Mol Cell Endocrinol.* 2010;323(1):35-54.

[14] Alt B, Elsalini OA, Schrumpf P, Haufs N, Lawson ND, Schwabe GC, et al. Arteries define the position of the thyroid gland during its developmental relocalisation. *Development.* 2006;133(19):3797-3804.

[15] Opitz R, Maquet E, Zoenen M, Dadhich R, Costagliola S. TSH Receptor Function Is Required for Normal Thyroid Differentiation in Zebrafish. *Mol Endocrinol.* 2011.

[16] Olney RS, Grosse SD, Vogt RF, Jr. Prevalence of congenital hypothyroidism--current trends and future directions: workshop summary. *Pediatrics.* 2010;125 Suppl 2:S31-36.

[17] Deladoey J, Ruel J, Giguere Y, Van Vliet G. Is the incidence of congenital hypothyroidism really increasing? A 20-year retrospective population-based study in quebec. *J Clin Endocrinol Metab.* 2011;96(8):2422-2429.
[18] Loeber JG. Neonatal screening in Europe; the situation in 2004. *J Inherit Metab Dis.* 2007;30(4):430-438.
[19] Grosse SD, Van Vliet G. Prevention of intellectual disability through screening for congenital hypothyroidism: how much and at what level? *Arch Dis Child.* 2011;96(4):374-379.
[20] Oken E, Braverman LE, Platek D, Mitchell ML, Lee SL, Pearce EN. Neonatal thyroxine, maternal thyroid function, and child cognition. *J Clin Endocrinol Metab.* 2009;94(2):497-503.
[21] Tillotson SL, Fuggle PW, Smith I, Ades AE, Grant DB. Relation between biochemical severity and intelligence in early treated congenital hypothyroidism: a threshold effect. *BMJ.* 1994;309(6952):440-445.
[22] Rapaport R. Congenital hypothyroidism: an evolving common clinical conundrum. *J Clin Endocrinol Metab.* 2010;95(9):4223-4225.
[23] Pollitt RJ. New technologies extend the scope of newborn blood-spot screening, but old problems remain unresolved. *Acta Paediatr.* 2010;99(12):1766-1772.
[24] Dussault JH. The anecdotal history of screening for congenital hypothyroidism. *J Clin Endocrinol Metab.* 1999;84(12):4332-4334.
[25] Delange F, Camus M, Winkler M, Dodion J, Ermans AM. Serum thyrotrophin determination on day 5 of life as screening procedure for congenital hypothyroidism. *Arch Dis Child.* 1977;52(2):89-96.
[26] La Gamma EF, van Wassenaer AG, Golombek SG, Morreale de Escobar G, Kok JH, Quero J, et al. Neonatal thyroxine supplementation for transient hypothyroxinemia of prematurity : beneficial or detrimental? *Treat Endocrinol.* 2006;5(6):335-346.
[27] Delange F, Dalhem A, Bourdoux P, Lagasse R, Glinoer D, Fisher DA, et al. Increased risk of primary hypothyroidism in preterm infants. *J Pediatr.* 1984;105(3):462-469.
[28] Chanoine JP, Pardou A, Bourdoux P, Delange F. Withdrawal of iodinated disinfectants at delivery decreases the recall rate at neonatal screening for congenital hypothyroidism. *Arch Dis Child.* 1988;63(10):1297-1298.
[29] Andersen HJ. Studies of hypothyroidism in children. *Acta Paediatr Suppl.* 1961;50(Suppl 125):1-150.
[30] Van Vliet G, Larroque B, Bubuteishvili L, Supernant K, Leger J. Sex-specific impact of congenital hypothyroidism due to thyroid dysgenesis on skeletal maturation in term newborns. *J Clin Endocrinol Metab.* 2003;88(5):2009-2013.
[31] Larson C, Hermos R, Delaney A, Daley D, Mitchell M. Risk factors associated with delayed thyrotropin elevations in congenital hypothyroidism. *J Pediatr.* 2003;143(5):587-591.
[32] Woo HC, Lizarda A, Tucker R, Mitchell ML, Vohr B, Oh W, et al. Congenital hypothyroidism with a delayed thyroid-stimulating hormone elevation in very premature infants: incidence and growth and developmental outcomes. *J Pediatr.* 2011;158(4):538-542.
[33] Mengreli C, Kanaka-Gantenbein C, Girginoudis P, Magiakou MA, Christakopoulou I, Giannoulia-Karantana A, et al. Screening for congenital hypothyroidism: the

significance of threshold limit in false-negative results. *J Clin Endocrinol Metab.* 2010;95(9):4283-4290.

[34] Corbetta C, Weber G, Cortinovis F, Calebiro D, Passoni A, Vigone MC, et al. A 7-year experience with low blood TSH cutoff levels for neonatal screening reveals an unsuspected frequency of congenital hypothyroidism (CH). *Clin Endocrinol (Oxf).* 2009;71(5):739-745.

[35] Korada M, Pearce MS, Ward Platt MP, Avis E, Turner S, Wastell H, et al. Repeat testing for congenital hypothyroidism in preterm infants is unnecessary with an appropriate thyroid stimulating hormone threshold. *Arch Dis Child Fetal Neonatal Ed.* 2008;93(4):F286-288.

[36] Vincent MA, Rodd C, Dussault JH, Van Vliet G. Very low birth weight newborns do not need repeat screening for congenital hypothyroidism. *J Pediatr.* 2002;140(3):311-314.

[37] van Trotsenburg AS, Vulsma T, van Santen HM, Cheung W, de Vijlder JJ. Lower neonatal screening thyroxine concentrations in down syndrome newborns. *J Clin Endocrinol Metab.* 2003;88(4):1512-1515.

[38] Harris KB, Pass KA. Increase in congenital hypothyroidism in New York State and in the United States. *Mol Genet Metab.* 2007;91(3):268-277.

[39] Pearce MS, Korada M, Day J, Turner S, Allison D, Kibirige M, et al. Increasing Incidence, but Lack of Seasonality, of Elevated TSH Levels, on Newborn Screening, in the North of England. *J Thyroid Res.* 2010;2010:101948.

[40] Hertzberg V, Mei J, Therrell BL. Effect of laboratory practices on the incidence rate of congenital hypothyroidism. *Pediatrics.* 2010;125 Suppl 2:S48-53.

[41] Leonardi D, Polizzotti N, Carta A, Gelsomino R, Sava L, Vigneri R, et al. Longitudinal study of thyroid function in children with mild hyperthyrotropinemia at neonatal screening for congenital hypothyroidism. *J Clin Endocrinol Metab.* 2008;93(7):2679-2685.

[42] Wilson JM, Jungner YG. [Principles and practice of mass screening for disease]. *Bol Oficina Sanit Panam.* 1968;65(4):281-393.

[43] Kemper AR, Ouyang L, Grosse SD. Discontinuation of thyroid hormone treatment among children in the United States with congenital hypothyroidism: findings from health insurance claims data. *BMC Pediatr.* 2010;10:9.

[44] Krude H, Blankenstein O. Treating patients not numbers: the benefit and burden of lowering TSH newborn screening cut-offs. *Arch Dis Child.* 2010;96(2):121-122.

[45] Hoffmann GF, Cornejo V, Pollitt RJ. Newborn screening-progress and challenges. *J Inherit Metab Dis.* 2010;33(Suppl 2):S199-200.

[46] Alm J, Hagenfeldt L, Larsson A, Lundberg K. Incidence of congenital hypothyroidism: retrospective study of neonatal laboratory screening versus clinical symptoms as indicators leading to diagnosis. *Br Med J (Clin Res Ed).* 1984;289(6453):1171-1175.

[47] Wolter R, Noel P, De Cock P, Craen M, Ernould C, Malvaux P, et al. Neuropsychological study in treated thyroid dysgenesis. *Acta Paediatr Scand Suppl.* 1979;277:41-46.

[48] Effects of neonatal screening for hypothyroidism: prevention of mental retardation by treatment before clinical manifestations. New England congenital hypothyroidism collaborative. *Lancet.* 1981;2(8255):1095-1098.

[49] Song SI, Daneman D, Rovet J. The influence of etiology and treatment factors on intellectual outcome in congenital hypothyroidism. *J Dev Behav Pediatr.* 2001;22(6):376-384.

[50] Simoneau-Roy J, Marti S, Deal C, Huot C, Robaey P, Van Vliet G. Cognition and behavior at school entry in children with congenital hypothyroidism treated early with high-dose levothyroxine. *J Pediatr.* 2004;144(6):747-752.

[51] Selva KA, Harper A, Downs A, Blasco PA, Lafranchi SH. Neurodevelopmental outcomes in congenital hypothyroidism: comparison of initial T4 dose and time to reach target T4 and TSH. *J Pediatr.* 2005;147(6):775-780.

[52] Castanet M, Lyonnet S, Bonaiti-Pellie C, Polak M, Czernichow P, Leger J. Familial forms of thyroid dysgenesis among infants with congenital hypothyroidism. *N Engl J Med.* 2000;343(6):441-442.

[53] Stoppa-Vaucher S, Van Vliet G, Deladoey J. Variation by ethnicity in the prevalence of congenital hypothyroidism due to thyroid dysgenesis. *Thyroid.* 2011;21(1):13-18.

[54] Castanet M, Sura-Trueba S, Chauty A, Carre A, de Roux N, Heath S, et al. Linkage and mutational analysis of familial thyroid dysgenesis demonstrate genetic heterogeneity implicating novel genes. *Eur J Hum Genet.* 2005;13(2):232-239.

[55] Dentice M, Cordeddu V, Rosica A, Ferrara AM, Santarpia L, Salvatore D, et al. Missense mutation in the transcription factor NKX2-5: a novel molecular event in the pathogenesis of thyroid dysgenesis. *J Clin Endocrinol Metab.* 2006;91(4):1428-1433.

[56] Deladoey J, Vassart G, Van Vliet G. Possible non-mendelian mechanisms of thyroid dysgenesis. *Endocr Dev.* 2007;10:29-42.

[57] Breedveld GJ, van Dongen JW, Danesino C, Guala A, Percy AK, Dure LS, et al. Mutations in TITF-1 are associated with benign hereditary chorea. *Hum Mol Genet.* 2002;11(8):971-979.

[58] Krude H, Schutz B, Biebermann H, von Moers A, Schnabel D, Neitzel H, et al. Choreoathetosis, hypothyroidism, and pulmonary alterations due to human NKX2-1 haploinsufficiency. *J Clin Invest.* 2002;109(4):475-480.

[59] Clifton-Bligh RJ, Wentworth JM, Heinz P, Crisp MS, John R, Lazarus JH, et al. Mutation of the gene encoding human TTF-2 associated with thyroid agenesis, cleft palate and choanal atresia. *Nat Genet.* 1998;19(4):399-401.

[60] Castanet M, Park SM, Smith A, Bost M, Leger J, Lyonnet S, et al. A novel loss-of-function mutation in TTF-2 is associated with congenital hypothyroidism, thyroid agenesis and cleft palate. *Hum Mol Genet.* 2002;11(17):2051-2059.

[61] Macchia PE, Lapi P, Krude H, Pirro MT, Missero C, Chiovato L, et al. PAX8 mutations associated with congenital hypothyroidism caused by thyroid dysgenesis. *Nat Genet.* 1998;19(1):83-86.

[62] Szinnai G, Lacroix L, Carre A, Guimiot F, Talbot M, Martinovic J, et al. Sodium/iodide symporter (NIS) gene expression is the limiting step for the onset of thyroid function in the human fetus. *J Clin Endocrinol Metab.* 2007;92(1):70-76.

[63] Amendola E, De Luca P, Macchia PE, Terracciano D, Rosica A, Chiappetta G, et al. A mouse model demonstrates a multigenic origin of congenital hypothyroidism. *Endocrinology.* 2005;146(12):5038-5047.

[64] Amendola E, Sanges R, Galvan A, Dathan N, Manenti G, Ferrandino G, et al. A locus on mouse chromosome 2 is involved in susceptibility to congenital hypothyroidism

and contains an essential gene expressed in thyroid. *Endocrinology.* 2010;151(4):1948-1958.

[65] Manley NR, Capecchi MR. Hox group 3 paralogs regulate the development and migration of the thymus, thyroid, and parathyroid glands. *Dev Biol.* 1998;195(1):1-15.

[66] Fagman H, Grande M, Gritli-Linde A, Nilsson M. Genetic deletion of sonic hedgehog causes hemiagenesis and ectopic development of the thyroid in mouse. *Am J Pathol.* 2004;164(5):1865-1872.

[67] Carre A, Rachdi L, Tron E, Richard B, Castanet M, Schlumberger M, et al. Hes1 is required for appropriate morphogenesis and differentiation during mouse thyroid gland development. *PLoS One.* 2011;6(2):e16752.

[68] Martinez Barbera JP, Clements M, Thomas P, Rodriguez T, Meloy D, Kioussis D, et al. The homeobox gene Hex is required in definitive endodermal tissues for normal forebrain, liver and thyroid formation. *Development.* 2000;127(11):2433-2445.

[69] Fagman H, Liao J, Westerlund J, Andersson L, Morrow BE, Nilsson M. The 22q11 deletion syndrome candidate gene Tbx1 determines thyroid size and positioning. *Hum Mol Genet.* 2007;16(3):276-285.

[70] Cooley MA, Kern CB, Fresco VM, Wessels A, Thompson RP, McQuinn TC, et al. Fibulin-1 is required for morphogenesis of neural crest-derived structures. *Dev Biol.* 2008;319(2):336-345.

[71] Bachiller D, Klingensmith J, Shneyder N, Tran U, Anderson R, Rossant J, et al. The role of chordin/Bmp signals in mammalian pharyngeal development and DiGeorge syndrome. *Development.* 2003;130(15):3567-3578.

[72] Ohuchi H, Hori Y, Yamasaki M, Harada H, Sekine K, Kato S, et al. FGF10 acts as a major ligand for FGF receptor 2 IIIb in mouse multi-organ development. *Biochem Biophys Res Commun.* 2000;277(3):643-649.

[73] Devos H, Rodd C, Gagne N, Laframboise R, Van Vliet G. A search for the possible molecular mechanisms of thyroid dysgenesis: sex ratios and associated malformations. *J Clin Endocrinol Metab.* 1999;84(7):2502-2506.

[74] El Kholy M, Fahmi ME, Nassar AE, Selim S, Elsedfy HH. Prevalence of Minor Musculoskeletal Anomalies in Children with Congenital Hypothyroidism. *Horm Res.* 2007;68(6):272-275.

[75] Alt B, Reibe S, Feitosa NM, Elsalini OA, Wendl T, Rohr KB. Analysis of origin and growth of the thyroid gland in zebrafish. *Dev Dyn.* 2006;235(7):1872-1883.

[76] Elsalini OA, Rohr KB. Phenylthiourea disrupts thyroid function in developing zebrafish. *Dev Genes Evol.* 2003;212(12):593-598.

[77] Wendl T, Adzic D, Schoenebeck JJ, Scholpp S, Brand M, Yelon D, et al. Early developmental specification of the thyroid gland depends on han-expressing surrounding tissue and on FGF signals. *Development.* 2007;134(15):2871-2879.

[78] Carre A, Szinnai G, Castanet M, Sura-Trueba S, Tron E, Broutin-L'Hermite I, et al. Five new TTF1/NKX2.1 mutations in brain-lung-thyroid syndrome: rescue by PAX8 synergism in one case. *Hum Mol Genet.* 2009;18(12):2266-2276.

[79] Maquet E, Costagliola S, Parma J, Christophe-Hobertus C, Oligny LL, Fournet JC, et al. Lethal respiratory failure and mild primary hypothyroidism in a term girl with a de novo heterozygous mutation in the TITF1/NKX2.1 gene. *J Clin Endocrinol Metab.* 2009;94(1):197-203.

[80] Senee V, Chelala C, Duchatelet S, Feng D, Blanc H, Cossec JC, et al. Mutations in GLIS3 are responsible for a rare syndrome with neonatal diabetes mellitus and congenital hypothyroidism. *Nat Genet.* 2006;38(6):682-687.

[81] Dimitri P, Warner JT, Minton JA, Patch AM, Ellard S, Hattersley AT, et al. Novel GLIS3 mutations demonstrate an extended multisystem phenotype. *Eur J Endocrinol.* 2011;164(3):437-443.

[82] Castanet M, Polak M, Bonaiti-Pellie C, Lyonnet S, Czernichow P, Leger J. Nineteen years of national screening for congenital hypothyroidism: familial cases with thyroid dysgenesis suggest the involvement of genetic factors. *J Clin Endocrinol Metab.* 2001;86(5):2009-2014.

[83] Ismail D, Smith VV, de Lonlay P, Ribeiro MJ, Rahier J, Blankenstein O, et al. Familial focal congenital hyperinsulinism. *J Clin Endocrinol Metab.* 2011;96(1):24-28.

[84] Giurgea I, Bellanne-Chantelot C, Ribeiro M, Hubert L, Sempoux C, Robert JJ, et al. Molecular mechanisms of neonatal hyperinsulinism. *Horm Res.* 2006;66(6):289-296.

[85] Girirajan S, Rosenfeld JA, Cooper GM, Antonacci F, Siswara P, Itsara A, et al. A recurrent 16p12.1 microdeletion supports a two-hit model for severe developmental delay. *Nat Genet.* 2010;42(3):203-209.

[86] Robertson SP, Thompson S, Morgan T, Holder-Espinasse M, Martinot-Duquenoy V, Wilkie AO, et al. Postzygotic mutation and germline mosaicism in the otopalatodigital syndrome spectrum disorders. *Eur J Hum Genet.* 2006;14(5):549-554.

[87] Vadlamudi L, Dibbens LM, Lawrence KM, Iona X, McMahon JM, Murrell W, et al. Timing of de novo mutagenesis--a twin study of sodium-channel mutations. *N Engl J Med.* 2010;363(14):1335-1340.

[88] Erlich Y. Blood ties: chimerism can mask twin discordance in high-throughput sequencing. *Twin Res Hum Genet.* 2011;14(2):137-143.

[89] Baranzini SE, Mudge J, van Velkinburgh JC, Khankhanian P, Khrebtukova I, Miller NA, et al. Genome, epigenome and RNA sequences of monozygotic twins discordant for multiple sclerosis. *Nature.* 2010;464(7293):1351-1356.

14

Consideration of Congenital Hypothyroidism as the Possible Cause of Autism

Xiaobin Xu[1], Hirohiko Kanai[2], Masanori Ookubo[3], Satoru Suzuki[4], Nobumasa Kato[5] and Miyuki Sadamatsu[6]

[1]*Center For Neuropsychiatric Disorders, Institute of Life Science, Nanchang University 330031,*
[2]*Dept. Psychiatry, Shiga Univ. Med. Sci., Shiga,*
[3]*Dept. Psychiatry, Minakuchi Hosp., Koka City, Shiga,*
[4]*Dept. Aging Med. and Geriatrics, Shinshu Univ., Nagano,*
[5]*Dept. of Psychiatry, Karasuyama Hospital, Showa Univ. Sch.of Med., Tokyo,*
[6]*Dept. Psychiatry, Nara Med. Univ. Nara,*
[1]*China*
[2,3,4,5,6] *Japan*

1. Introduction

Autism is a behaviorally defined disorder associated with characteristic impairments in social interactions and communication, as well as restricted and repetitive behaviors and interest. Its prevalence was thought to be 2 in 10,000, but recently, several large reviews on autism prevalence revealed that the rate of occurrence is approximately 30 in 10,000. While autism has been considered a developmental disorder, little is known about its causes.

The genetic component clearly plays an important role in the pathophysiology of this disorder. However, environmental factors can also cause developmental disabilities. Case reports of autism associated with environmental factors, such as rubella virus, valproic acid, and thalidomide exposure during pregnancy, led to the hypothesis that nongenetic mechanisms may also produce an autistic syndrome (Chess 1977).

Thyroid hormone is essential for brain development and maintenance of basal metabolic rates. Manipulation of the thyroid hormone in laboratory animals typically increases activity levels and decreases performance during motivated learning tasks. It is well known that hypothyroidism during the critical period of brain development induces irreversible dysfunction of the central nervous system (CNS). The timing of thyroid hormone manipulation plays a critical role in the degree to which developmental sequelae are expressed. Lactating rats receiving 0.02% propylthiouracil (PTU) in their drinking water transfer the goitrogenic effect to the offspring through their milk. This treatment induces a temporary mild hypothyroid condition in the pups (Van Middlesworth 1980). We conducted experiments to investigate the effects of temporary neonatal PTU-induced hypothyroidism on behavior of rats. Rat pups were treated with 0.02% PTU in drinking water which was given to dams from day 0 through day 19 post partum (Kato 1982). The serum T4 level was depressed below the limit of detection at 2 weeks of age, but recovered to the normal level at 4 weeks of age (Akaike 1991). The open field test was conducted at 3, 6, and 9 weeks of age. At 3 weeks of age, the number of ambulations did not differ between PTU-treated rats and controls. At 6 and 9 weeks of age, the number of ambulations of PTU-treated rats was significantly higher than that of control rats. Kato et al. reported extensive hyperactivity (Akaike 1991; Akaike 1997) and attenuated habituation in the open field test in PTU-treated rats after maturation, as shown in Fig 1 (Kato 1992).

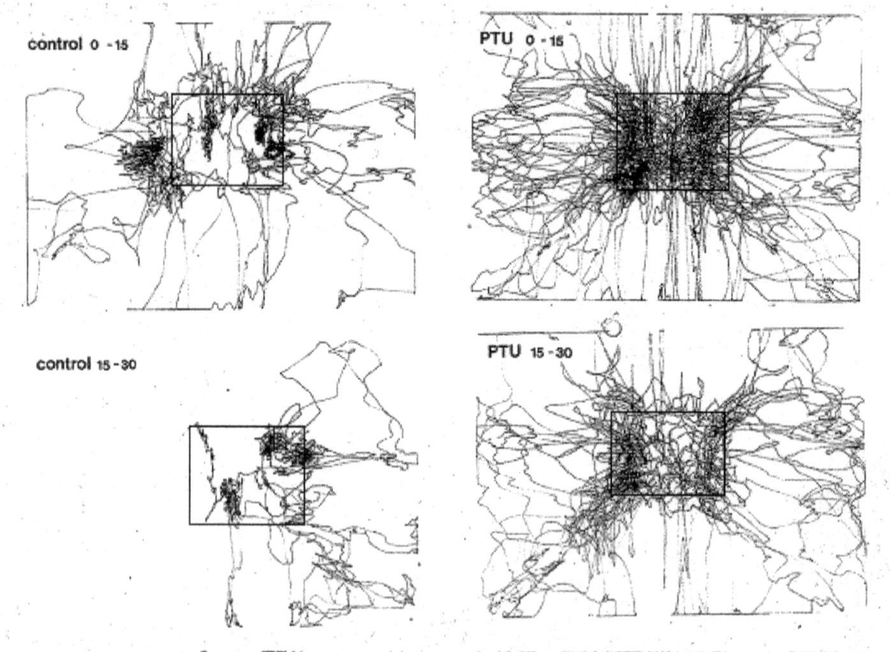

Fig. 1. Comparison of spontaneous movement in a propylthiouracil (PTU)-treated rat (right) and its littermate control (left), as detected by a multidimensional behavioral analyzer (Animex II) at the age of 10 weeks. The device recorded the linear locomotion activity of the animal for 2 consecutive 15-min periods. The rectangle in the centre of each figure indicates the base of the cage and traces outside the rectangle indicate rearing (Kato 1992).

The functions of thyroid hormones in brain are mediated by 2 isoforms of thyroid hormone receptors (TRs), TR-α and TR-β (Leonard JL 1994). TR-α and TR-β are expressed in a cell- and region-specific manner and differentially control a wide array of gene expression throughout the prenatal and postnatal periods (Mellström B 1991; Bradley 1992). While TR-α expression is widely distributed during the prenatal period, the distribution of TR-β expression is more restricted and almost overlaps with that of TR-α before birth; however, TR-β expression is more widely distributed and increases after birth(Mellström B 1991; Bradley 1992).

In the rodent brain, the striatum and hippocampus, 2 important regions in the limbic system, have the highest expression of both TRs throughout the prenatal and neonatal period, and high TR expression levels are maintained into adulthood (Bradley 1992). Because developmental program and function acquisition are strictly controlled, it has been hypothesized that lack of TR-signaling in the critical period causes permanent functional abnormalities related to TR-expressing regions (Manzano J 2007). Dramatic cytoarchitectural maturation seems to occur 2-3 weeks after birth in the normal caudate. Neonatal hypothyroidism in a PTU model causes a marked maturational delay in caudate neuronal proliferation, elaboration of neuronal networks, and attainment of mature synaptic contacts in rat pups (Lu EJ 1977). However, the internal supply of thyroid hormones after the lactating period results in a rapid "catch-up" phenomenon of caudate synaptogenesis (Lu EJ 1977). Repression of thyroid function does not entirely prevent development of the caudate nucleus, but it allows a fairly extensive, though critically incomplete, degree of maturation. Similarly, neonatal thyroid hormone deficiency has been reported to interfere with the contact between mossy fibers and dendritic excrescences of CA3 pyramidal cells of the rat hippocampus (Madeira MD 1993). Although the change in the total number of synapse enabled a complete "catch-up," synaptic reorganization was not fully achieved, as revealed by the reduction in the size of the synaptic sites (Madeira MD 1993). However, the critical mechanisms, as well as the role of TR signaling, remain unclear in such permanent behavioral abnormalities.

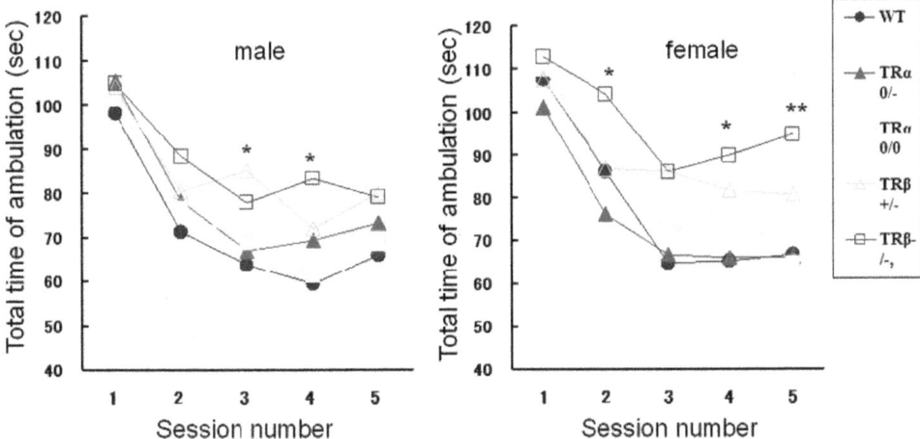

Fig. 2. The locomotor activity in male and female thyroid hormone receptor (TR)-mutant mice. Whereas the wild-type mice habituated over multiple sessions, TR-$\beta^{+/-}$ mice and TR-$\beta^{-/-}$ mice exhibited significant hyperactivity. Gender difference is not statistically significant. (ANOVA, *$p < 0.01$, **$p < 0.001$).

TRs bind to thyroid hormone response elements in the promoter region and regulate a wide array of genes (Zhang J 2000; Jeyakumar M 2007). N-CoR (nuclear receptor corepressor), SMRT (silencing mediator of retinoid and thyroid hormone receptors), and histone deacetylase 3 form large complexes with unliganded TRs, and these complexes mediate the basal transcriptional regulation both positively and negatively. In the presence of T3, corepressor complexes are released from liganded TRs that, in turn, associate with coactivator complexes containing SRC (steroid receptor coactivators), CBP (cAMP response element-binding protein-binding protein), and P/CAF (Zhang J 2000; Jeyakumar M 2007). Thus, gene regulation mediated by TRs involves histone modification, and therefore, raises the possibility that TR-gene disruption induces chronic epigenetic changes in the TR-related brain regions.

Genetic disruption of TRs causes distinct behavioral impairments in humans and in animal models. TR-β knock-in mice (TR-β^{PV} mice) show hyperactivity with lack of habituation, which is similar to findings observed in a PTU-treated model (Wong R 1997; Siesser WB 2005; Siesser WB 2006). Methylphenidate is a psychostimulant drug approved for treatment of attention deficit hyperactivity disorder (ADHD), and is known to paradoxically decrease hyperactivity in ADHD children. This drug is effective in reducing hyperactivity of TR-β^{PV} mice as well (Wong R 1997). In contrast, TR-α mutant mice were reported to show memory impairment and an increased anxiety profile (Wallis K 2008). In humans, an inherited syndrome caused by the mutated TR-β gene, resistance to thyroid hormone (RTH), has been described, whereas lack of TR-α is thought to be lethal. Most patients with RTH are heterozygous, carrying only 1 mutated gene. A generalized form of RTH is characterized by reduced responsiveness of the pituitary and peripheral tissues to thyroid hormones and has a high ratio of comorbid ADHD which reaches up to 40-70% (Siesser WB 2005). Although disruption of TR signaling is transient in a PTU-treated model, disruption of the TR-β gene appears to cause common behavioral abnormalities. In addition to its important roles in behavior, various alterations of the monoaminergic systems have been reported either in TR-gene disrupted animal models or in a PTU-treated model. To investigate the roles of TR-signaling in behavioral changes, we performed behavioral tests in TR-gene disrupted mice. In addition, we determined dopamine and serotonin concentrations in the striatum and hippocampus of male TRs mutant mice by using high performance liquid chromatography. We measured the striatal and hippocampal expressions of proteins, including acetylated histone H3, an epigenetic marker, and glial fibrillary acidic protein (GFAP), a marker of proliferation and maturation of astrocytes.

We used the following 5 strains (N = 5 or 6 each): TR-$\alpha^{0/0}$, TR-$\alpha^{0/-}$, TR-$\beta^{+/-}$, TR-$\beta^{-/-}$, and wild-type mice (Forrest D 1996; Gauthier K 2001). In addition to learning impairments, the characteristic behavioral abnormality in a PTU-treated model is hyperactivity. We used an open field test to compare locomotor activities in each mouse strain of both genders (Fig 1). As results of the open field tests, TR-$\alpha^{0/0}$ mice did not show any apparent difference compared to wild-type mice with regard to total time of ambulation and other indicators, eg, number of rearing. TR-$\alpha^{0/0}$ mice exhibited a slightly increased tendency of mean latency to enter novel areas compared with that of wild-type mice (data not shown). In contrast, TR-$\beta^{+/-}$ mice and TR-$\beta^{-/-}$ mice exhibited significant hyperactivity. Since TR-β^{PV} mice have been reported to exhibit hyperactivity, our results were likely to confirm the relationship between hyperactivity and TR-β gene in another mutant mouse strain. Dopamine concentrations were significantly increased in the striatum and slightly, but not statistically significant, increased in the hippocampus of TR-$\beta^{+/-}$ mice and TR-$\beta^{-/-}$ mice (Fig 3). Serotonin concentrations in the striatum and hippocampus did not differ among all strains (data not shown). As results of western blotting analysis, acetylation of histone H3 in the striatum was significantly increased in TR-$\beta^{+/-}$ mice and slightly increased in TR-$\beta^{-/-}$ mice, suggesting the possibility of epigenetic changes in gene expression (Fig 4). These findings emphasize the possibility of a functional alteration of the dopaminergic system in the striatum. In the hippocampus, there was no change in the concentrations of dopamine and serotonin among the strains, but elevated GFAP expression was noted in TR-α$^{0/0}$ and TR-α$^{0/-}$ mice, indicating the possible involvement of minimal neuronal loss and reactive gliosis there (Fig 4). Both T3 and T4 can be transported into the CNS, and T4 can be converted to bioactive T3 and subsequently metabolized mainly in astrocytes (Leonard JL 1994; Guadaño-Ferraz A 1997). In addition specific neuronal loss, the activation and/or proliferation of astrocytes per se might indirectly contribute to changes in hippocampal TR signaling.

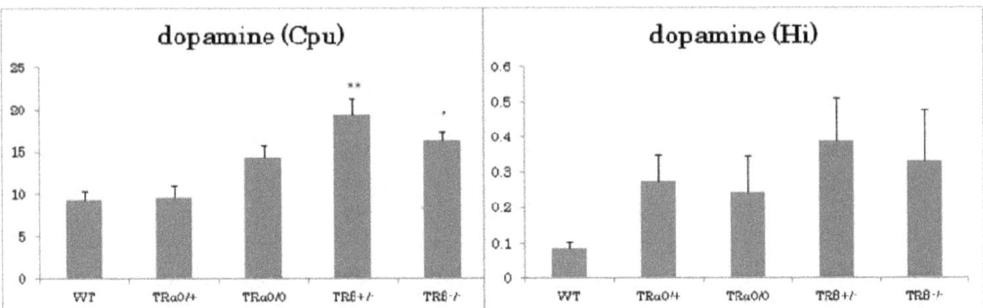

Fig. 3. Dopamine concentrations in the striatum (Cpu) and hippocampus (Hi) of thyroid hormone receptor (TR)-mutant mice. Dopamine concentrations in TR-β$^{+/-}$- and TR-β$^{-/-}$-mutant mice were significantly elevated in the striatum, but not in the hippocampus. (*p < 0.01, **p < 0.001)

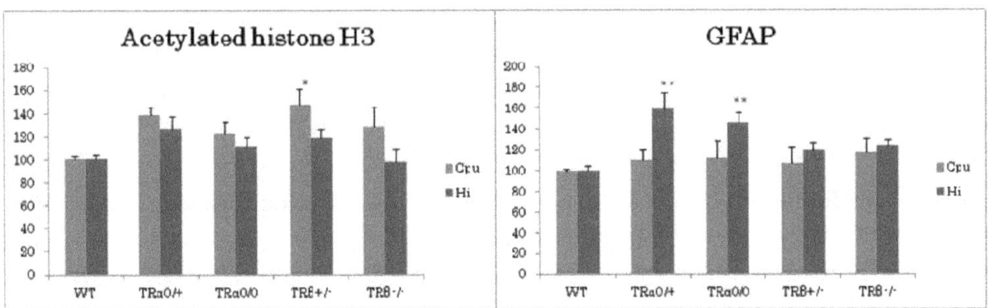

Histone modification and glial marker expression in the striatum and hippocampus. Acetylation of histone H3 was significantly increased in the striatum of TR-β$^{+/-}$ mice. GFAP expressions were significantly elevated in the hippocampus of TR-α$^{0/0}$ and TR-α$^{0/-}$ mice. (*p < 0.01, **p < 0.001)

Fig. 4. Serum free thyroxine (T4) levels after bisphenol A (BPA) exposure
(A) Serum free T4 of dams. (B) Serum free T4 of pups.

Thyroid hormones are known to modulate a number of neurotransmitter systems, including monoamines (Ahmed OM 2010; Tousson E 2011). Genetic studies imply that variants of both dopamine and serotonin systems may frequently occur in ADHD for neurotransmitter uptake, synthesis, and breakdown functions. The prefrontal cortex, hippocampus, and striatum are strongly involved in executive functions such as planning and novelty-related decision making, as well as in the reward system (Rinaldi A 2010). These regions are densely innervated by serotonergic afferents from the raphe complex and dopaminergic afferents from the substantia nigra and the ventral tegmental area. Learning and memory are robustly modulated by serotonin and dopamine neurotransmitter activity at the synaptic level, and in some cases, they interact interdependently to sustain the psychobiological organization of these cognitive processes (González-Burgos I 2008). In fact, several experimental models of neurotransmitter activity, including a PTU-treated model, have identified a close association between serotonin-dopamine imbalance and cytoarchitectonic changes underlying learning and memory impairment (González-Burgos I 2008).

Recent research has demonstrated that epigenetic mechanisms, which regulate gene activity without altering the DNA code, have long-lasting effects within mature neurons (Colvis CM 2005; Tsankova N 2007). The existence of sustained epigenetic mechanisms of gene regulation in neurons has been implicated in the regulation of complex behavior, including abnormalities in mental disorders (eg, autism and ADHD) (Colvis CM 2005; Tsankova N 2007). Recently, Tousson et al. (Tousson E 2011) demonstrated that coadministration of folate ameliorated monoamine concentration changes in a PTU-treated model. Since folate participates in the enzymatic demethylation of histones, this micronutrient could play a role in the epigenetic control of gene expression. Lakshmy et al. have reported that histone acetylation sustained during the neonatal period in the whole brain of PTU-treated rats (Lakshmy R 1999). Although TRs interact histone protein complexes, the local changes of histone acetylation within regions that highly express TRs have remained unclear. In this study, we found the striatum as a region with specific increase in histone acetylation in TR-$\beta^{+/-}$ mutant mice. In addition, we demonstrated increased dopaminergic contents and unchanged serotonin contents in the same region of TR-β-mutant mice. Although these results imply the possibility of a relationship between the increase in histone acetylation and the change in serotonin-dopamine balance in the striatum, further studies should be aimed at elucidating more close relationships between histone modifications and outcomes either in monoaminergic systems or in distinct hyperactivity, caused by TR-β gene disruption.

As many publications demonstrated that a large number of toxic chemicals might affect human health, the thyroid gland and hormones secreted by it are targets of environmental contaminants as well. Beginning in the early 1960s, the mink industry, which had been prospering around the Great Lakes, began to falter–not because the demand for mink was decreasing but because of mysterious reproductive problems. Dr. Jacobson and his wife reported that the children of women who had regularly eaten Great Lakes fish polluted by poly chlorinated biphenyl (PCB), a family of synthetic chemicals used to insulate electrical equipment, showed abnormalities in cognitive and behavioral development such as visual recognition memory and short-term memory (Jacobson 1985; Jacobson JL 1991), which tend to predict later IQ. It is reported that PCBs impair the normal thyroid function, which plays a key role in brain development; thus, a delay in neurological development may be caused by perinatal exposure to PCBs (Porterfield 2000). Of course, there are other endocrine-disrupting chemicals which have also been shown to disrupt the normal thyroid function, eg, dioxins (Sher ES 1998). Some experts stated that these contaminants "contribute to learning disabilities, including ADHD and perhaps other neurological abnormalities" (Colborn 2004).

Our research team focused on another synthetic chemical, bisphenol A (BPA), because it is widely used in the manufacture of dental sealants, linings of metal cans for preserved foods, and items such as baby bottles and the clear plastic cages to house laboratory animals. In rats, perinatal exposure to BPA has been implicated in abnormal brain development, characterized by hyperactivity and impaired cognition, even at or below the tolerable daily intake (TDI, http://www.bisphenol-a.org/health/exposure/consumer/research.html, 50 μg·kg^{-1}·day^{-1} in humans) (Kubo 2001; Carr R 2003). While BPA is known to have mixed estrogen agonist/antagonist properties, several studies have shown that the thyroid function can be impaired by BPA. In an in vitro study, Moriyama et al. demonstrated that BPA binds to TRs and disrupts thyroid action (Moriyama 2002), while an in vivo study conducted by Zoeller et al. showed that BPA increases serum thyroxine levels and alters the expression of its responsive gene RC3/neurogranin in the developing rat brain (Zoeller 2005).

We housed female Sprague-Dawley rats individually in metal cages from gestation day 7, and provided water in glass bottles. BPA was administered to these rats by dissolving it in drinking water at both doses of 0.1 and 50 mg/L from gestation day 11 to postnatal day 21. From day 21 after birth, the offspring were housed by sex and randomly selected for T4 measurement, behavioral tests, and real time polymerase chain reaction (PCR) analysis.

T4 levels in the whole blood of dams and pups were monitored. Interestingly, low-dose BPA treatment (0.1 mg/L) reduced serum T4 levels in the dams in the first week after delivery, whereas high-dose BPA treatment (50 mg/L) showed no effect on serum T4 levels in the dams at all days tested. Maternal BPA exposure of different doses caused different changes in male pups; however, no changes were seen in female pups. Low-dose BPA exposure significantly increased serum T4 levels in male pups at day 7 after birth, while high-dose BPA exposure decreased T4 levels in male pups at day 21 after birth (Fig 5). As a positive

A

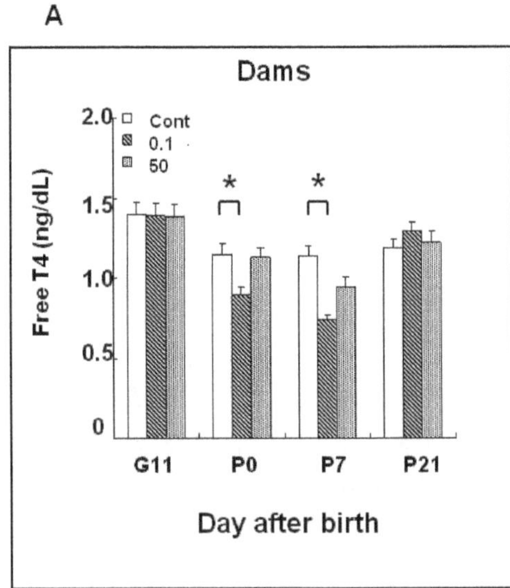

B

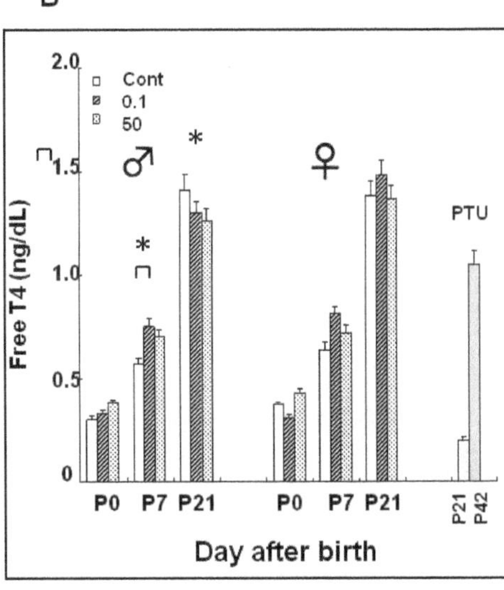

Fig. 5. Locomotor activity (left) and rearing activity (right) in the open field test.

control, we used pups perinatally treated with 0.02% PTU through their mother's milk and their T4 values are shown in Fig 1. A severe decrease in T4 levels was induced by PTU treatment at day 21 after birth, while the value was almost that of the controls at day 42.

With regard to the transient hyperthyroidism of pups at day 7 after birth, one can hypothesize that the thyroid gland of male pups initially compensates against the hypothyroid effect of maternal BPA, resulting in transient hyperthyroidism, and, thereafter, succumbs to the toxic effect of BPA following sustained treatment with BPA through the mother's milk.

The open field test was performed in 6-week-old pups. The open field apparatus was a round field with a 0.8-m diameter and its bottom was divided by lines into 25 regions. To avoid confounding effects due to time differences, the test was performed from 1:00 pm to 4:00 pm every day. Each rat was placed in the central region and allowed to move freely for 3 min. Movement from one region to another was counted as 1 ambulation, and 1 rearing was defined as the rat standing on its hind legs with both front feet were off the ground. The total numbers of ambulation and rearing were manually recorded to evaluate locomotor activity and exploratory behavior, respectively. The open field was cleaned between each subject to prevent olfactory cues from affecting the behavior of subsequently tested rats.

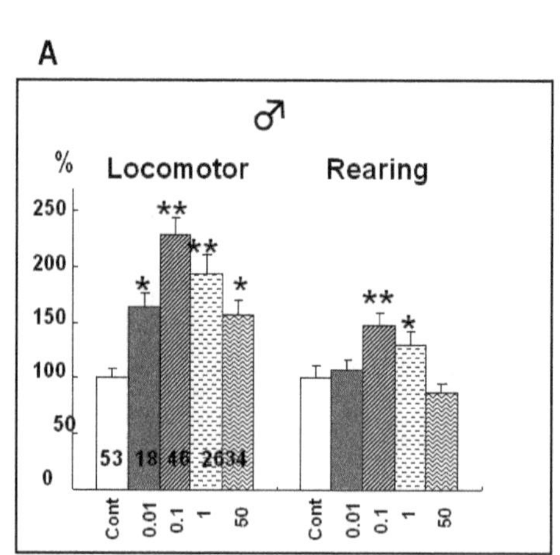

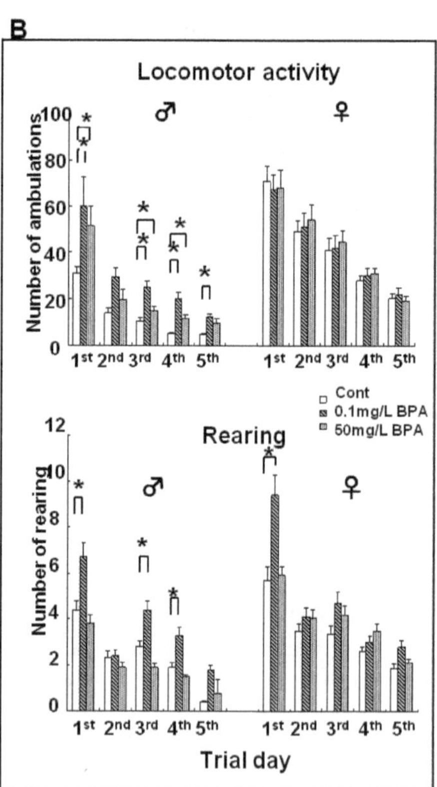

Fig. 6. Latency time in the Morris water maze test.

Male pups of the low-dose BPA (0.1 mg/L) group showed more locomotor activity and more frequent rearing than control male pups, whereas those from the high-dose BPA group did not show differences in rearing activity, except a less marked but significant increase in locomotor activity. Female pups, in contrast, showed no change in either locomotor or rearing activity at either BPA dose (Fig 6).

The Morris water maze test was carried out at 10 weeks of age. The apparatus was a circular pool (diameter = 1.5 m) of water maintained at a temperature of 25 ± 1°C. The pool was divided into 4 sectors (ie, N, S, E, and W) and a transparent resin goal platform, 10 cm in diameter, was placed approximately 1.5 cm below the water surface about halfway between the edge and the center of the pool in the S sector. Each experimental animal performed 2 trials per day for 5 days, and the maximum time permitted for 1 trial was 120 s. If the animal had not reached the goal by the end of the trial, it was led to the goal platform and left on it for 15 s. The escape time of every trial was recorded manually. After every trial, any visible feces were removed from the pool (Fig 7).

Morris water maze

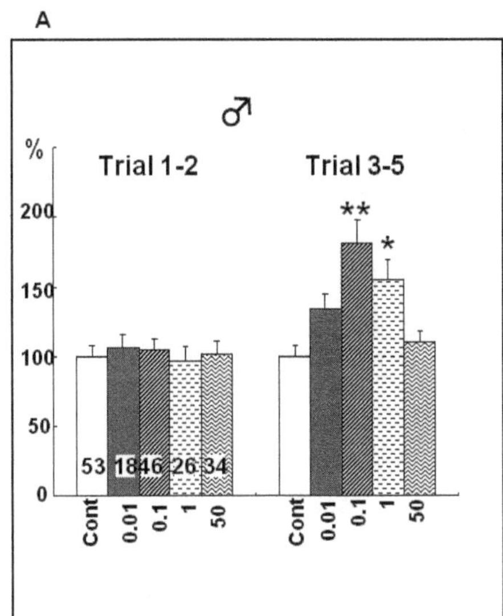

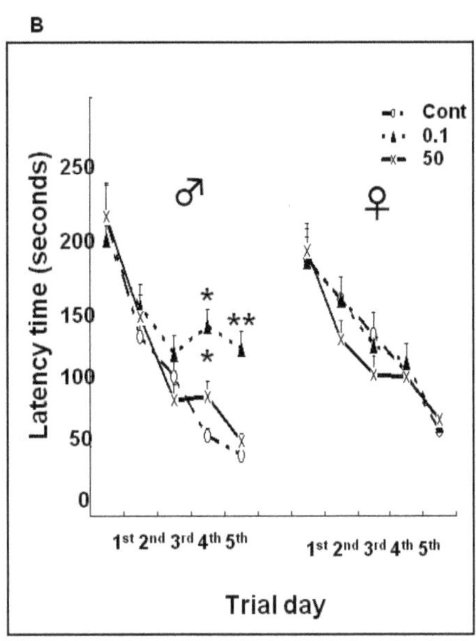

Fig. 7. Effect of 0.1 mg/L bisphenol A (BPA) on thyroid hormone receptor (TR)-α expression in the male hippocampus.

The results of the water maze test were similar to those of the open field test. Male offspring from the low-dose BPA group required about 2.2-fold more time to reach the goal compared to controls on days 4 and 5 of the trial. The effect of high-dose BPA treatment was less obvious than that of low-dose BPA treatment. Female offspring from both BPA-treated groups showed no impairment of spatial learning at all.

These behavioral outcomes paralleling the results of the quantitative determination of serum T4 levels suggest that perinatal BPA exposure disturbs normal thyroid function, consequently leading to irreversible neurological deficits. Why were the males predominantly affected by perinatal BPA exposure? What is the underlying mechanism? We performed further studies to address these critical questions and to unravel the mystery.

Firstly, to assess the thyroid hormone pathway, we investigated the expression of TR-α, -β, RC3/neurogranin, and SRC-1 in the developing hippocampus, a region deeply involved in cognition. The CA1 region of the hippocampus where memory is encoded, consolidated, and stored by synaptic plasticity plays a more crucial role for spatial learning (Huang YY 1995; Vara H 2003). TR-α was highly expressed in the CA1-2 region and dentate gyrus at day 7 after birth (Fig 8), while RC3/neurogranin showed high mRNA levels in the hippocampus from days 7 to 42 after birth. However, BPA treatment did not cause differences in TR-α or RC3/neurogranin levels compared to controls. TR-β was not expressed in the hippocampus throughout the period tested.

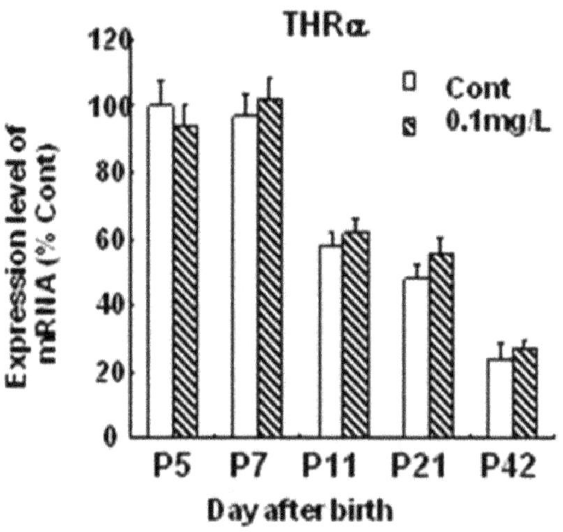

Fig. 8. Effect of 0.1 mg/L bisphenol A (BPA) on RC3/neurogranin expression in the male hippocampus.

Although no change was observed in the expressions of TR-α, β, and the thyroid responsive gene RC3/neurogranin of BPA-treated male pups, SRC-1 levels were significantly up-regulated in the CA1-2 region of the hippocampus by BPA treatment from days 5 to 7 after birth (Fig 9). SRC-1 is a member of the growing family of cellular proteins that act as "amplifiers" of transcription mediated by nuclear receptors upon ligand binding. Therefore, its expression is also regulated by the expression levels of nuclear receptors. Our findings indicate that perinatal BPA exposure at a very low level may influence thyroid function and, consequently, affects brain development only in male pups, while TR itself seems unlikely to be involved. Since SRC-1 is a common transcription cofactor for thyroid hormone as well as other steroid hormones, the involvement of gonadal hormones and their receptors should be taken into account. In this regard, a very clear gender difference of BPA disruption on thyroid function and behavior outcome would support, at least in part, this assumption. However, further investigation is needed.

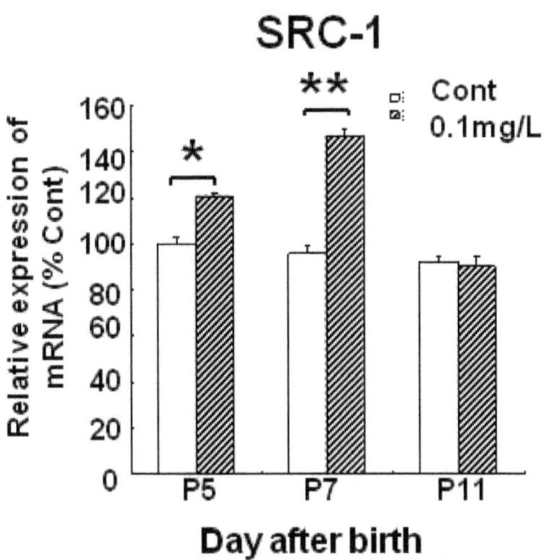

Fig. 9.

The results of our other study support the hypothesis that BPA disturbs brain development via the gonadal hormone pathway. Because there is a significant sexual difference for sweet taste in rats, ie, female rats prefer sweetness more than male rats, we treated maternal rats with 0.1 mg/L BPA (supplied in the drinking water from gestational day 11 until day 21 after delivery). Then, the offspring were supplied with water containing 15% sucrose. We found that BPA-treated male rats liked sucrose more than control rats, while BPA-treated female rats showed less preference for sucrose than control rats. Sexual differentiation of sweet taste was weakened by BPA treatment (Xu X 2011). This finding further suggests involvement of the gonadal hormone pathway in BPA-mediated disruption.

Gonadal hormone receptors and TRs are members of the nuclear receptor superfamily that bind low-molecular-weight ligands (gonadal hormone and thyroid hormone, respectively). They transduce these signals in gene regulatory events. These receptors have a modular protein structure with high homology in the central DNA binding domain. It has been well documented that there is cross-talk between members of the nuclear receptor superfamily which can multiply the theoretically possible modes of gene regulation, leading to a greater and more flexible array of transcriptional responses to environmental changes (Vasudevan N 2002). BPA may influence thyroid function via the gonadal hormone pathway, consequently affecting sexual differentiation and impairing brain development modulated by the thyroid.

Convincing evidence showed widespread exposure to BPA in 95% of urine samples from people in the United States examined by the Centers for Disease Control and Prevention. Furthermore, BPA has recently been shown to be present in the serum during pregnancy as well as in fetal serum and full-term amniotic fluid, confirming its passage through the placenta. These findings translate into an increasing threat to public health. Because the neonatal period of rats is equivalent to the midgestation period in humans, the present study may provide a warning that BPA exposure to fetuses may lead to behavioral abnormalities and cognitive dysfunction in the hippocampus in humans, especially in case of boys. At present, there is no direct evidence linking the increasing number of children with ADHD and autism to large consumption of chemical compounds. Therefore, carefully controlled studies examining this association are urgently needed.

2. References

Ahmed OM, A. E.-T. S., Ahmed RG. (2010). "Effects of experimentally induced maternal hypothyroidism and hyperthyroidism on the development of rat offspring: I. The development of the thyroid hormones-neurotransmitters and adenosinergic system interactions." *Int J Dev Neurosci.* 28(6): 437-454.

Akaike, M., Kato, N. (1997). "Abnormal behavior, spatia learning impairment and neuropeptides caused by temporary neonatal hypothyroidism." *Recent Res, Dev, Neuroendo.*: 39-48.

Akaike, M., Kato, N., Ohno, H., Kobayashi, T. (1991). "Hyperactivity and spatial maze learning impairment of adult rats with temporary neonatal hypothyroidism." *Neurotoxicol Teratol.* 13(3): 317-322.

Bradley, D., Towle, HC., Young III, WS. (1992). "Spatial and temporal expression of a- and b-thyroid hormone receptor mRNAs, including the b2-subtype, in the developing mammalian nervous system." *J. Neurosci.* 12(6): 2288-2302.

Carr R, B. F., Betancourt A, Bowers S, Gandy BS, Ryan P, Willard S. (2003). "Effect of neonatal rat bisphenol a exposure on performance in the Morris water maze." *J Toxicol Environ Health A.* 66(21): 2077-2088.

Chess, S. (1977). "Follow-up report on autism in congenital rubella." *J Autism Child Schizophr.* 7(1): 69-81.

Colborn, T. (2004). "Neurodevelopment and endocrine disruption." *Environ. Health Perspect.* 112(9): 944-949.

Colvis CM, P. J., Goodman RH, Impey S, Dunn J, Mandel G, Champagne FA, Mayford M, Korzus E, Kumar A, Renthal W, Theobald DE, Nestler EJ. (2005). "Epigenetic mechanisms and gene networks in the nervous system." *J Neurosci.* 25(45): 10379-10389.

Forrest D, H. E., Smeyne RJ, Everds N, Stewart CL, Wehner JM, Curran T. (1996). "Recessive resistance to thyroid hormone in mice lacking thyroid hormone receptor beta: evidence for tissue-specific modulation of receptor function." *EMBO J.* 15(12): 3006-3015.

Gauthier K, P. M., Harvey CB, Williams GR, Weiss RE, Refetoff S, Willott JF, Sundin V, Roux JP, Malaval L, Hara M, Samarut J, Chassande O. (2001). "Genetic analysis reveals different functions for the products of the thyroid hormone receptor alpha locus." *Mol Cell Biol.* 21(14): 4748-4760.

González-Burgos I, F.-V. A. (2008). "Serotonin/dopamine interaction in memory formation." *Prog Brain Res.* 172: 603-623.

Guadaño-Ferraz A, O. M., St Germain DL, Bernal J. (1997). "The type 2 iodothyronine deiodinase is expressed primarily in glial cells in the neonatal rat brain." *Proc Natl Acad Sci U S A.* 94(19): 10391-10396.

Huang YY, K. E., Varshavsky L, Brandon EP, Qi M, Idzerda RL, McKnight GS, Bourtchouladze R. (1995). "A genetic test of the effects of mutations in PKA on mossy fiber LTP and its relation to spatial and contextual learning." *Cell* 83(7): 1211-1222.

Jacobson JL, J. S. (1991). "Assessment of teratogenic effects on cognitive and behavioral development in infancy and childhood." *NIDA Res Monogr.* 114: 248-261.

Jacobson, S., Fein, GG., Jacobson, JL., Schwartz, PM., Dowler, JK. (1985). "The effect of intrauterine PCB exposure on visual recognition memory." *Child Dev.* 56(4): 853-860.

Jeyakumar M, L. X., Erdjument-Bromage H, Tempst P, Bagchi MK. (2007). "Phosphorylation of thyroid hormone receptor-associated nuclear receptor corepressor holocomplex by the DNA-dependent protein kinase enhances its histone deacetylase activity." *J Biol Chem.* 282(13): 9312-9322.

Kato, N., Akaike, M., Masui, A., Naruse, H. (1992). *Brain somatostatin in possible animal models of infantile autism.*, Elsevier Science Publishers.

Kato, N., Sundmark, VC., Van Middlesworth, L., Havlicek, V., Friesen, HG. (1982). "Immunoreactive somatostatin and beta-endorphin content in the brain of mature rats after neonatal exposure to propylthiouracil." *Endocrinology* 110(6): 1851-1855.

Kubo, K., Arai, O., Ogata, R., Omura, M., Hori, T., Aou, S. (2001). "Exposure to bisphenol A during the fetal and suckling periods disrupts sexual differentiation of the locus coeruleus and of behavior in the rat." *Neurosci. Lett.* 304(1-2): 73-76.

Lakshmy R, K. M., Das BC, Shah P, Ammini AC. (1999). "Effect of PTU treatment on histone acetylation pattern in the developing rat brain." *Endocr Res.* 25(11): 75-88.

Leonard JL, F. A., Yen PM, Chin WW, Stula M. (1994). "Differential expression of thyroid hormone receptor isoforms in neurons and astroglial cells." *Endocrinology.* 135(2): 548-555.

Lu EJ, B. W. (1977). "An electron microscopic study of the developing caudate nucleus in euthyroid and hypothyroid states." *Anat Embryol (Berl).* 150(3): 335-364.

Madeira MD, P.-B. M. (1993). "Reorganization of mossy fiber synapses in male and female hypothyroid rats: a stereological study." *J Comp Neurol.* 337(2): 334-352.

Manzano J, B. J., Morte B. (2007). "Influence of thyroid hormones on maturation of rat cerebellar astrocytes." *Int J Dev Neurosci.* 35(3): 171-179.

Mellström B, N. J., Santos A, Gonzalez AM, Bernal J. (1991). "Independent expression of the alpha and beta c-erbA genes in developing rat brain." *Mol Endocrinol.* 5(9): 1339-1350.

Moriyama, K., Tagam, T., Akamizu, T., Usui, T., Saijo, M., Kanamoto, N., Hataya, Y., Shimatsu, A., Kuzuya, H., Nakao, K. (2002). "Thyroid hormone action is disrupted by bisphenol A as an antagonist." *J. Clin. Endocrinol. Metab.* 877(11): 5185-5190.

Oades, R. (2008). "Dopamine-serotonin interactions in attention-deficit hyperactivity disorder (ADHD)." *Prog Brain Res.* 172(543-565).

Porterfield, S. (2000). "Thyroidal dysfunction and environemntal chemicals: potential impact on brain development." *Environ. Health Perspect.* 108(suppl3): 433-438.

Rinaldi A, R. S., Agustín-Pavón C, Oliverio A, Mele A. (2010). "Distinct patterns of Fos immunoreactivity in striatum and hippocampus induced by different kinds of novelty in mice." *Neurobiol Learn Mem.* 94(3): 373-381.

Sher ES, X. X., Adams PM, Craft CM, Stein SA. (1998). "The effects of thyroid hormone level and action in developing brain: are these targets for the actions of polychlorinated biphenyls and dioxins?" *Toxicol Ind Health.* 14(1-2): 121-158.

Siesser WB, C. S., McDonald MP. (2005). "Hyperactivity, impaired learning on a vigilance task, and a differential response to methylphenidate in the TRbetaPV knock-in mouse." *Psychopharmacology (Berl).* 181(4): 653-663.

Siesser WB, Z. J., Miller LR, Cheng SY, McDonald MP. (2006). "Transgenic mice expressing a human mutant beta1 thyroid receptor are hyperactive, impulsive, and inattentive." *Genes Brain Behav.* 5(3): 282-297.

Tousson E, I. W., Arafa N, Akela MA. (2011). "Monoamine concentrations changes in the PTU induced hypothyroid rat brain and the ameliorating role of folic acid." *Hum Exp Toxicol.* Apr.

Tsankova N, R. W., Kumar A, Nestler EJ. (2007). "Epigenetic regulation in psychiatric disorders." *Nat Rev Neurosci.* 8(5): 355-367.

Van Middlesworth, L., Norris, CH. (1980). "Audiogenic seizures and cochlear damage in rats after perinatal antithyroid treatment." *Endocrinology* 106(6): 1686-1690.

Vara H, M.-C. J., Colino A. (2003). "Age-dependent alterations of long-term synaptic plasticity in thyroid-deficient rats." *Hippocampus.* 13(7): 816-825.

Vasudevan N, O. S., Pfaff D. (2002). "Estrogen and thyroid hormone receptor interactions: physiological flexibility by molecular specificity." *Physiol Rev.* 82(4): 923-944.

Wallis K, S. M., van Hogerlinden M, Silberberg G, Fisahn A, Nordström K, Larsson L, Westerblad H, Morreale de Escobar G, Shupliakov O, Vennström B. (2008). "Locomotor deficiencies and aberrant development of subtype-specific GABAergic interneurons caused by an unliganded thyroid hormone receptor alpha1." *J Neurosci.* 28(8): 1904-1915.

Wong R, V. V., Ting YT, Kutler DI, Willingham MC, Weintraub BD, Cheng S. (1997). "Transgenic mice bearing a human mutant thyroid hormone beta 1 receptor manifest thyroid function anomalies, weight reduction, and hyperactivity." *Mol Med.* 3(5): 303-314.

Xu X, T. L., Himi T, Sadamatsu M, Tsutsumi S, Akaike M, Kato N. (2011). "Changed preference for sweet taste in adulthood induced by perinatal exposure to bisphenol A-A probable link to overweight and obesity." *Neurotoxicol Teratol.* June.

Zhang J, L. M. (2000). "The mechanism of action of thyroid hormones." *Annu Rev Physiol.* 62(439-466).

Zoeller, R., Bansal, R., Parris, C. (2005). "Bisphenol-A, an environmental contaminant that acts as a thyroid hormone receptor antagonist in vitro, increases serum thyroxine, and alters RC3/neurogranin expression in the developing rat brain." *Endocrinology* 146(2): 697-612.

Permissions

The contributors of this book come from diverse backgrounds, making this book a truly international effort. This book will bring forth new frontiers with its revolutionizing research information and detailed analysis of the nascent developments around the world.

We would like to thank Drahomira Springer, for lending her expertise to make the book truly unique. She has played a crucial role in the development of this book. Without her invaluable contribution this book wouldn't have been possible. She has made vital efforts to compile up to date information on the varied aspects of this subject to make this book a valuable addition to the collection of many professionals and students.

This book was conceptualized with the vision of imparting up-to-date information and advanced data in this field. To ensure the same, a matchless editorial board was set up. Every individual on the board went through rigorous rounds of assessment to prove their worth. After which they invested a large part of their time researching and compiling the most relevant data for our readers. Conferences and sessions were held from time to time between the editorial board and the contributing authors to present the data in the most comprehensible form. The editorial team has worked tirelessly to provide valuable and valid information to help people across the globe.

Every chapter published in this book has been scrutinized by our experts. Their significance has been extensively debated. The topics covered herein carry significant findings which will fuel the growth of the discipline. They may even be implemented as practical applications or may be referred to as a beginning point for another development. Chapters in this book were first published by InTech; hereby published with permission under the Creative Commons Attribution License or equivalent.

The editorial board has been involved in producing this book since its inception. They have spent rigorous hours researching and exploring the diverse topics which have resulted in the successful publishing of this book. They have passed on their knowledge of decades through this book. To expedite this challenging task, the publisher supported the team at every step. A small team of assistant editors was also appointed to further simplify the editing procedure and attain best results for the readers.

Our editorial team has been hand-picked from every corner of the world. Their multi-ethnicity adds dynamic inputs to the discussions which result in innovative outcomes. These outcomes are then further discussed with the researchers and contributors who give their valuable feedback and opinion regarding the same. The feedback is then collaborated with the researches and they are edited in a comprehensive manner to aid the understanding of the subject.

Apart from the editorial board, the designing team has also invested a significant amount of their time in understanding the subject and creating the most relevant covers. They scrutinized every image to scout for the most suitable representation of the subject and create an appropriate cover for the book.

The publishing team has been involved in this book since its early stages. They were actively engaged in every process, be it collecting the data, connecting with the contributors or procuring relevant information. The team has been an ardent support to the editorial, designing and production team. Their endless efforts to recruit the best for this project, has resulted in the accomplishment of this book. They are a veteran in the field of academics and their pool of knowledge is as vast as their experience in printing. Their expertise and guidance has proved useful at every step. Their uncompromising quality standards have made this book an exceptional effort. Their encouragement from time to time has been an inspiration for everyone.

The publisher and the editorial board hope that this book will prove to be a valuable piece of knowledge for researchers, students, practitioners and scholars across the globe.

List of Contributors

Osama M. Ahmed
Physiology Division, Zoology Department, Faculty of Science, Beni-Suef University, Egypt

R. G. Ahmed
Lab of Comparative Endocrinology, Catholic University, Leuven, Belgium

R. G. Ahmed
Zoology Department, Faculty of Science, Beni-Suef University, Egypt

Francesco Massart and Giuseppe Saggese
St. Chiara University Hospital of Pisa, Italy

Pietro Ferrara
Sacro Cuore Catholic University of Rome, Italy

Noura Bougacha-Elleuch and Hammadi Ayadi
Unité Cibles pour le Diagnostic et la Thérapie, Centre de Biotechnologie de Sfax, Tunisia

Mouna Mnif-Feki, Nadia Charfi-Sellami and Mohamed Abid
Service Endocrinologie, CHU Hédi Chaker, Sfax, Tunisia

Julieta Gerenova, Irena Manolova and Veselina Gadjeva
Medical Faculty, Trakia University, Stara Zagora, Bulgaria

Arvin Parvathaneni, Daniel Fischman and Pramil Cheriyath
Pinnacle Health System-Harrisburg Hospital Harrisburg, Pennsylvania, USA

Ljiljana Saranac and Hristina Stamenkovic
Pediatric Clinic, Faculty of Medicine Nis, University of Nis, Serbia

Eliska Potlukova, Jan Jiskra, Zdenek Telicka and Zdenka Limanova
3rd Department of Medicine, General University Hospital and 1st Faculty of Medicine, Charles University in Prague, Czech Republic

Drahomira Springer
Institute of Clinical Biochemistry and Laboratory Diagnostics, General University Hospital, Prague, Czech Republic

Teresa M. Bailey
Ferris State University College of Pharmacy, USA

Elpis Vlachopapadopoulou
Dept. of Growth and Development, Children's Hosp. "P.A. Kyriakou", Greece

Vassilios Papadakis, Georgia Avgerinou and Sophia Polychronopoulou
Dept. of Pediatric Hematology-Oncology, "Agia Sofia" Children's Hosp Athens, Greece

Susana Ares and José Quero
Neonatology Unit, Hospital LA PAZ, Madrid, Spain

Belén Sáenz-Rico de Santiago
Department of Didactics and school Organization of the Faculty of Education of the Complutense University of Madrid, Spain

Gabriela Morreale de Escobar
Instituto de Investigaciones Biomédicas, Universidad Autónoma de Madrid Spanish Preterm Thyroid Group, Spain

S.M.L. Chamindrani Mendis-Handagama
Department of Biomedical and Diagnostic Sciences, The University of Tennessee College of Veterinary Medicine, Knoxville, Tennessee, USA

Minjing Zou and Yufei Shi
Dept. of Genetics King Faisal Specialist Hospital and Research Centre Riyadh, Saudi Arabia

Johnny Deladoey
CHU Sainte-Justine, University of Montreal, Canada

Xiaobin Xu
Center For Neuropsychiatric Disorders, Institute of Life Science, Nanchang University 330031, China

Hirohiko Kanai
Dept. Psychiatry, Shiga Univ. Med. Sci., Shiga, Japan

Masanori Ookubo
Dept. Psychiatry, Minakuchi Hosp., Koka City, Shiga, Japan

Satoru Suzuki
Dept. Aging Med. and Geriatrics, Shinshu Univ., Nagano, Japan

Nobumasa Kato
Dept. of Psychiatry, Karasuyama Hospital, Showa Univ. Sch.of Med., Tokyo, Japan

Miyuki Sadamatsu
Dept. Psychiatry, Nara Med. Univ. Nara, Japan